Handbook on
MANAGING INFERTILITY

AOFOG

Asia & Oceania Federation of Obstetrics & Gynaecology

Handbook on MANAGING INFERTILITY

(Meeting the Challenges in Low-Resource Settings)

Jaideep Malhotra MD FICOG FICMCH
Editor-in-Chief SAFOMS Journal
Treasurer Indian Menopause Society
National Coordinater Club 35 Plus
Vice President FOGSI 2010
Governing Council Member of ASPIRE, ISAR, ICOG and IFUMB
Agra, Uttar Pradesh, India
jaideepmalhotraagra@gmail.com

Rohana Haththotuwa
Consultant Obstetrician and Gynecologist
Chairman
Ninewells CARE Mother and Baby Hospital
55/1, Kirimandala Mawatha
Colombo, Sri Lanka

Jaydeep D Tank MD DNB DGO FCPS MICOG
Consultant
Jupiter Hospital Centre for IVF
Joint Clinical Secretary
Mumbai Obstetric and Gynecological Society (MOGS)
Ashwini Maternity and Surgical Hospital
Center for Advanced Endoscopy and IVF

Forewords

PC Ho
Walfrido W Sumpaico

An AOFOG Publication

JAYPEE BROTHERS MEDICAL PUBLISHERS (P) LTD

New Delhi • Panama City • London

Jaypee Brothers Medical Publishers (P) Ltd.

Headquarter

Jaypee Brothers Medical Publishers (P) Ltd
4838/24, Ansari Road, Daryaganj
New Delhi 110 002, India
Phone: +91-11-43574357
Fax: +91-11-43574314
Email: jaypee@jaypeebrothers.com

Overseas Offices

J.P. Medical Ltd.,
83 Victoria Street London
SW1H 0HW (UK)
Phone: +44-2031708910
Fax: +02-03-0086180
Email: info@jpmedpub.com

Jaypee-Highlights Medical Publishers Inc.
City of Knowledge, Bld. 237, Clayton
Panama City, Panama
Phone: 507-317-0160
Fax: +50-73-010499
Email: cservice@jphmedical.com

Website: www.jaypeebrothers.com
Website: www.jaypeedigital.com

Inquiries for bulk sales may be solicited at: jaypee@jaypeebrothers.com

Handbook on Managing Infertility (Meeting the Challenges in Low-Resource Settings)

First Edition : 2012

ISBN 978-93-5025-595-7

Printed at Sanat Printers, Kundli.

Contributors

Asma Munir MD
Gynecologist and IVF Consultant
Karachi, Pakistan

Bharat Joshi MSc
Laboratory Director and Chief Embryologist
Pulse Women's Hospital
Ahmedabad, Gujarat, India

Bhavna Sharma MBBS DGO
Consultant Obstetrics and Gynecology
KM and KDJ Hospital
Gwalior, Madhya Pradesh, India

Bhola Rijal MRTCOG
Chief Consultant and Chairman of Om Hospital and Research Center, and Nepal Medical College
Founder of IVF unit in Om Hospital and Research Center, Kathmandu

Derek F Lok MBChB PhD (Adel) FRANZCOG, CREI
Senior Clinical Lecturer, University of Sydney
Consultant Gynecologist, RPAH, Westmead and Liverpool Hospital, Geneva
Liverpool, NSW 2170, Australia

Ernest Hung Yu NG
Department of Obstetrics and Gynecology
The University of Hong Kong
Queen Mary Hospital, Hong Kong

Hang Wun Raymond LI
Department of Obstetrics and Gynecology
The University of Hong Kong
Queen Mary Hospital, Hong Kong

Haroon Latif Khan MBBS FSC
Embryologist/Chief Executive
Lahore Institute of Fertility and Endocrinology (LIFE)
Lahore, Pakistan

Hrishikesh Pai MD FCPS FICOG MSc (USA)
Treasurer of FOGSI; Vice President ISAR
Past President
Mumbai OBGYN Society
Past Senior Vice President FOGSI
Past President Indian Society of Gynecological Endoscopist
Consultant (IVF Expert)
Fortis Bloom IVF Centre
and at Lilavati Hospital
Mumbai
Maharashtra, India

Ian S Fraser AO MD BSc (Hons) ChB FRANZCOG FRCOG CREI DUa
Professor in Reproductive Medicine
University of Sydney, NSW, Australia
Visiting Medical Officer, Royal Prince Alfred Hospital, Sydney, NSW, Australia
Honorary Secretary, FIGO

Ivan Rizal Sini MD FRANZCOG GDRM SpOG
Clinical Director of Morula IVF Jakarta and Chairman of Indonesian Reproductive Science Institute
Morula IVF Jakarta
The BIC, 1st Floor
Jl. Teuku Cik Ditiro 12
Menteng
Jakarta 10310

Jaideep Malhotra MD FICOG FICMCH
Editor in Chief SAFOMS Journal
Treasurer Indian Menopause Society
National Coordinater Club 35 Plus
Vice President FOGSI 2010
Governing Council Member of ASPIRE, ISAR, ICOG and IFUMB
Agra
Uttar Pradesh, India

Jaydeep D Tank MD DNB DGO FCPS MICOG
Consultant
Jupeter Hospital Centre for IVF
Joint Clinical Secretary
Mumbai Obstetric and Gynecological Society (MOGS)
Ashwini Maternity and Surgical Hospital
Center for Advanced Endoscopy and IVF
Mumbai, Maharashtra, India

JP Rao MD
Consulting Sonologist
Malhotra Nursing and Maternity Home
Agra, Uttar Pradesh, India

Kamini A Rao DGO DORCP FRCOG FICOG FNAMS
Obstetrics and Gynaecology (Infertility Specialist)
Director
Bangalore Assisted Conception Center
Bengaluru, Karnataka, India

Lakhwinder Singh MS FAIS FMAS FIAGES
Laparoscopic Surgeon and Andrologist
Genesis Fertility and Surgical Center
Jalandhar, Punjab, India
Malhotra Test Tube Baby Center
Agra, Uttar Pradesh, India

Manish Banker MD
Director and Infertility Specialist
Pulse Women's Hospital, Ahmedabad
President Elect, Indian Society for Assisted Reproduction [ISAR]
Chairman, Infertility Committee
Federation of Obstetrics and Gynecological Societies of India [FOGSI] [2007 – 2010]

Nandan Roongta DNB, DGO, DFP
Clinical Associate
Lilavati Hospital IVF Centre
Mumbai, Maharashtra, India

Nandita Palshetkar MD FCPS FICOG
Present Senior Vice President of FOGSI
Clinical secretary of Mumbai OBGYN Society
Treasurer of Indian association of Gynecological Endoscopy
Member of the Managing Committee of ISAR
Consultant IVF Expert at Fortis Bloom IVF Centre
New Delhi/mohali/vashi and At Lilavati Hospital
Mumbai
Maharashtra, India

Narendra Malhotra MBBS MD FICMCH FIAJAGO FICOG FICMU FRSH
Consultant, Obstetrician, Gynecologist and IVF Specialist, Malhotra Hospital
Agra, Uttar Pradesh, India
Honorary Professor Indian College of Maternal and Child Health (ICMCH Kolkata)
Consultant and Co-ordinator, Department of Obstetrics and Gynecology Apollo Pankaj Hospitals
Agra, Uttar Pradesh, India
President FOGSI, 2008
Dean, Indian College of Ultrasound (ICMU) 2008
Chairman, AOFOG YGAA and Publication Committee

Neharika Malhotra MD
Consultant, Obstetrician
Gynecologist and IVF Specialist
Malhotra Hospital
Agra, Uttar Pradesh, India

Parikshit Tank MD DNB FCPS DGO DFP MNAMS MICOG MRCOG
Honorary Clinical Associate Obstetrics and Gynecology, Nowrosjee Wadia Maternity Hospital
Mumbai, Maharashtra, India
Consultant, Ashwini Maternity and Surgical Hospital
Center for Endoscopy and ART
Mumbai
Maharashtra, India

PC Ho
President, Asia & Oceania Federation of Obstetrics and Gynaecology (AOFOG)
Department of Obstetrics and Gynaecology, Queen Mary Hospital, 6th Floor
Professorial Block, 102 Pokfulam Road
Hong Kong

Priya Sivadas
Fellow, Sydney IVF
Liverpool, NSW 2170
Australia

Ragweshwar Jyoti MBBS MD
Gynecologist
Deen Dayal Upadhyay Zonal Hospital
Shimla, Himachal Pradesh, India

Rajat Gyaneshwar MBBS MHEd FRANZCOG
Professor of Obstetrics and Gynecology
College of Medicine Nursing and Health Sciences
Fiji National University
Fiji

Rajesh Chaudhary MD
Lecturer in Department of Obstetrics and Gynecology, Nepal Medical College
Research Officer
Om Hospital and Research Center
Kathmandu, Nepal

Rishma Pai MD DNB DGO FCPS FICOG
Past Senior Vice President FOGSI; Treasurer of Indian Society of Assisted Reproduction
Convenor DNB
Jaslok Hospital, Member of Managing Committee
Mumbai, Maharashtra, India
OBGYN Societies and IAGE
Consultant IVF Expert at Fortis Bloom IVF Centre and at Lilavati Hospital
Mumbai
Maharashtra, India

RJ Norman BSc (Hons) MBChB (Hons) MD FRANZCOG FRCPA FRCPath FRCOG CREI
Director
The Robinson Institute
The University of Adelaide
Ground floor, Norwich Centre
55 King William Road
North Adelaide
South Australia 5006

Rohana Haththotuwa
Chairman
Ninewells CARE Mother and Baby Hospital
Colombo 05
Sri Lanka

Rutvij Dalal
Fellow in Reproductive Biology
Lilavati Hospital Research Centre
Mumbai
Maharashtra, India

Sabina Pradhan MD
Consultant
IVF Unit
Om Hospital and Research Center
Kathmandu, Nepal

Sakshi Tomar MBBS MD
Consulting Radiologist
Lakimpur, India

Sanjay Gupte MD DGO FICOG FRCOG LLB
Director
Gupte Hospital
Pune, Maharashtra, India
President of FOGSI (2009-2010)

Seung-Yup Ku MD
Department of Obstetrics and Gynecology
Seoul National University Hospital
Seoul, Korea

Shee-Uan Chen MD
Gynecologist (Infertility specialist)
Department of Obstetrics and Gynecology
National Taiwan University Hospital
Taipei, Taiwan

Sheila Loh
Clinical Director
Raffles Fertility Centre
Raffles Hospital
Singapore

Shin Yong Moon MD PhD
Professor
Department of Obstetrics and Gynecology
Seoul National University College of Medicine
Director, Institute of Reproductive Medicine and Population, Seoul National University
Seoul, Korea
Director, Laboratory of *In Vitro* Fertilization
Seoul National University Hospital
Seoul, Korea

Shivanand Sakhare MS DNB FCPS
National Board Fellow in Reproductive Medicine
Clinical Assistant Bloom IVF Centre
Mumbai, Maharashtra, India

Shyam V Desai MD DGO DFP FCPS MNAMS FICOG
Honorary Professor Obstetrics and Gynecology
Mumbai University
Postgraduate Teacher
Port Trust Hospital, Mumbai
Consultant Obstetrics
Gynecology and Endoscopic Surgeon
Dr Balabhai Nanavati Hospital
Hinduja Healthcare Surgical
Seven Hills Hospital and Dr LH Hiranandani Hospital, Mumbai, Maharashtra, India

Sonal Karia MBBS MD FRANZCOG
Obstetrician, Gynaecologist and Fertility Specialist
Sydney, NSW, Australia
CREI fellow, Sydney IVF and Royal Prince Alfred Hospital
Sydney, NSW
Australia

Tomoko Inoue MD PhD
Director
IVF Namba Clinic
Okaka

Upul Senarath MBBS MD
Senior Lecturer in Community Medicine
Faculty of Medicine
University of Colombo
Colombo, Sri Lanka

Vijay Kulkarni MS
Consultant Andrologist and Microsurgeon
Mumbai, Maharashtra, India

Walfrido W Sumpaico MD
Dean
College of Medicine
Manila Central University
Secretary General, AOFOG
President/CEO of the
United Doctors Medical Center

Yin Yin Yong
Senior Embryologist (resp)
Raffles Fertility Centre
Raffles Hospital
Singapore

Yoshiharu Morimoto MD PhD
IVF Namba Clinic
1-17-28, Minamihorie, Nishi-ku
Osaka, Japan

Yu-Shih Yang MD PhD
Department of Obstetrics and Gynecology
National Taiwan University Hospital
No. 7 Chung-Shan South Road, Taipei, Taiwan

Foreword

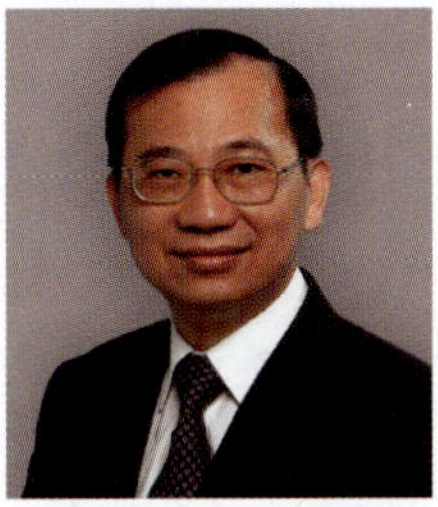

Infertility is a common gynecological condition. Although it is not a life-threatening condition, but infertility is a stigma in many countries in this region, leading to a lot of distress in the infertile couples. In the recent few decades, many significant advances have been made especially in the area of assisted reproduction and more infertile couples can now achieve a successful pregnancy. However, many of the new methods of infertility treatment are expensive and may not be affordable to patients in low-resource settings. Despite the rapid economic advances of many countries in the Asia-Oceania region, many patients in this region still cannot afford the expenses involved in infertility treatment. I would like to congratulate Dr Jaideep Malhotra, Dr Rohana Haththotuwa and Dr Jaydeep D Tank for organizing the *Handbook on Managing Infertility* which concentrates on the infertility management in low-resource settings. This book will be useful to many gynecologists in this region as a practical guide in their management of infertile couples.

PC Ho
President
Asia & Oceania Federation of
Obstetrics and Gynaecology (AOFOG)

Foreword

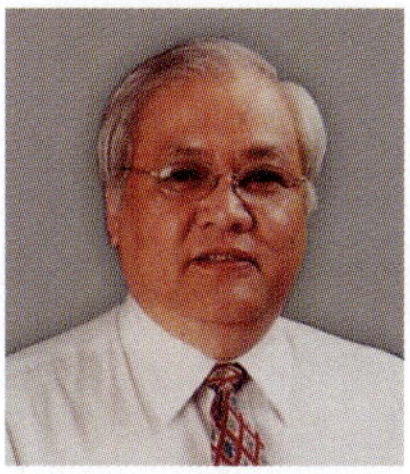

From the earliest days, man has always sought companionship with woman. They profess undying love for each other and promise to look after each other's welfare till death do they part. But, in addition, they also promise to take care of the children, they will be blessed with. And we have all been witness to the joy and contentment in the births of beloved descendants.

This is the central core of the problem of infertility—it fulfills the goal of companionship between man and woman but frustrates their goal of continuity. One must, therefore, look not only on the medical aspects of the problem for much greater might be the personal and social aspects of infertility.

Handbook on Managing Infertility is unique because it is written from an *"eastern"* perspective, a bit different from what has been written in current literature. Moreover, it is authored by persons with great personal experience and expertise on the topic. Finally, it fulfills AOFOGs main thrust of education for it is members and the population they serve. I am grateful for the privilege of writing this foreword. Daunting as the task may have been, I congratulate the editors and contributors for their effort, time and talent in producing this handbook. I wish the reader satisfaction in reading the handbook.

Walfrido W Sumpaico
Dean, College of Medicine
Manila Central University
Secretary General, AOFOG
President/CEO of the United Doctors Medical Center

Preface

What do we gift a person who cannot hear..., a hearing aid, may be?, or a wheelchair to someone who cannot walk.., but what do we give to the infertile couples of developing world, struggling with their nutritional and infrastructural needs, have humungous maternal and neonatal mortality and morbidity, are high on dependency and definitely low on faith...

Yes. It is a 'child' the most precious gift to mankind for its continuity, perpetuation and prosperity! The birth of Louise Brown in 1978, a remarkable beginning, one of its kinds, rarest of all...but the most celebrated one so far, gave hope and happiness to millions in this world. This was regarded as the beginning of a new era of assisted reproductive technology (ART). Since then, the field of ART has seen innumerable new discoveries and technological advances which has led to increasing indications, which otherwise were unthinkable and beyond the reach of common man.

Today, the world boasts of 4 million IVF babies, but still 80 million couples are childless and either have no access to the fertility services or cannot afford them.

Even though ART today is an accepted treatment modality, the simplification of setting up labs and technology has led to mushrooming of ART centers even in developing countries, but the lack of expertise, adequately trained clinicians and technical personnel has made it a bit compromised. Also, sheer amiss of laws (only guidelines) has made 3rd party reproduction more lucrative business and the West is looking towards this region for oocyte donors and surrogates.

In our more than two decades of obstetric and gynecological practice in this region, we have been frustrated enough for not being able to offer, fertility services to our infertile couples because of sheer lack of accessibility or affordability.

This endeavor of ours is to equip ourselves with the least possible resources most effectively and enduringly! This small effort of ours is, indeed an attempt to highlight the special problems and hurdles these low-resourced countries face on their way to successive implementation of high end technological implications and their increasingly unmet need for an intensive and expensive infrastructure for it to support, this package of technological advancement.

Our main aim is to throw light on those specific areas, which can be and should be tackled with a little foresight and care, so as to maximize all available resources with time and cost effectiveness, ensuring higher results in lower input areas as well. We are sure that this book will be a great help to all practitioners looking for viable and workable solutions.

The journey continues...!

We would like to express our deep sense of gratitude to Professor Walfrido W Sumpaico, for his motivation for this first ever AOFOG publication. Sincere thanks to Prof PC Ho for his constant support and guidance, deep sense of appreciation to all our esteemed contributors for burning the midnight oils to get this manuscript ready on time, and have no words for Shri Jitendar P Vij (Chairman and Managing Director) and his team, for the untiring help and effort to get this publication ready, lastly to all our spouses and children for bearing with us in our endeavor.

Jaideep Malhotra
Rohana Haththotuwa
Jaydeep D Tank

Contents

Chapter 1

History of Human Assisted Reproductive Technology

Parikshit Tank, Narendra Malhotra, Neharika Malhotra

The history of IVF dates back, actually to the understanding of oocyte maturation *in vitro*. The first known studies on maturation of mammalian oocytes *in vitro* were done by George Pincus (inventor of the contraceptive pill). He was the first to show *in vitro* expulsion of the first polar body and also studied human oocytes.[1,2]

Trying to fertilize oocytes *in vitro* was unsuccessful even in animals till the 1960s. Various reasons like sperm capacitation (Austin and Chang 1969).[3] In the 1950s Robert Edwards, Mervyn Runner and Ruth Fowler (Edward's wife) tried to use mare's serum (PMS) to induce ovulation and estrus in mice.[4-6]

In USA at around 1950s, a lot of genetic work on identifying chromosomes was being done and also at this time Stein and Levinthal described polycystic ovarian syndrome and described "wedge" resection as a treatment.

Robert Edwards used to study these wedges, which were provided to him by gynecologist Molly Rose and he studied various stages of oocyte development.[7]

Maturation of oocytes at 36 hours after insemination was also described by Edwards here. And also stem cell development was documented by John Paul.[8]

Robert Edwards was first to classify the stages of meiosis in human oocyte and this had a clinical significance of 2nd polar body extrusion 37 hours after injection of human chorionic gonadotropin (hCG). The first attempts to fertilize oocytes removed 36 hours after injection of hCG were tried and failed at this stage (sperm capacitation and use of epididymal sperms).

The work of Prof Robert Edwards at this stage in United Kingdom raised many questions in the medical, social and religious circles on ethics, abnormal babies, sexing and cloning. Professor Robert Geoffrey Edwards, born in Leeds on the September 27, 1925, is presently the Chief Editor of Reproductive BioMedicine Online. As a young science graduate from the University of Wales, he began his PhD at the Edinburgh University in 1951. His early work was on altering chromosomal content of mouse embryos. This gave him a strong background in embryology and reproductive physiology of mice. He teamed up with a colleague (and his future wife), Ruth Fowler to study the induction of multiple ovulations in mice with pregnant mares' serum (PMS) which was rich in gonadotropins. They were able to induce oocyte maturation and meiosis *in vitro* as early as 1957. Edwards traveled to California to widen his horizons into molecular biology and genetics. He returned to London and spent two years working intensely on immunology until his curiosity retuned to oocyte maturation and fertilization.

In vivo and *in vitro* experiments with gonadotropins confirmed the earlier success with rabbit, hamster and rat oocytes which matured within 12 hours of administering hCG followed by insemination. However, oocytes from cows, sheep and monkeys showed no signs of maturity when inseminated at 12 hours. Similarly, human oocyte maturation was also thought to be impossible *in vitro*. Molly Rose, the gynecologist who had delivered two of his daughters, agreed to provide him with human ovarian tissue. He worked with oocytes harvested from slithers or wedges of human ovaries removed from patients with Stein-Leventhal syndrome. The results from the first two years of his work were disappointing. A common basis of his failure, as well of other workers who had experimented in this field, was the early work by Pincus et al which proposed that human oocytes matured at 12 hours after hCG administration.[8] Having exhausted a number of options such as changing culture media, adding higher doses of hormones and sera, Edwards decided that there might be some difference in mammalian species regarding the time to oocyte maturation. This was a vital breakthrough and he was finally able to demonstrate meiosis between 24 and 48 hours. This was further refined and the time of ovulation for human oocytes was identified as 36 hours. Pig oocytes were closest to humans, requiring 37 hours![9] Edwards moved to Cambridge where he further explored and optimized incubators, media and cell line cultivation.

Patrick Christopher Steptoe was born on June 9, 1913 in Oxfordshire, England. His father was a church organist, while his mother served as a social worker. Steptoe studied medicine at the University of London's St. George Hospital Medical School. After qualifying, his medical career was interrupted by World War II. Steptoe volunteered as a naval surgeon. He was captured with his shipmates by Italian forces in 1941 after their ship sank in the Battle of Crete. Initially granted special privileges in prison because he was a physician, Steptoe was placed in solitary confinement after officials detected his efforts to help fellow prisoners escape. Following the war, Steptoe completed additional studies in obstetrics and gynecology. In 1948, he became a member of the Royal College of Obstetricians and Gynecologists and moved to Manchester to set-up a private practice. In 1951, Steptoe began working at Oldham General and District Hospital in northeast England. While at Oldham General and District Hospital, Steptoe pursued his interest in fertility problems. He was a pioneer of laparoscopy in England, having trained with Palmer in Paris and Frangenheim in Germany. In the early part of his career he had trouble convincing the profession about its utility. Five years passed before Steptoe published his first paper on laparoscopy. He also described laparoscopy at ovulation and the ability to collect oocytes from the ovaries.[10] This drew attention from all quarters of the medical profession and included Robert Edwards.

The historic collaboration began with a phone call from Edwards to Steptoe and flourished at the Oldham and District General Hospital and later at the Kershaw's Hospital. They set-up a small laboratory at Oldham. Women were stimulated with purified urinary human menopausal gonadotropin (hMG) and ovulation triggered with hCG. Oocytes were aspirated 36 hours later via laparoscopy. Human embryo formation was routinely achieved. Once again, there were disappointing results in the first three years with no pregnancies. One of the mistakes that was identified was the use of Primolut depot as a form of luteal support. It was later found to be a luteolytic and abortifacient. They switched to hCG and progesterone thereafter. The pressures from critics, ethicists and colleagues were mounting. The patients, however, remained loyal and a steady stream ensured that work progressed. Much of the early work was funded by Edwards and Steptoe themselves. More bad news was in store. Though a clinical pregnancy was established in 1976, it turned out to be an ectopic which had to be removed at about 10 weeks.[11] Working against the odds, Steptoe and Edwards experimented with various stimulation protocols and natural cycle IVF. Lesley and John Brown were the second entrants in the natural IVF group. Lesley had no oviducts, having lost them to ectopic pregnancies earlier. This proved to be a valuable discussion to critics who would later claim that the pregnancy was a fraud.

After seven years of work at Oldham, the positive pregnancy test in a natural cycle was a major milestone. Louise Brown was born at 11:47 pm on July 25th 1978 at Oldham, through a planned caesarean section delivered by registrar John Webster. She weighed 5 pounds, 12 ounces (2.608 kg) at birth. Her younger sister, Natalie Brown, was also conceived through IVF, four years later, and became the world's fortieth IVF baby, and the first one to give birth herself, naturally, in 1999. Louise Brown also has a son, conceived naturally and born in 2006, with Professor Edwards in attendance. Steptoe and Edwards published their early results in 1980 with four pregnancies out of 32 embryo transfers.[12]

The Oldham team wound up the small laboratory and set-up a private clinic at Bourn Hall. Criticism and plaudits were earned in equal measure until the late 1980s when IVF became an international phenomenon and was widely accepted in clinical practice and the public view. Patrick Steptoe died from cancer in 1988. Professor Robert Edwards continues to work on the genetic aspects controlling human reproduction and the ethics of assisted reproduction.[13]

Assisted reproductive technologies (ART) have enabled millions of people in the world to have biological children who otherwise would not have been able to do so. According to the European Society for Human Reproduction and Embryology, more than three million babies have been born using ART worldwide in the last 30 years, enabling infertile women and men; single women and men; and lesbian, gay, and transgender couples to form genetically-related families.

These new technologies have transformed the way we view reproduction. While they have created new hopeful possibilities, they also require that we pay attention to issues of health, ethics, law, and policy. Key concerns include: lack of access; health effects on women and children; potential for devaluation of the lives of people with disabilities; limitations on use by lesbian, gay, bisexual, transgender, questioning, and intersex (LGBTQI) individuals and couples; dangers of selecting characteristics of children; the commercial environment surrounding ART; and the nature of regulation in the US and other countries.

Some of the major milestones which happened over the last 30 years are as follows:

MAJOR MILESTONES OF THE PROCESS

The History of *In Vitro* Fertilization (IVF)—The Milestones

The history of *in vitro fertilization* (IVF) and embryo transfer (ET) dates back as early as the 1890s when Walter Heape a professor and physician at the University of Cambridge, England, United Kingdom, who had been conducting research on reproduction in a number of animal species, reported the first known case of embryo transplantation in rabbits, long before the applications to human fertility were even suggested.

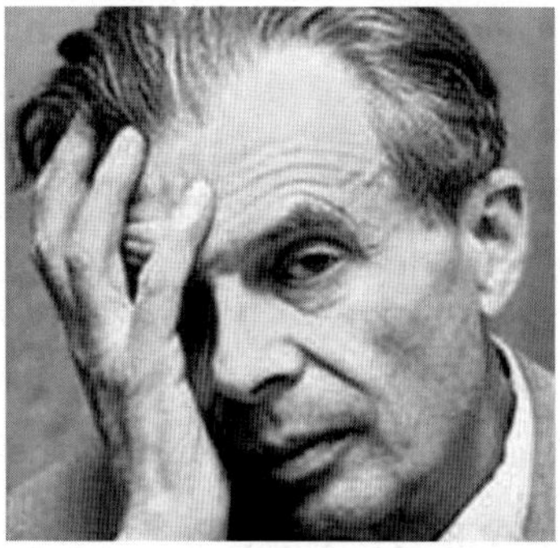

Aldous Huxley

In 1932, 'Brave New World' was published by Aldous Huxley. In this science fiction novel, Huxley realistically described the technique of IVF as we know it. Five years later in 1937, an editorial appeared in the New England Journal of Medicine (NEJM 1937, 21 October) which is note worthy.

"Conception in a watch glass: The 'Brave New World' of Aldous Huxley may be nearer realization. Pincus and Enzmann have started one step earlier with the rabbit, isolating an ovum, fertilizing it in a watch glass and reimplanting it in a doe other than the one which furnished the oocyte and have thus successfully inaugurated pregnancy in the unmated animal. If such an accomplishment with rabbits were to be duplicated in the human being, we should in the words of 'flaming youth' be 'going places'.

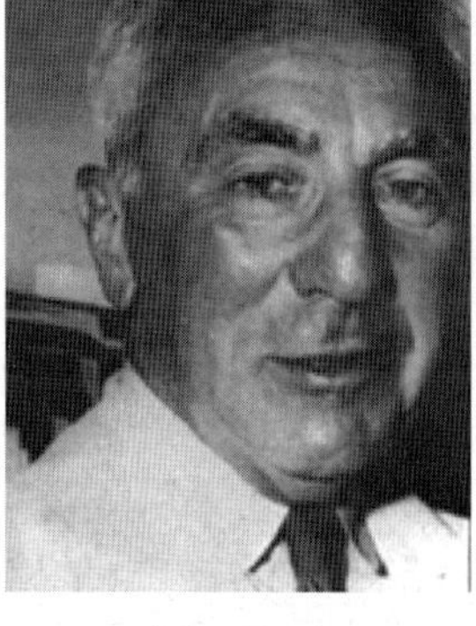

John Rock

In 1934, Pincus and Enzmann, from the Laboratory of General Physiology at Harvard University, published a paper in the Proceedings of the National Academy of Sciences of the USA, raising the possibility that mammalian eggs can undergo normal development *in vitro*. Fourteen years later, in 1948, Miriam Menken and John Rock retrieved more than 800 oocytes from women during operations for various conditions. One hundred and thirty-eight of these oocytes were exposed to spermatozoa *in vitro*. In 1948, they published their experiences in the American Journal of Obstetrics and Gynecology.

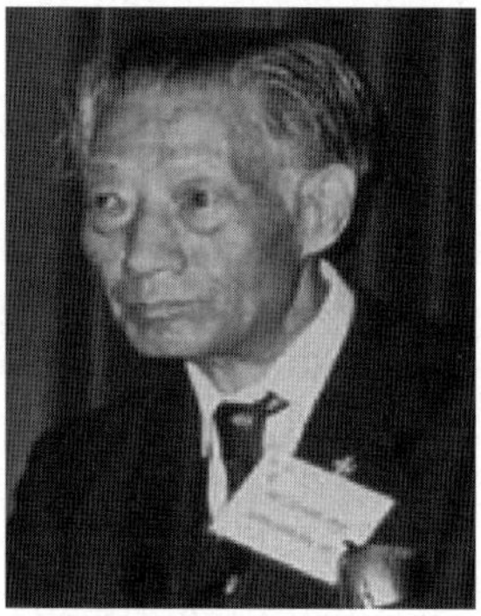

MC Chang

However, it was not until 1959 that indisputable evidence of IVF was obtained by Chang (Chang M. Nature 1959;184:466) who was the first to achieve births in a mammal (a rabbit) by IVF. The newly-ovulated eggs were fertilized, *in vitro* by incubation with capacitated sperm in a small Carrel flask for 4 hours, thus opening the way to assisted procreation.

Professionals in the fields of microscopy, embryology, and anatomy laid the foundations for future achievements. The recent rapid growth of IVF-ET and related techniques worldwide are further supported by the social and scientific climate which favors their continuation.

Through the years numerous modifications have been made in the development of IVF-ET in humans: Refinement of fertilization and embryo culture media; earlier transfer of the embryo; improvements in equipment; use of a reduced number of spermatozoa in the fertilization dish and embryo biopsy among others.

The purpose of this introduction is to acknowledge those who initiated new steps in the development of the treatment protocols and techniques that we now use facilitating such simple and promising IVF-ET procedures.

1961 Palmer from France described the first retrieval of oocytes by laparoscopy.

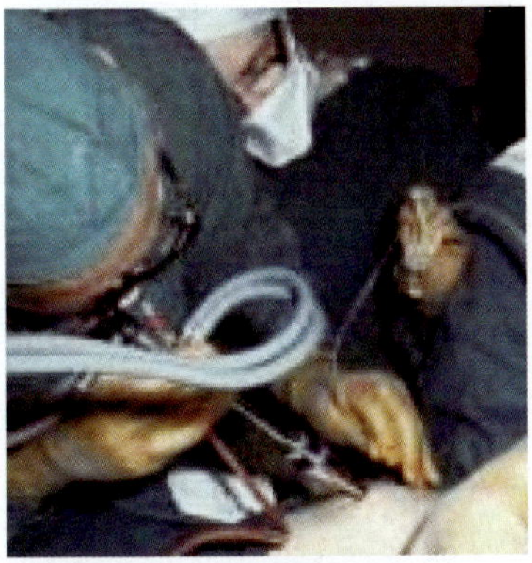

Laparoscopic retrieval

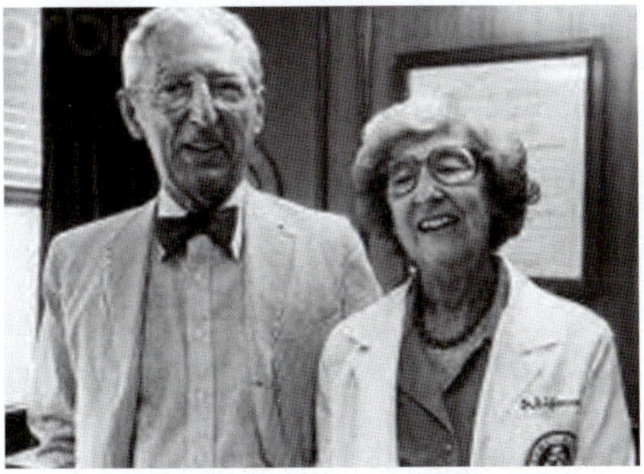

Georgeanna and Howard Jones

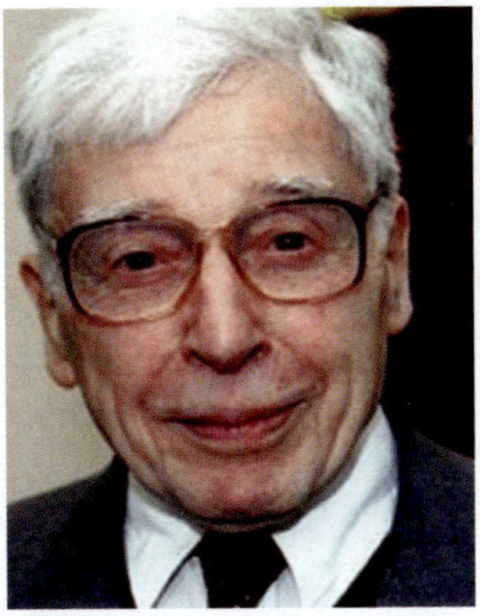

Robert Edwards

1965 In 1965, Robert Edwards together with Georgeanna and Howard Jones at Johns Hopkins Hospital in the USA attempted to fertilize human oocytes *in vitro* (Edwards et al. Am J Obstet Gynecol 1966;96:192).

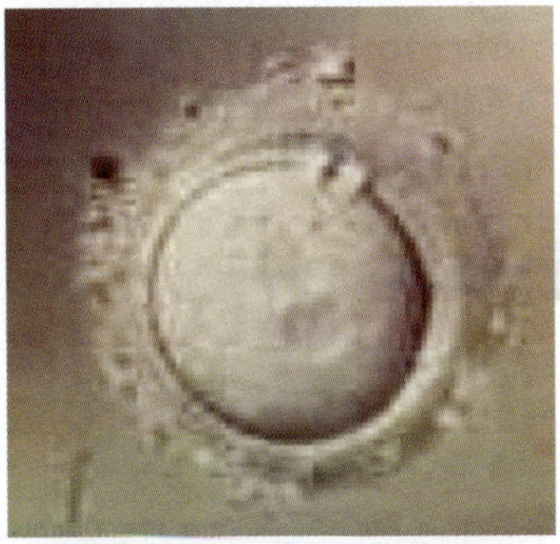

Fertilized human oocyte

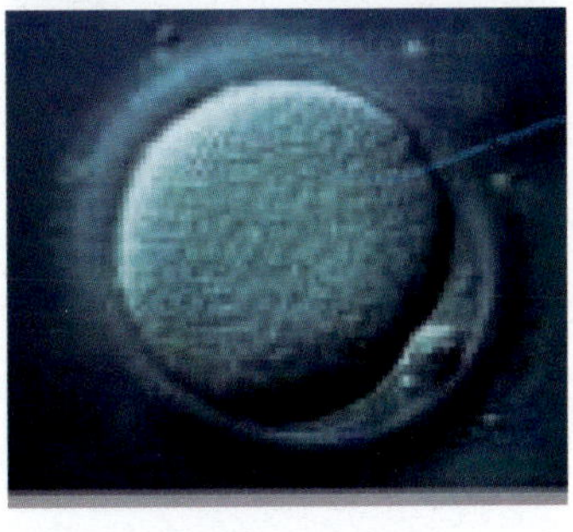

Human oocyte

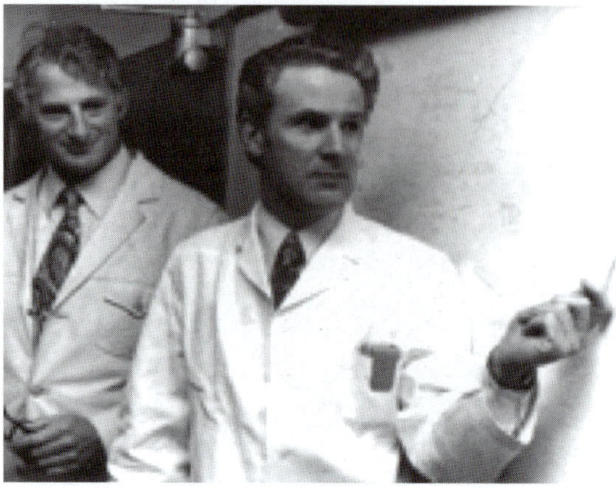

Carl Wood and John Leeton

1973 The first IVF pregnancy was reported by the Monash research team of Professors Carl Wood and John Leeton in Melbourne, Australia. Unfortunately, this resulted in early miscarriage (deKretzer et al. Lancet 1973;2:728).

1976 Y Menezo developed the world's first B2 culture medium, known as 'the French medium'. This specific medium reflected the follicular, tubal and uterine environments of the sheep, rabbits and humans.

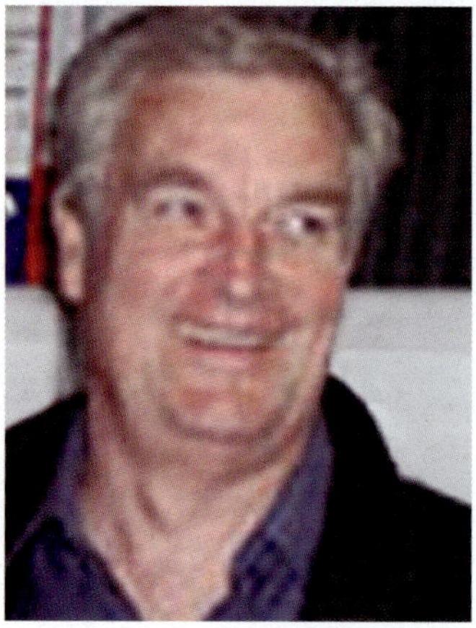

Yves Menezo

Steptoe and Edwards published a report on an ectopic pregnancy following transfer of a human embryo at the late morulae /early blastocyst stage. (Steptoe and Edwards. Lancet 1976;1:880).

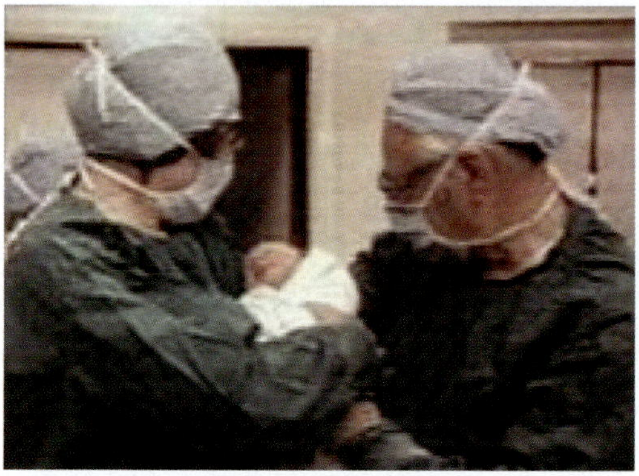

Birth of Louise Brown

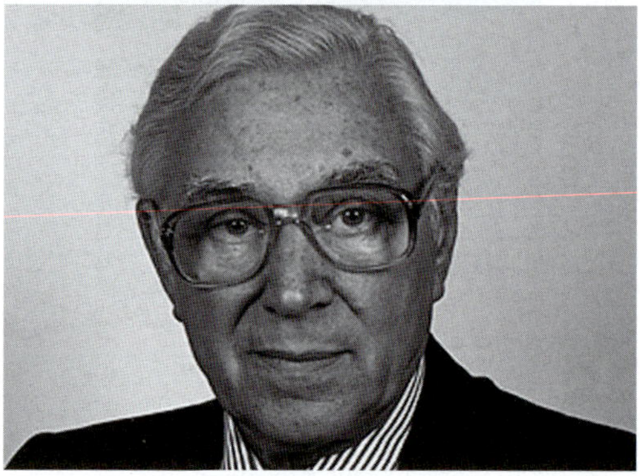

Patrick Steptoe

1978 The first ever IVF birth occurred in Oldham, England on July 25, 1978. This birth was the result of the collaborative work of Patrick Steptoe and Robert Edwards (Steptoe and Edwards. Lancet 1978;312:366).

1979 Pez et al began tracking the growth of follicles by ultrasound. They showed an appreciable relationship between the echographic and laparoscopic observations (Pez et al. 1979, 17° soirée gynéco-obstricale de St Maurice le 9.10.79).

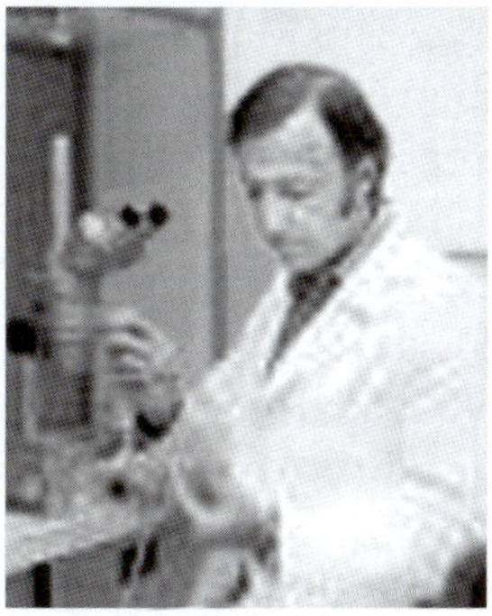

Alex Lopata

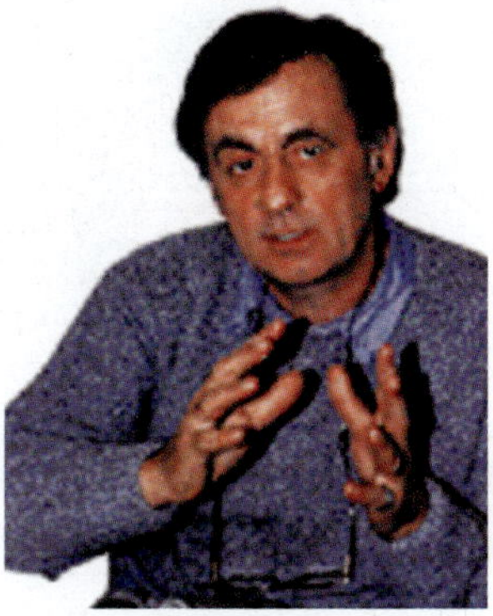

Jacques Testart

1980 The first IVF birth in Australia to the joint Victorian Monash-Melbourne team occurred at RWH (Lopata et al. Fertil Steril 1980;33:117).

1981 Howard and Georgianna Seegar Jones announced the delivery of the first IVF baby in the United States. This first IVF birth in the USA was achieved with the use of hMG.

Introduction of Clomiphene Citrate and hMG in the IVF treatment protocol (Trounson et al. Science 1981;212:681).

The Clamart group in France developed an LH assay (LH-SIR0) which could detect the initial LH rise in plasma allowing accurate prediction of the ideal time for the retrieval of oocytes (Testart et al. Fertil Steril 1981;36:50).

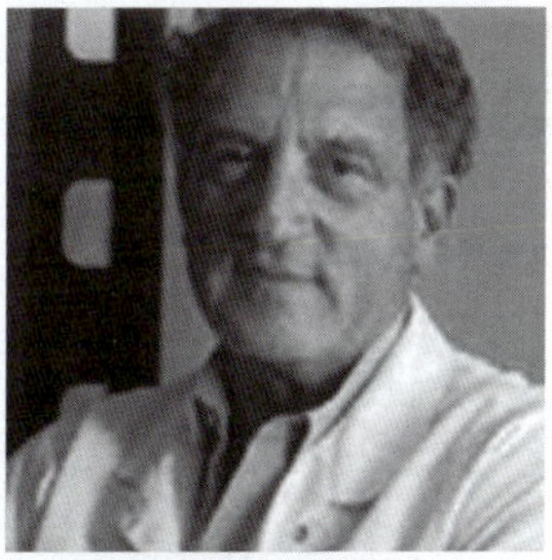

Rene Frydman

1982 The first French IVF birth occurred in Clamart, France by the group of Frydman and Testart. The first IVF birth in Sweden (Hamberger et al. Acta Med Rom 1982;20:370-8).

The first frozen embryo twins were born in Australia.

The introduction of culture medium (Mohr and Trounson. J Reprod Fertil 1980;58:189).

The first report of the need for a delay between oocyte collection and insemination to allow oocytes collected to complete maturation (Trounson et al. J Reprod Fertil 1982;64:285).

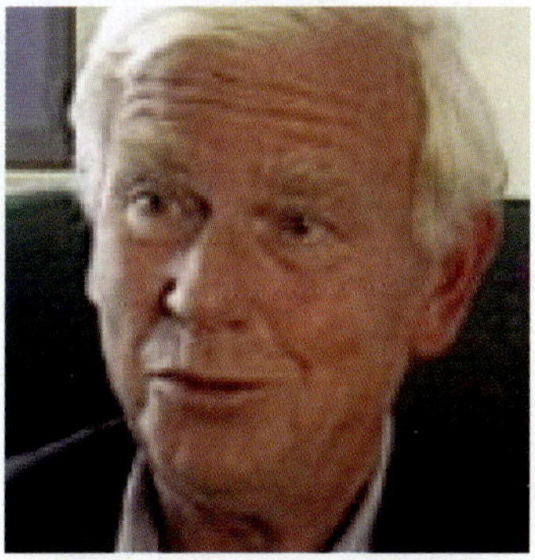

Lars Hamberger

Susan Lenz and Jörgen G Lauritsen demonstrated transabdominal transvesical oocyte aspiration using an ultrasound-guided needle (Lenz and Lauritsen. Fertil Steril 1982;38:673).

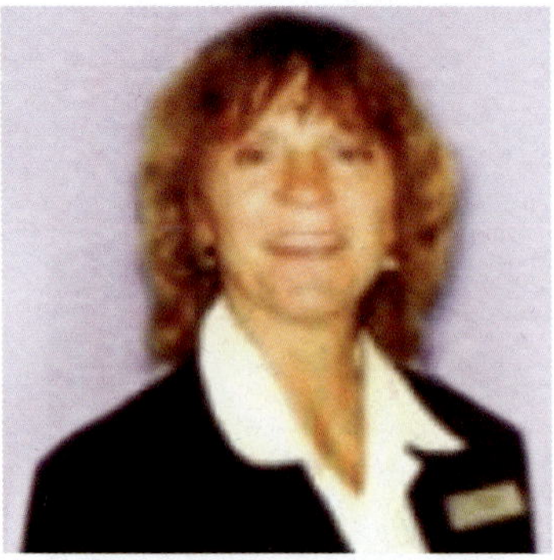

Susan Lenz

1983 *Donor egg*: The Monash IVF team achieved the first birth by a woman without ovaries by using donor eggs creating of artificial menstrual cycles and a special hormonal formula for the first 10 weeks of pregnancy (Trounson et al. Br Med J 1983;286:835).

Monash IVF team reported on the birth of the first frozen embryo baby (Embryo freezing developed in Cambridge, England on cattle – minor adaptations to adjust to humans). (Trounson and Mohr. Nature 1983;305:707).

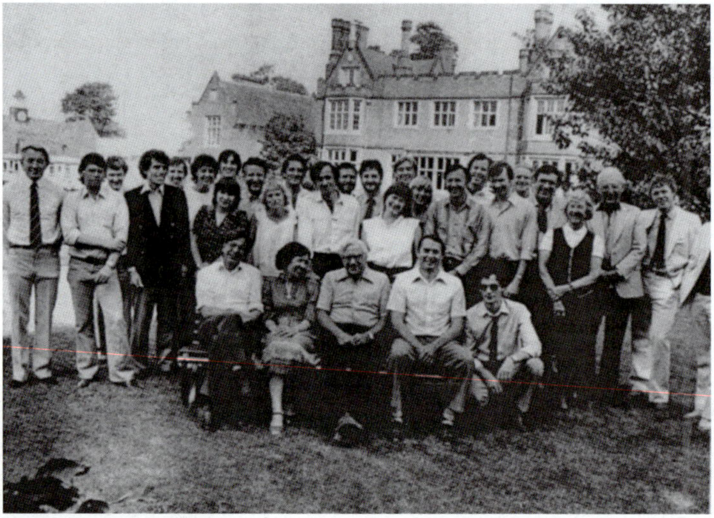

Bourne Hall—World's first IVF Conference

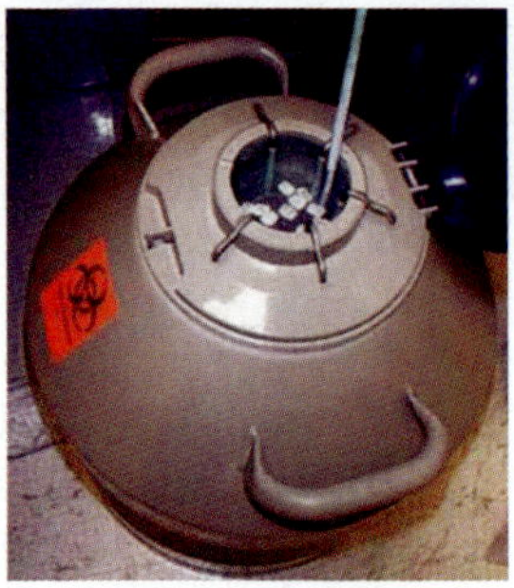

Frozen embryos

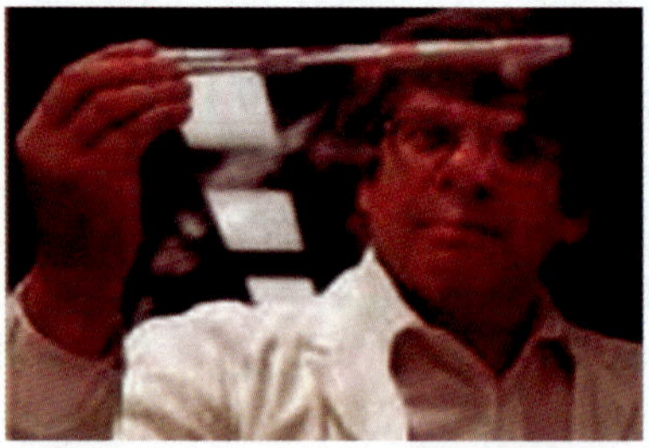

Alan Trounson

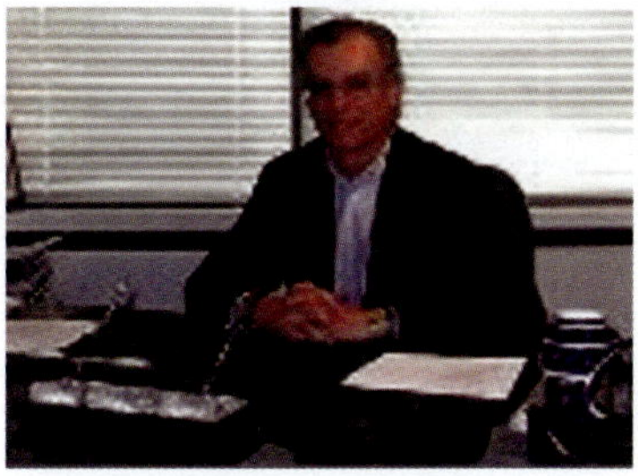

Robert Casper

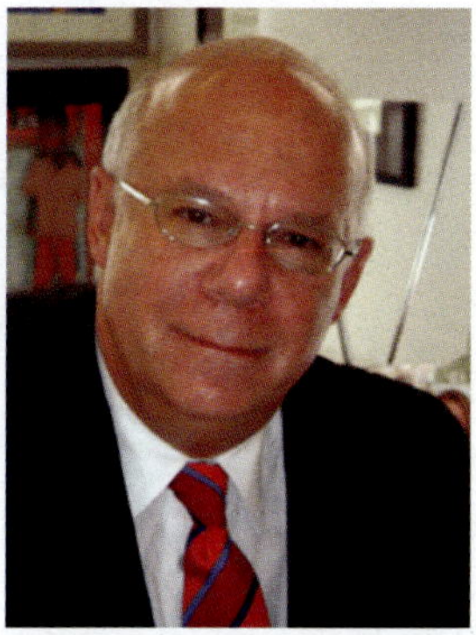

Norbert Gleicher

Maturation and fertilization of morphologically immature human oocytes in a program of *in vitro* fertilization (Veek et al. Fertil Steril 1983;39:594).

First pregnancy after oocyte donation. (Trounson et al. Br Med J 1983;286:835).

First successful delivery following egg donation. (Buster et al. Lancet 1983;2:223).

Gleicher and his group reported the first vaginal egg retrieval using an abdominal ultrasound (Gleicher et al. Lancet 1983;2:508).

1984 The Government of Victoria established a review of IVF research and practice which led to the proclamation of the research.

First surrogacy embryo transfer baby born in California.

First report on pregnancy following trans-laparoscopic gamete intrafallopian transfer (GIFT) procedure (Asch et al. Lancet 1984; 2(8410):1034).

The first report on pregnancy following IVF and egg donation in a woman with primary ovarian failure (Lutien et al. Nature 1984;307(5947):174).

Introduction of GnRH agonists to the IVF treatment protocol (Porter et al. Lancet 1984;2:1284).

A report of pregnancy following transfer of intact frozen-thawed embryos (Zeilmaker et al. Fertil Steril 1984;42:293).

An unusual report of the possibility that abnormal spermatozoa could be enriched and give rise to healthy babies (Cohen et al. Lancet 1984; 1(8388):1239-40).

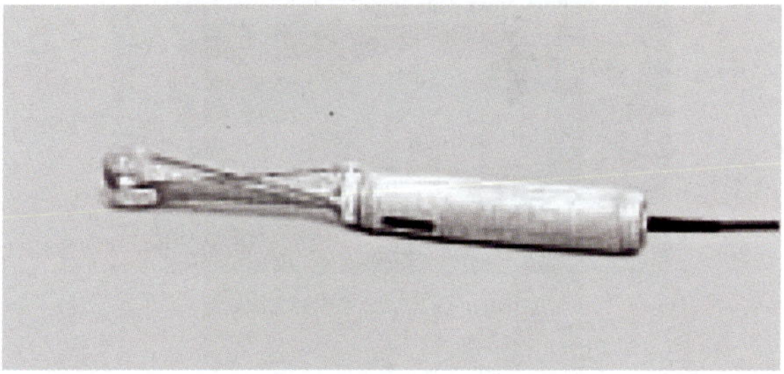

Kretztechnik's mechanical rotary vaginal scanner in 1985 with puncture attachment

Casper and his colleagues were the first to described the use of low dose hCG for support of the luteal phase in ART cycles (Casper et al. Lancet 1983;2:1191).

1985 Human pregnancy by *in vitro* fertilization (IVF) using sperm aspirated from the epididymis. (Temple-Smith. J *In Vitro* Fert Embryo Trans 1985;2:119).

Jacqueline Mandelbaumm with Dan Szollosi described the microstructures of the human oocyte, which became known as 'oocyte dysmorphia' (Szollosi et al. J *In Vitro* Fertil Embryo Trans 1986;3:232).

Matts Wikland in Gothenburg, Sweden, described the possibility of using a vaginal sector

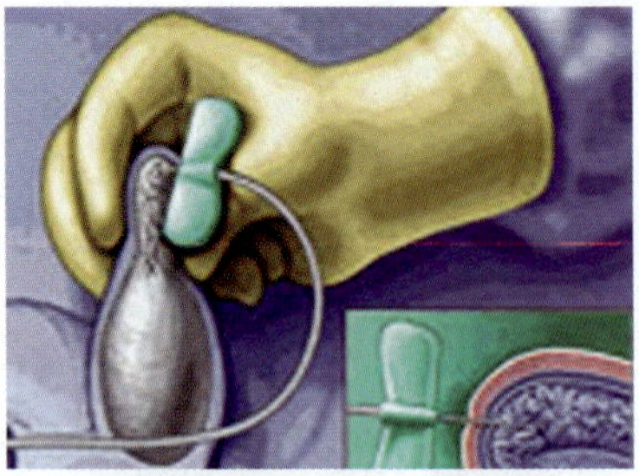

Epididymis sperm aspiration

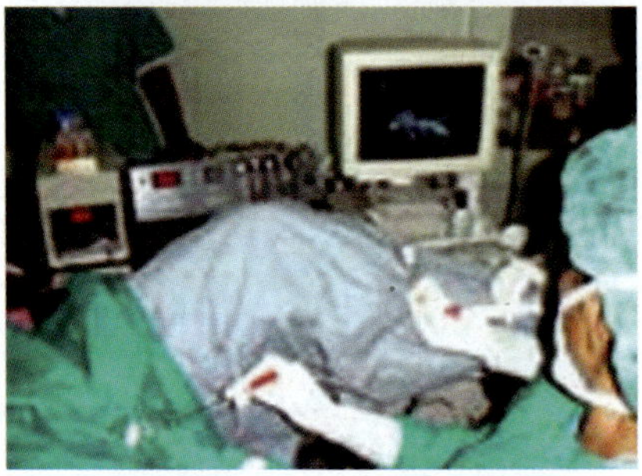

Vaginal oocyte aspiration

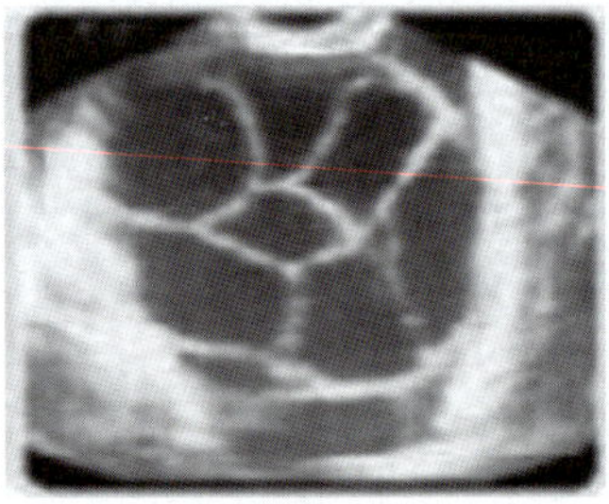

Ultrasound image of follicles

scanner (transvaginal technique) for oocyte aspiration (Wikland et al. Ann NY Acad Sci 1985; 442:182).

First report of the use of abdominal ultrasound guidance for embryo transfer (Strickler et al. Fertil Steril 1985;43:54).

The first reported birth after replacement of hatching blastocyst cryopreserved at expanded blastocyst stage (Cohen et al. Lancet 1985;1(8429): 647).

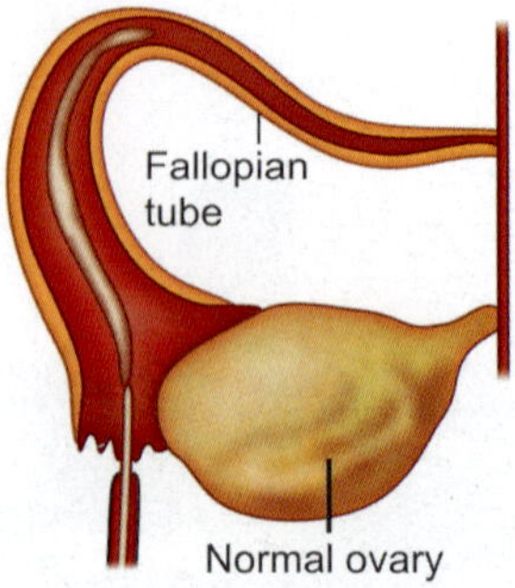

Gamete intrafallopian transfer (GIFT) procedure

First report about the Canadian IVF baby by the group of Victor Gomel at the University of British Columbia (Young S Moon et al. Gamete Research 1985;11:289).

In 1985, Quinn and Warnes published a formula entitled Human Tubal Fluid (HTF) which mimics the *in vivo* environment to which the embryo is exposed (Quinn P, Kerin JF, Warnes GM. Fertil Steril 1985;1985:493).

1986 Harsha Chawda, the first baby to be conceived from IVF in India is born. This was achieved by the work of Indira Hinduja at the Seth GS Medical College and KEM Hospital, Mumbai. Earlier reports (1978) of a birth from IVF conception in Kolkata through the work of Subhash Mukhopadhyay exist, but documentation surrounding it is poor and it is still mired in controversy.

First description of transvaginal sector scan sonography for needle-guided transvaginal follicle aspiration (Fiechtinger and Kemeter. Fertil Steril 1986;45:722).

First pregnancy, following IVF donated oocytes, in a non-ovarian failure patient (Rosenwaks et al. Fertil Steril 1986;45:417).

Navot et al. reported the possibility to artificially induced endometrial cycles and

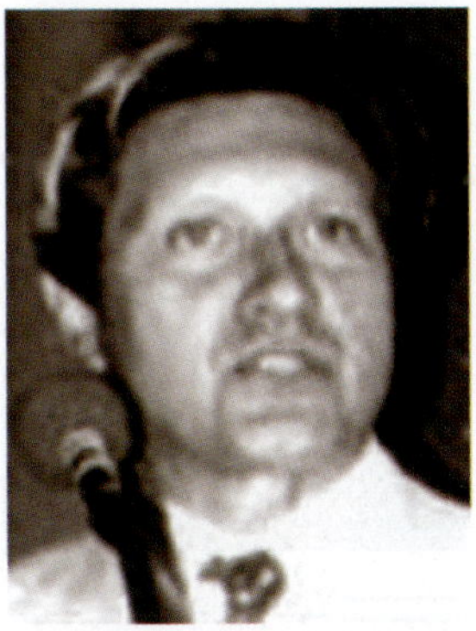

W Feichtinger

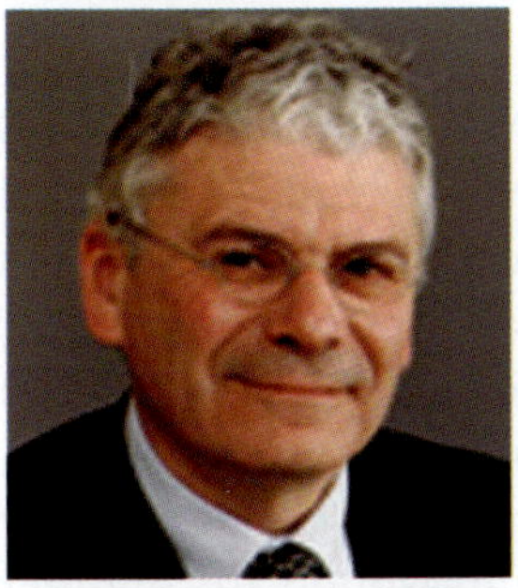

Paul Devroey

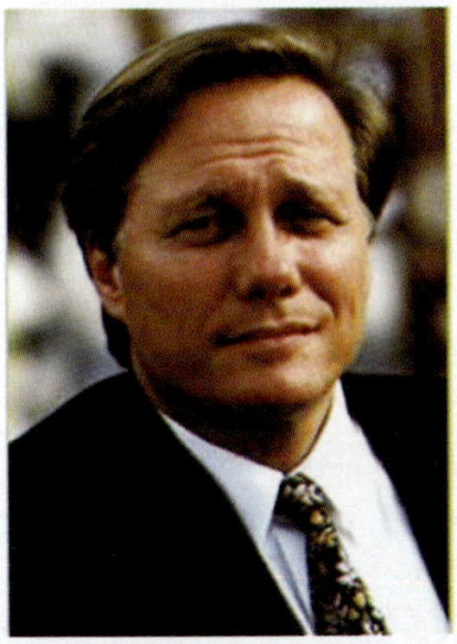

Zev Rosenwaks

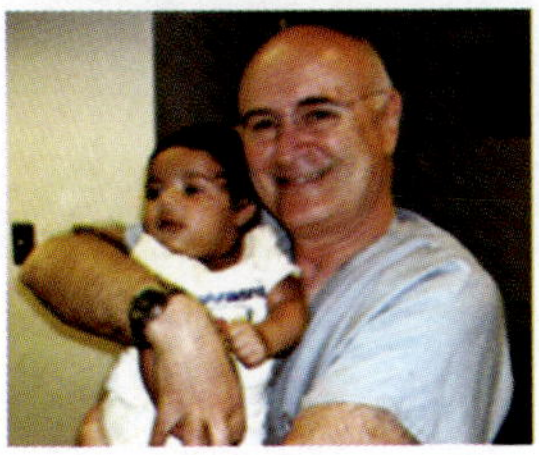

Daniel Navot

establishment of pregnancies in the absence of ovaries (Navot et al. NEJM 1986;314:806).

First report on pregnancy after trans-laparoscopic zygote intrafallopian transfer (Devroey et al. Lancet 1986;1(8493):1329).

1987 Fertilization of human oocytes by microinjection of a single sperm under the zona pellucida (Laws King et al. Fertil Steril 1987;48:637).

1988 Embryo biopsy technique was developed in mice by Professor Alan Trounson and Leeanda Wilton.

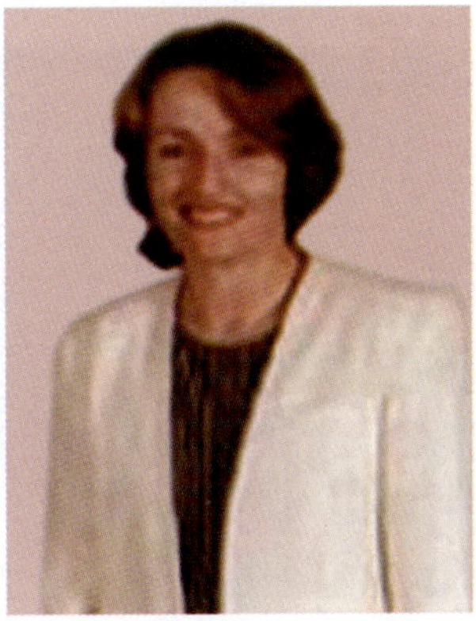

Leeanda Wilton

First two babies born after epididymal sperm aspiration for men with congenital absence of the vas deferens and naming of the technique MESA (Patrizio et al. Lancet 1988;2(8624):1364).

Australia's first IVF surrogate birth.

The first baby birth using subzonal sperm injection at National University of Singapore (Ng et al. Lancet 1988;2:790).

Pregnancy was obtained from micro-manipulation using zona drilling or mechanical partial zona dissection (Cohen et al. Lancet 1988;2(8603):162).

The death of Dr Patrick Steptoe—March 21 1988.

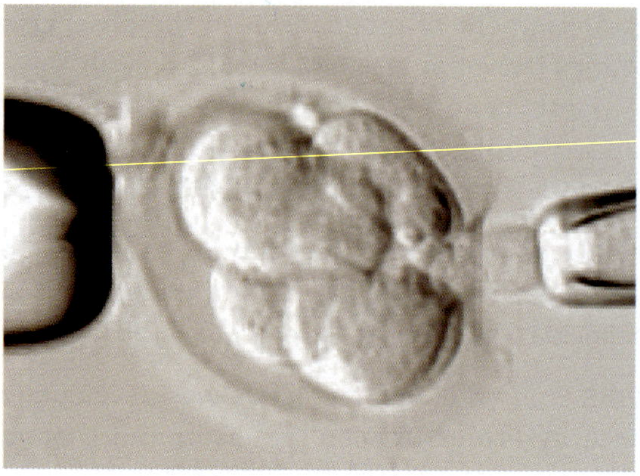

Biopsy of an embryo

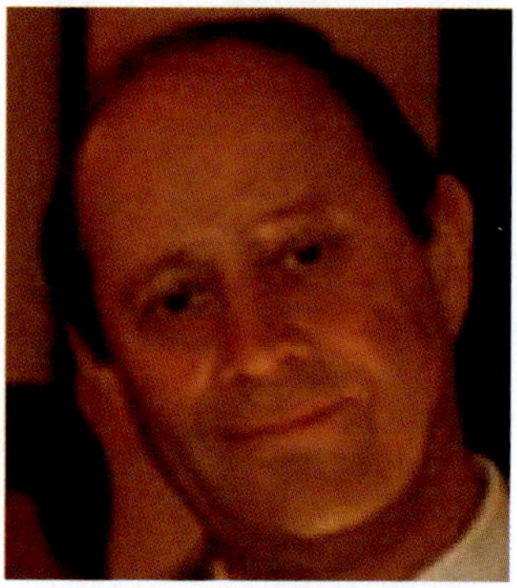

Yona Tadir

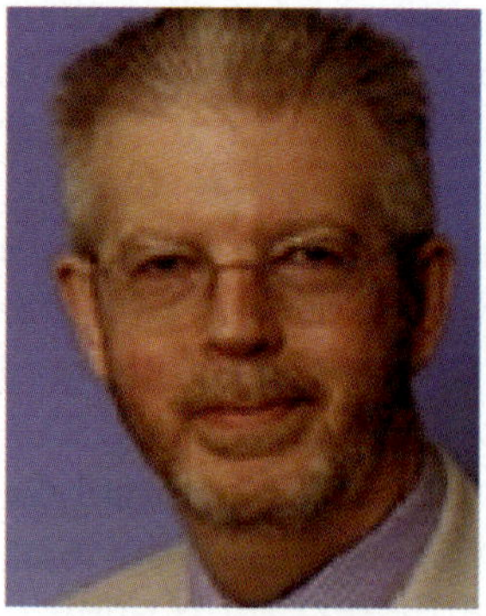

Alan Handyside

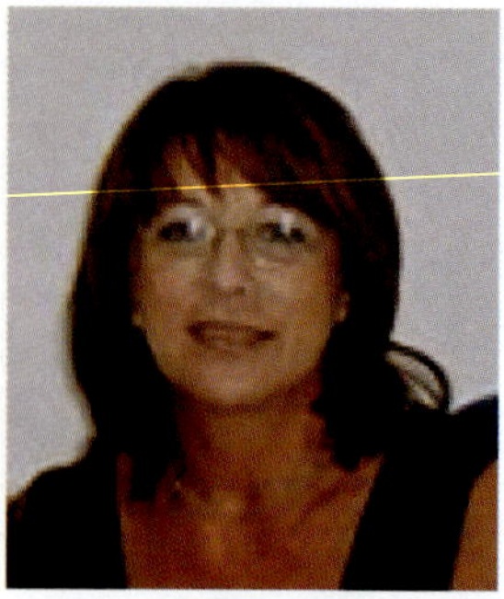

Yael Gonen

1989 First report on biopsy of human preimplantation embryos and sexing by DNA amplification (Handyside et al. Lancet 1989;1:347).

First report of the use of laser techniques in the field of assisted reproduction for application in gametes or embryos (Tadir et al. Fertil Steril 1989;52:870).

Gonen and her colleagues in Toronto pioneered the use of ultrasound for endometrial quality (thickness and pattern) related to IVF pregnancy. (Gonen et al. Fertil Steril 1989;52:446).

1990 The first successful human cleavage-stage embryo vitrification followed by a successful delivery (Gordts et al. Fertil Steril 1990;53:469).

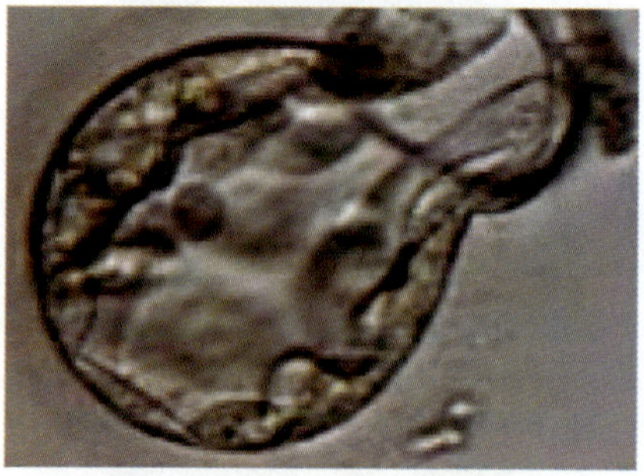

Hatching of a blastocyst

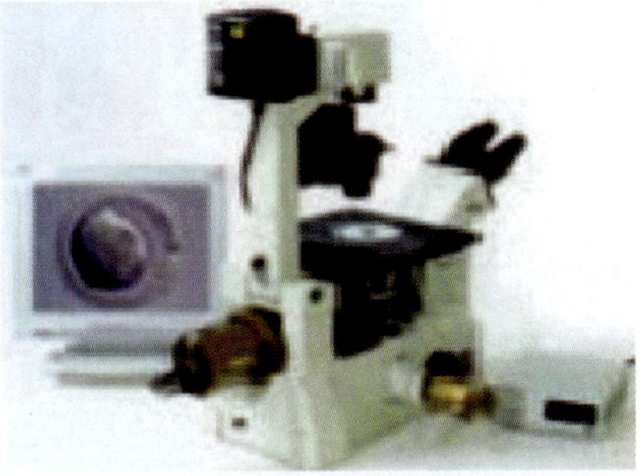

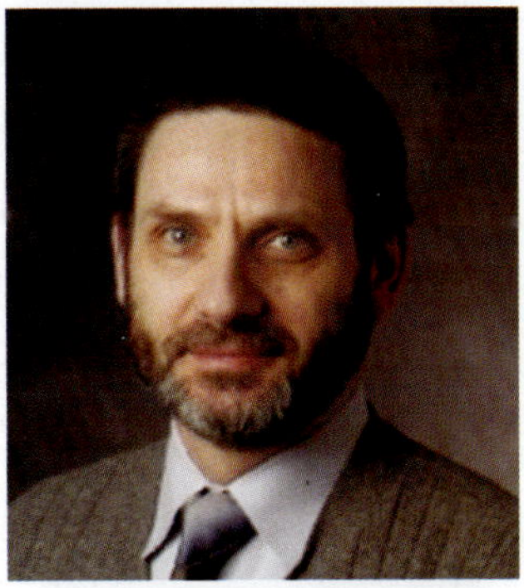

Daniel Palanker

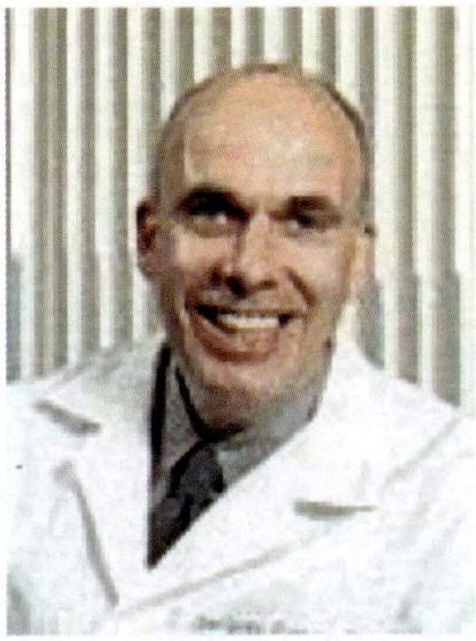

Jacques Cohen

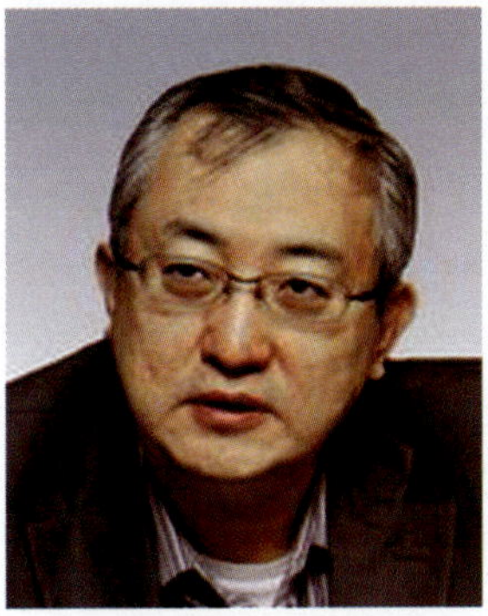

Kwang Ryul Cha

Pregnancies from biopsied human preimplantation embryos sexed by Y-specific DNA amplification (Handyside et al. Nature 1990; 344:768).

First report of assisted hatching in human embryos (Cohen et al. Human Reprod 1990;5:7).

The first report on polar body biopsy, transfer of the embryo and achieving pregnancy (Verlinsky et al. Hum Reprod 1990;7:826).

Gonen et al proposed the use of GnRH agonist in place of hCG as a means to trigger the gonadotropic surge for IVF (Gonen et al. J Clin Endocrinol Metab 1990;71:918).

Gonen, Jacobson and Casper pioneered the use of combined oral contraceptives for follicle synchronization and cycle scheduling in IVF (Gonen et al. Fertil Steril 1990;53:282).

1991 *In Vitro* Maturation (IVM) in unstimulated cycle resulted in pregnancy in a donor oocyte program (Cha et al. Fertil Steril 1991;55:109).

The first report suggesting the use of GnRH antagonist, Nal-Glue, to prevent premature LH rise and progesterone in controlled ovarian hyperstimulation treatment (Frydman et al. Fertil Steril 1991;56:932).

The first report on the use of a laser for Zona Pelucida drilling (Palanker et al. Laser Surg Med 1991;11:589).

Navot et al confirmed that the age-related decline in female fertility is attributable to oocyte quality (Navot et al. Lancet 1991;337(8754):137).

1992 Successful *in vitro* fertilization and embryo transfer after treatment with recombinant human

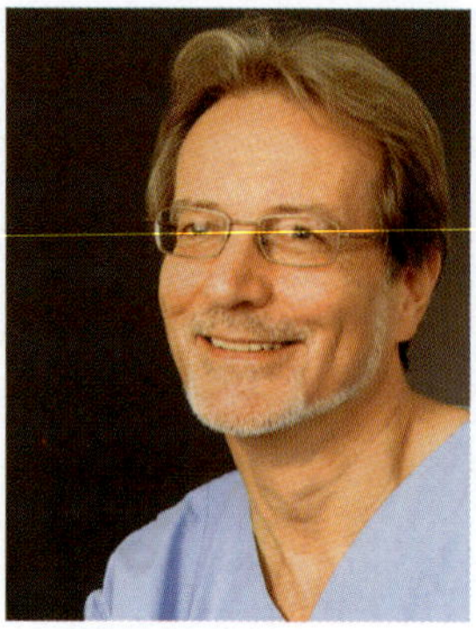

Marc Germond

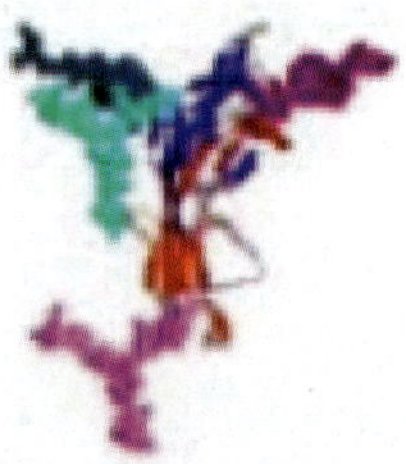

Recombinant FSH

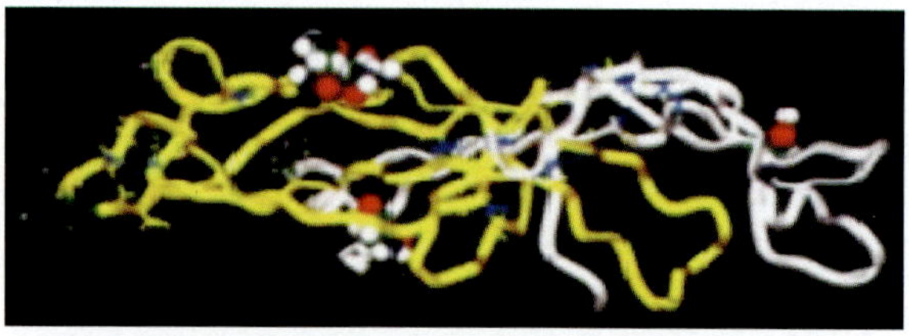

Three-dimensional model structure of follicle stimulating hormone (FSH)

follicle stimulating hormone (FSH). (Germond et al. Lancet 1992;9;339(8802):1170) (Devroey et al. Lancet 1992;9;339(8802):1170).

Assisted zona hatching was introduced in IVF programs to breach the zona pellucida and promote the natural process of hatching (Cohen et al. Hum Reprod 1992;7:685-91).

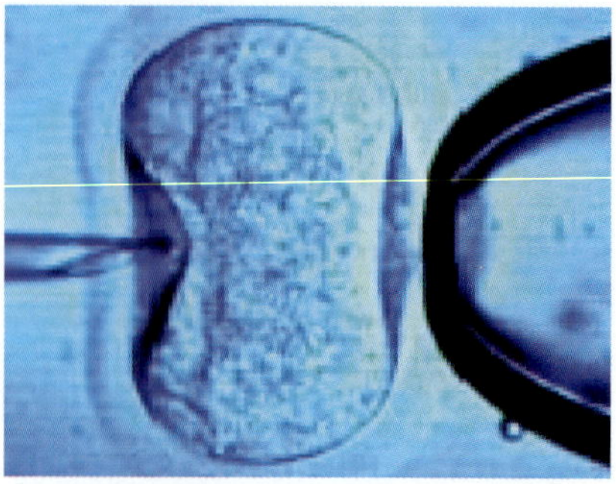

Intracytoplasmic sperm injection (ICSI) process

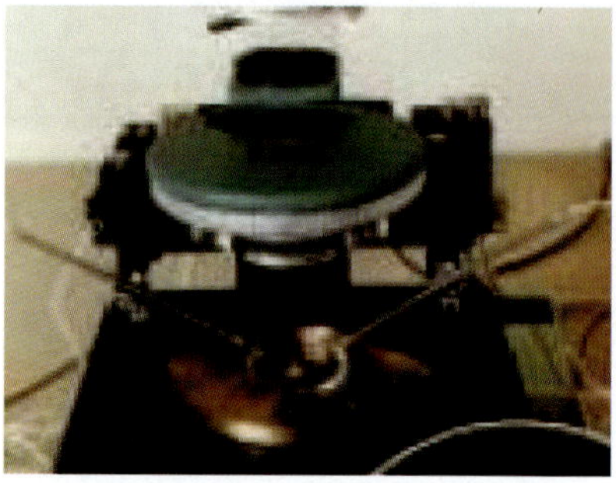

ICSI microscope

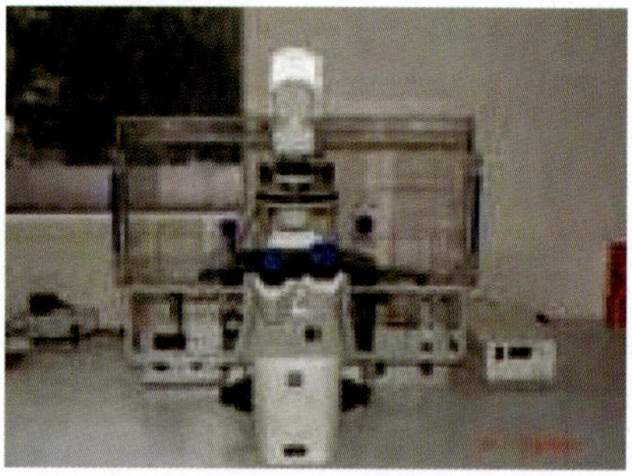

ICSI microscope

Discovery that men with congenital absence of the vas deferens have a mild form of cystic fibrosis: Two papers: (Anguiano et al. JAMA 1992;267(13): 1794) (Patrizio and Asch. Annals Acad Med Singapore 1992;21:533).

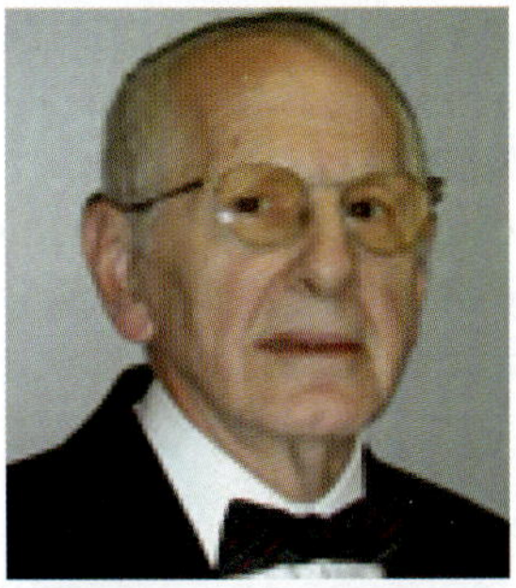

Andre Van-Steirtegham

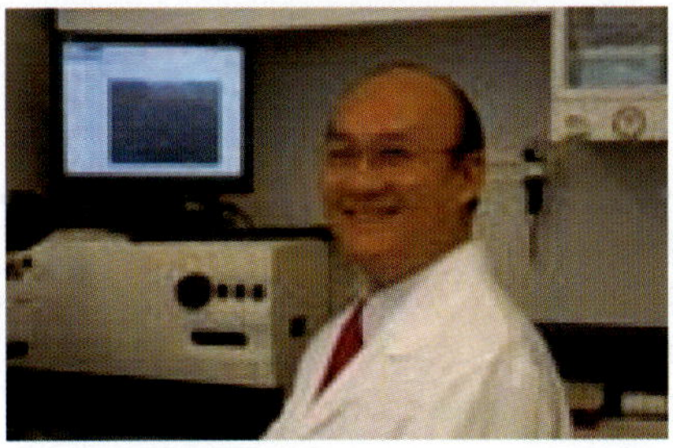

Seang Lin Tan

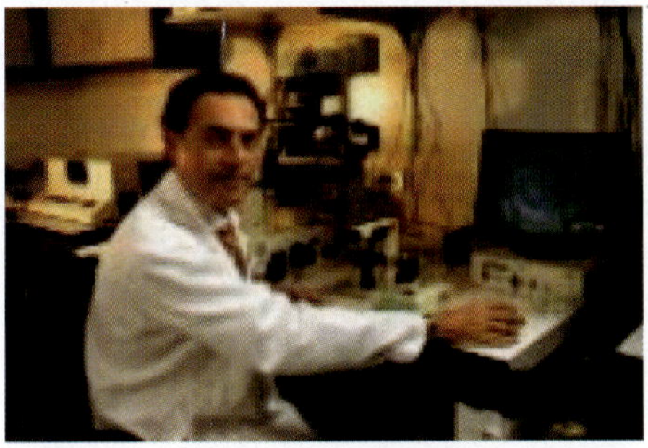

Gianpiero Palermo

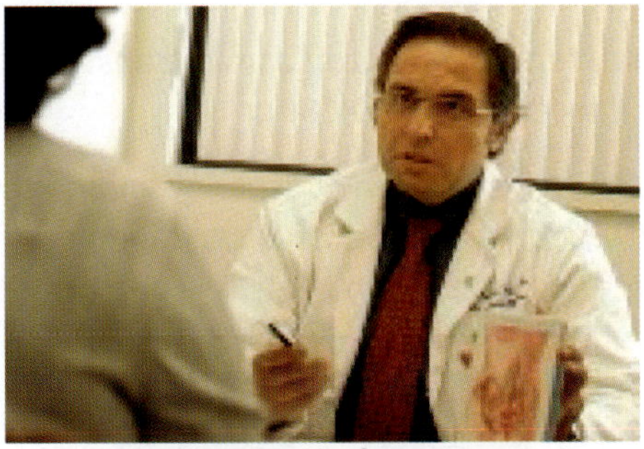

Pasquale Patrizio

Report of the first pregnancy after intracytoplasmic sperm injection (ICSI) by the group in Brussels (Palermo et al. Lancet 1992;2:17).

Pregnancy after embryo biopsy and coamplification of DNA from X and Y chromosomes (Gilbert et al. JAMA 1992;268:727).

Ovulation induction by endogenous LH released by the administration of an LHRH agonist after follicular stimulation for *in vitro* fertilization (Emperaire et al. J Gynecol Obstet Biol Reprod (Paris) 1992;21:489).

First report of cumulative conception and live-birth rates after IVF in relation to patient age and cause of infertility (Tan et al. Lancet 1992; 339:1390).

1993 The second term pregnancy after ICSI reported by a group in Sweden (Hamberger et al. In: Gordts S (Ed). Proceedings of European Symposium on Micromanipulation. Drukkerij Nauwelaerts, Leuven, Belgium 1993; p. 85).

Confirmation that men with congenital absence of the vas defference, have cystic fibrosis mutations which can be transmitted to the offspring (Patrizio P et al. Hum Reprod 1983;8:215).

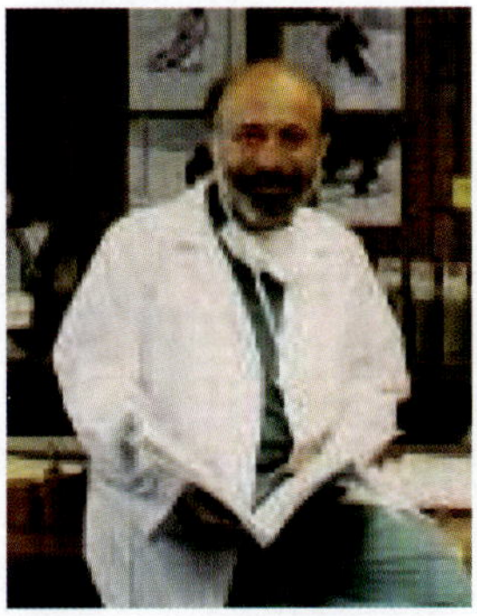

Sherman Silber

First report on the use of testicular sperm extraction (TESE) and ICSI (Silber et al. Hum Reprod 1994).

1994 The first livebirth as a result of IVM following transvaginal ultrasound-guided oocyte collection. (Trounson et al. Fertil Steril 1994;62:353).

First two births from replacement of frozen embryos produced with epididymal sperm (Patrizio et al. Hum Reprod 1992;7:652).

The first reported birth resulting a frozen-thawed oocyte and ICSI (Chen Lancet 1986;1:884).

1995 Pregnancies after testicular sperm extraction (TESE) and ICSI in nonobstructive azoospermia. (Devroey et al. Hum Reprod 1995;10:1457).

Birth after blastocyst development from IVM oocyte plus ICSI plus Assisted Hatching (Barnes et al. Hum Reprod 1995;10:3243) The first report of aneuploidy testing (Munné et al. Am J Obstet Gynecol 1995;172:1191).

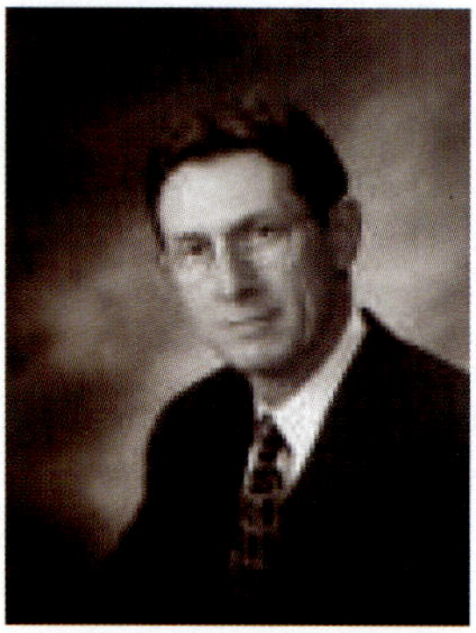

Frank Barnes

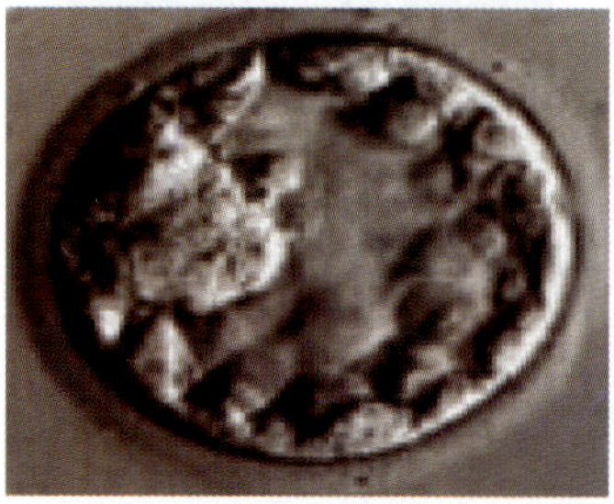

Blastocyst

Zenzes from the group of Casper in Toronto demonstrated adverse effects of cigarette smoking on nuclear spindle (Zenzes et al. Hum Reprod 1995;10:3213).

1996 The Valencia group reported on the first pregnancy employing cryopreserved testicular sperm following IVF-ICSI (Gil-Salom et al. Hum Reprod 1996;11:1309).

Discovery that some men with severe oligoasthenospermia have deletions in the Y-chromosome (Rejio et al. Lancet 1996;347(9011): 1290).

Jurisicova from the group of Casper was the first to recognize that preimplantation human embryo fragmentation involved programmed cell death. (Jurisicova et al. Mol Hum Reprod 1996;2:93).

Casper and his colleagues were the first to demonstrate and introduce the use of the hypo-osmotic swelling test for selection of immotile sperm for ICSI (Casper et al. Fertil Steril 1996; 65:972).

First report on Cytoplasmic transfer (Cohen et al. Lancet 1996;350:186).

1997 Sun, Jurisicova and Casper described the use of TUNEL for detection of DNA fragmentation in sperm and correlation with IVF outcome. They

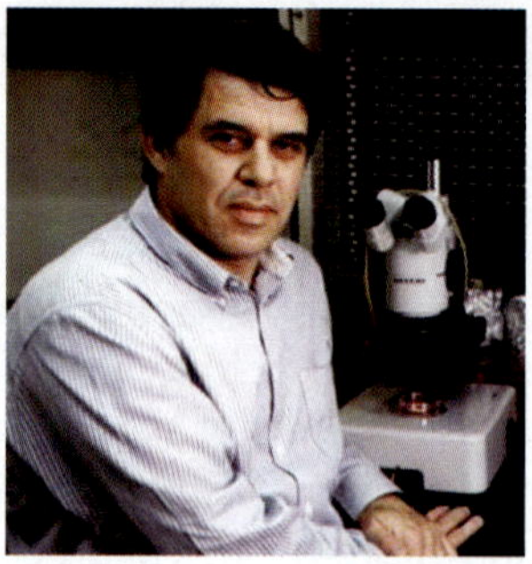

Joseph Itskovitz-Eldor

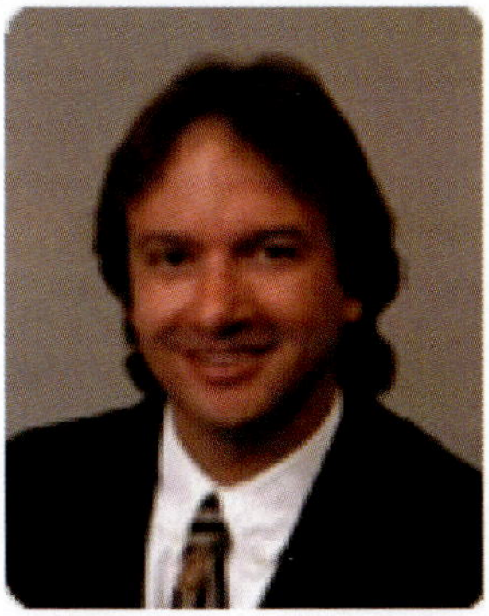

David Gardner

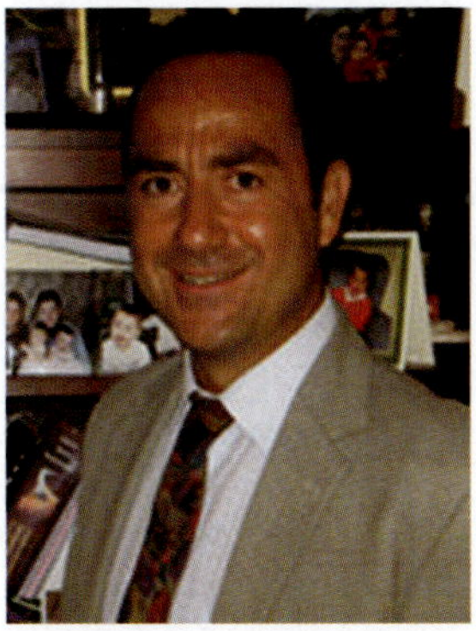

Kutluk Oktay

showed almost uniform presence of DNA fragmentation in round spermatids as explanation for failure to achieve pregnancy with these immature gametes (Sun et al. Biol Reprod 1997;56:602).

1998 First establish pregnancy using recombinant FSH and GnRH antagonist (Itskovitz-Eldor et al. Hum Reprod 1998;13:294).

Gardner introduced sequential media and blastocyst transfer which is now greatly assisting in the move to single embryo transfer (Gardner et al. Human Reproduction 1998;13:3434).

Births after intracytoplasmic injection of sperm obtained by testicular extraction from men with nonmosaic Klinefelter's sydrome (Palermo et al. N Engl J Med 1998;338:588).

First report on cytoplasmic transfer (Cohen et al. Lancet 1996;350(9072):186).

1999 First unaffected pregnancy using preimplantation genetic diagnosis for sickle cell anemia (Xu et al. JAMA 1999;281:1701).

Birth following vitrification of human oocyte (Kuleshova et al. Hum Reprod 1999;14:3077).

Chian et al demonstrated that hCG priming prior to immature oocyte retrieval in women with PCO increases the maturation rate and produces high pregnancy rates of 40 percent per IVM cycle started (Chian et al. N Eng J Med 1999;341:1624).

World's first IVF/ICSI pregnancy and livebirth after successful air transport of oocytes reported by the McGill Reproductive Center, enabling the creation of an airtransport IVF program in large countries with scattered populations or in areas remote from infertility centers (Buckett WM et al. Fertil Steril 1999;71:753).

2000 Oktay and Karlikaya were the first to report on ovarian tissue transplant after frozen storage (Oktay and Karlikaya. NEJM 2000;342:1919).

2001 First report using ultrasound for embryo transfer (Kojima et al. Hum Reprod 2001;16:2578).

Embryo transfer catheter is visualized by vaginal ultrasound.

Birth of an infant from cryopreserved embryos (zygotes) produced by IVM oocytes derived from an unstimulated patient with polycysticovary

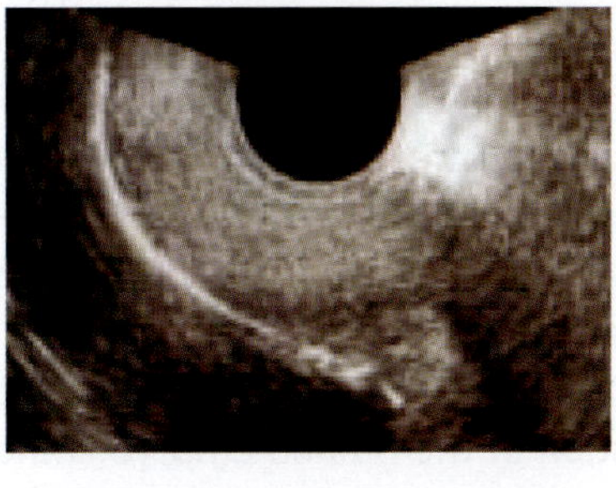

Embryo transfer catheter

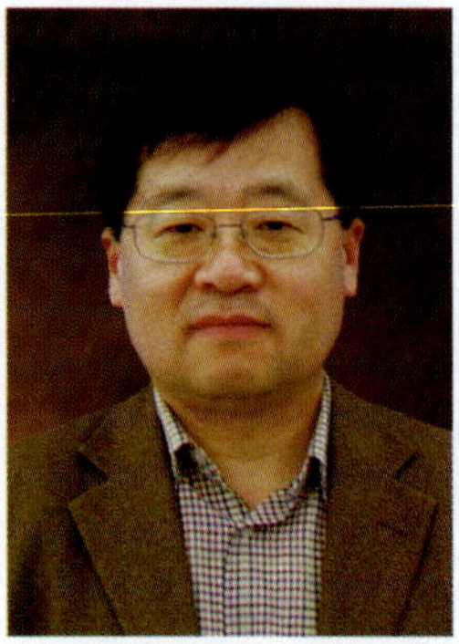

Ri-Cheng Chian

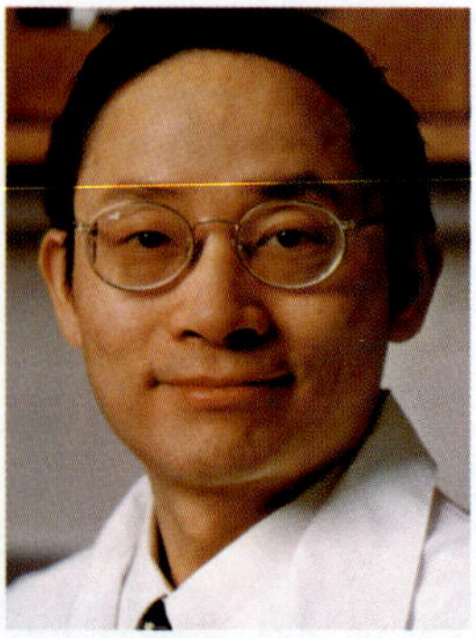

Ren-He Xu

syndrome (PCOS) (Chian et al. Hum Reprod 2001;16:1700).

Ongoing twin pregnancy after ICSI of PESA-retrieved spermatozoa into *in vitro* matured oocytes reported by the McGill group. (Ahmad Kamal Abdul-Jalil et al. Hum Reprod 2001;16:1424).

Livebirth after sperm retrieval from a moribund man (Belker et al. Fertil Steril 2001;76:841).

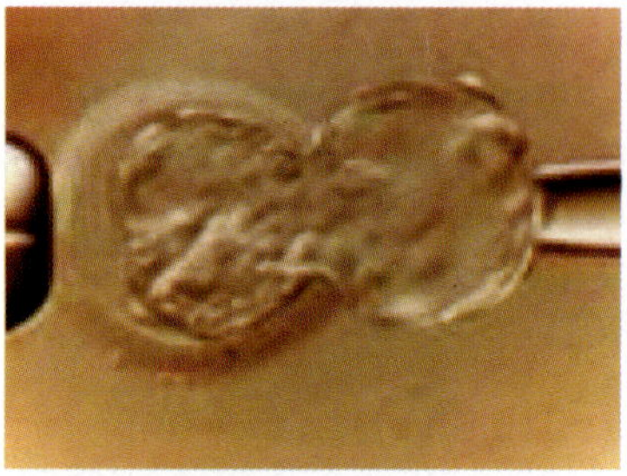

Blastocyst biopsy

2002 First livebirth following blastocyst biopsy and PGD analysis (De Boer et al. Reprod Biomed Online 2002;4:35).

First clinical application of comparative genomic hybridization and polar body testing for preimplantation genetic diagnosis of aneuploidy. (Wells et al. Fertil Steril 2002;78:543).

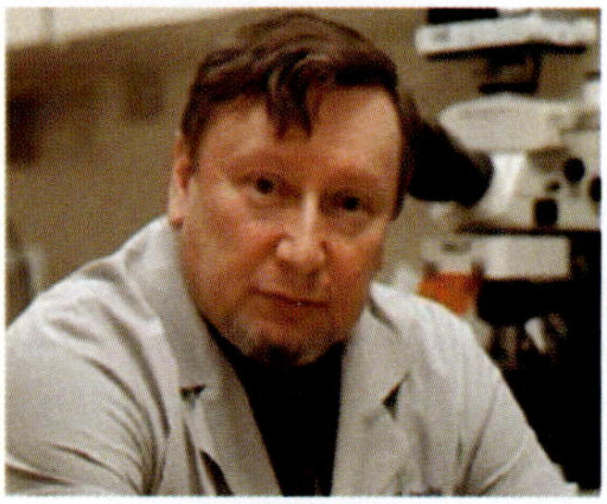

Yuri Verlinsky

2003 Livebirths after vitrification of oocytes in a stimulated *in vitro* fertilization–embryo transfer program (Yoon et al. Fertil Steril 2003;79:1323).

First livebirth after ovarian stimulation using a chimeric long-acting human recombinant follicle-stimulating hormone (FSH) agonist (recFSH-CTP) for *in vitro* fertilization (Beckers et al. Fertil Steril 2003;79:621).

The first reported liveborn following preimplantation genetic diagnosis for Retino-blastoma (Xu et al. Am J Opthalmol 2003;18) Implantation of the human embryo is the limiting factor in the success of IVF. Dr Barash and

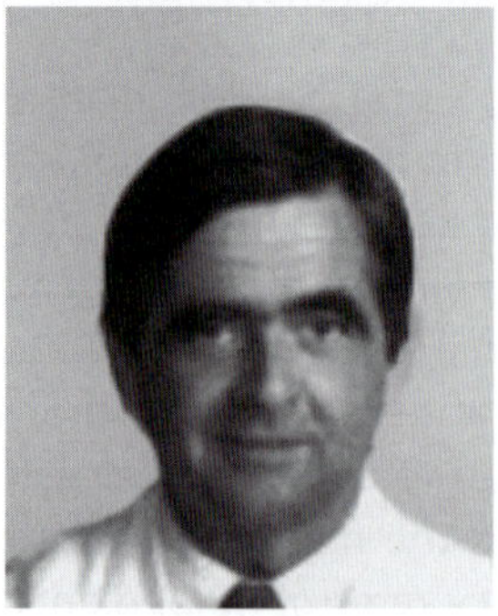

Jacques Donezz

Prof Dekel showed an increasing implantation rate following endometrial injury, performed by Pipelle curettage as a simple outpatient procedure. (Barash et al. Fertil Steril 2003;79:1317).

2004 Successful pregnancy and delivery following combined treatment of *in vitro* maturation (IVM) and testicular sperm extraction (TESE) (Fuchinoue et al. J of Assisted Reprod Genetics 2004;21:371).

Jaques Donnez reporting about the first Livebirth after orthotopic transplantation of cryopreserved ovarian tissue (Donnez et al. Lancet 2004;364(9443):1405).

Gardner and colleagues performed the world's first prospective single blastocyst trial, which showed the feasibility of SBT and in keeping high pregnancy rates (Gardner et al. Fertil Steril 2004; 81:551).

The first preimplantation HLA matching for stem cell transplantation to affected sibling (Verlinsky et al. JAMA 2004;291:2079).

First report of fertility preservation for cancer patients using IVM and oocyte vitrification (Rao et al. Lancet 2004;363:1829). First report on natural cycle in IVF combined with IVM as a potential approach to infertility treatment (Chian et al. Fertil and Steril 2004;82:1675).

2005 Pregnancies and livebirths after trophectoderm biopsy and preimplantation genetic testing of human blastocysts (McArthur et al. Fertil Steril 2005;84:1628).

First birth in Israel from thawed ovarian cortex re-transplants (Meirow et al. N Engl J Med 2005; 535(3):318).

2006 First successful pregnancy after preimplantation genetic diagnosis for aneuploidy screening in embryos generated from natural-cycle IVF combined with IVM (Ao et al. Fertil Steril 2006;85: 1510e).

Cryopreservation of intact human ovary with its vascular pedicle (Bedaiwy et al. Hum Reprod 2006;21:3258).

First successful pregnancy after preimplantation genetic diagnosis for aneuploidy screening in embryos generated from natural-cycle IVF combined with IVM achieved at the McGill Reproductive Centre (Ao et al. Fertil Steril 2006;85: 1510).

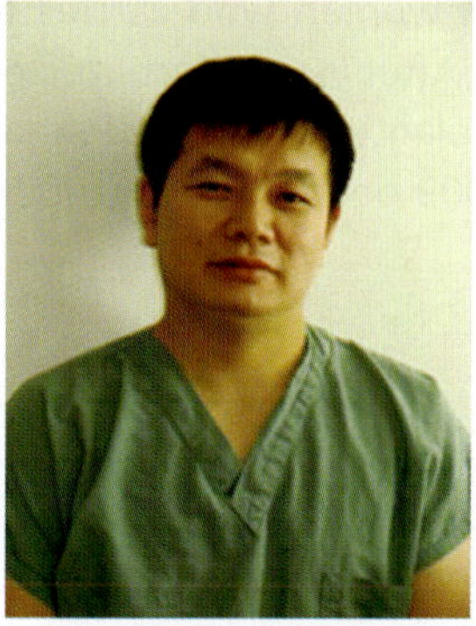

Weon-young Son

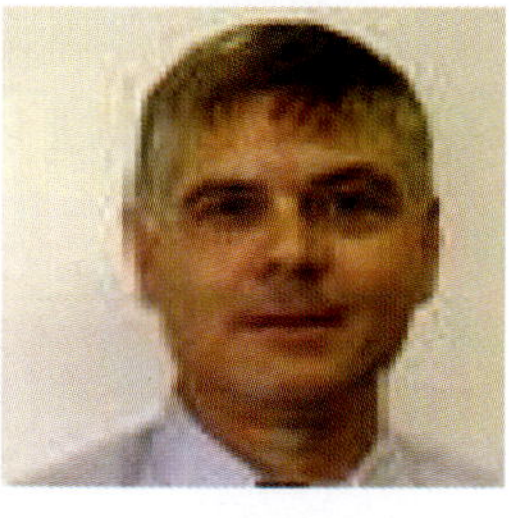

Dror Meirow

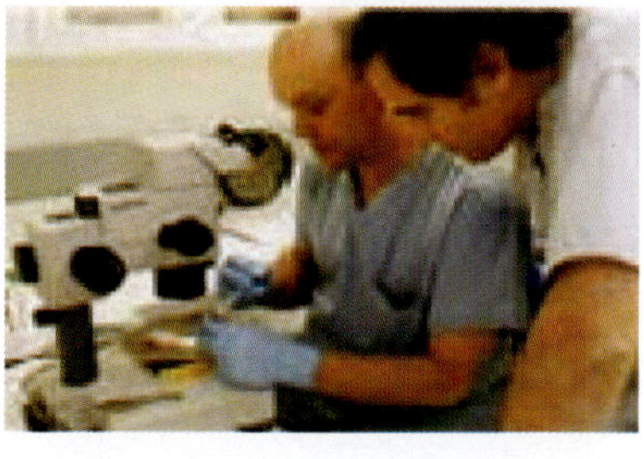

Amir Arav and Pasquale Patrizio

2007 Report from McGill Reproductive Center, Canada and Maria Infertility Hospital, Seoul, Korea on deliveries after transfer of human blastocysts derived from oocytes matured by *in vitro* maturation (IVM) (Weon-Young Son et al. Fertil Steril 2007;87:1491).

Introducing the concept of mild treatment strategy for IVF (Heijnen et al. Lancet 2007;369 (9563):743).

A novel multi-gradient freezing technique for the cryopreservation of the whole ovary. Thawing the ovary resulted in normal ovarian architecture and no damage to the vascular wall or intima (Arav and Pasquale. Yale Practice 2007;12:2).

First IVM egg donation pregnancy in North America achieved by McGill Reproductive Centre (Holzer et al. Fertil Steril 2007;88:62).

2008 Prof Laufer at the Hadassah Medical Center in Jerusalem reported on a viable pregnancy achieved in a woman who carries the defective BRCA2 genes. After *in vitro* fertilized embryos were tested and implanted (Sagi et al. Pernatal Diagnosis, Published, 2009 online DOI:10/1002/pd).

REFERENCES

1. Pincus G, Sanders B. Anat Rec 1939;75:537.
2. Menkin MF, Rock J. Am J obstet Gynecol 1949;55:440.
3. Chang MC. J Exp 2001 1955;128:379-405.
4. Runner M, Gates AH. J Hered 1954;45:51.
5. Gates AH. Nature 1954;177:754.
6. Fowler RE, Edwards RG. J Endocrinol 1957;15:374-84.
7. Edwards RG. Nature 1962;196:446-5.
8. Cole R, Edwards RG, Paul J. Cytodifferentiation and embryogenesis in cell colonises and tissue culture derived from ova and blastocyts of the rabbit. Devbiol 1966;13:385-407.
9. Pincus G, Saunders B. The comparative behavior of mammalian eggs in vivo and in vitro. VI. The maturation of human ovarian ova. Anat Rec 1939; 75:537-45.
10. Edwards RG. Maturation in vitro of mouse, sheep, cow, pig, rhesus monkey and human ovarian oocytes. Nature 1965;208:349-51.
11. Steptoe PC. Laparoscopy and ovulation. Lancet 1968; 2:913.
12. Steptoe PC, Edwards RG. Reimplantation of a human embryo with subsequent tubal pregnancy. Lancet 1976;1:880-2.
13. Steptoe PC, Edwards RG, Purdy JM. Clinical aspects of pregnancies established with cleaving embryos grown in vitro. BJOG 1980;87:757-68.

Chapter 2

Infertility in the Developing World

Rajat Gyaneshwar

Infertility is a common presentation at busy gynecology outpatient clinics throughout the world. Currently I work in such a setting in a resource poor country. The hospital serves a population of about 400,000 people in the Fiji Islands which has been marred by political instability for over two decades. The once thriving country is now similar to many developing countries the world over. The economy is struggling, there is an exodus of skilled professionals leaving for better opportunities. The infrastructure for virtually every government service has deteriorated. Health care in this setting competes with other essential services for scarce resources. Amongst patients with terminal gynecological cancers, new referral with cervical lesions and pelvic masses I saw a thirty five year old woman who has had several appointments over the last 15 years because of her failure to conceive. She has had the routine tests. The semen analysis was reported normal by the microbiology department. There is no specialized service for andrology. She has irregular cycles and perhaps not ovulating regularly. Hormonal assays cannot be done locally and must be sent abroad. She has had several unsuccessful courses of clomiphene at considerable relative cost when one looks at the couples uncertain meagre income. Tubal patency tests have not been done as laparoscopy is not available. Laparoscopy was introduced in the 1980's principally for tubal occlusion however the equipment no longer works due to poor maintenance. Hysterosalpingography is problematic as the radiology department can barely cope with the more urgent demands on their service. Seeing her for the first time I reviewed the notes and told her that her prognosis for a spontaneous conception was grim and that assisted reproductive interventions were not available unless she had funds to access this abroad. She burst into tears. She still could not come to terms with her failure to conceive and was reminded daily by the in-laws of her barrenness. She was a social pariah often treated as a bad omen when some special occasion like a wedding was being celebrated. She had visited most temples, consulted many doctors and attended many charlatans. Each had demanded their fee. The couple are poor like 24 percent of the population which meet the international criteria for poverty. She is a farm laborer with access to only seasonal work. She although a high school graduate had an arranged marriage to a man who had barely finished primary school. Her in-laws will not allow her to find a job as this will bring disgrace to the family. Her tears were for unfulfilled human potential and perception of inadequacy.

Fertility is essential for most of us. She was shedding tears because she was certain that she was to be blamed for her reproductive failure. She, in spite of her education thought that she deserved the social stigmata as just punishment. She would be happy for her husband to desert her for someone who could bear him children. I discussed the option of an adoption. There is no organized adoption service for couples such as this. They would not meet the economic criteria. She was put on the waiting list for a tubal patency test but it is likely that this will be normal. She will attend the clinic once again in three or four months like the many times before in the last 15 years.

My patient is probably one amongst 50 to 80 million others in the world who can not conceive. The global figures quoted estimate 8 to 12 percent infertility rates however accurate figures are difficult due to inconsistencies in definition. It is estimated that 5 percent of couples are unable to conceive due to anatomic, genetic, endocrinological and immunologic problems. Male and female factors are probably equally prevalent. Countries where sexually transmitted infections are prevalent have much higher rates of infertility.

There have been rapid advances in the management of known causes of infertility. For various reasons even in the developed world these services are more readily available in the private sector.

The limited capacity to manage infertility in developing countries is a result of several factors. Poverty is a key factor as this is linked with poor nutrition, and poor health indicators overall. The first three millennium development goals recognize the impact of poverty, lack of education and gender based inequalities as key to social development. Developing countries are faced with competing priorities. Rapid population growth, high birth rates and fertility reduction are high on the global development agenda. However, as valid as this might be economically the plight of infertile couples is about basic human rights. Any other condition which is as prevalent would attract huge donor attention. The donors remain immune to the silent suffering of these couples who do not have recourse to adequate assessment and care. As with many services which are necessary to human enjoyment of life the poor remain deprived. Equity of access remains a challenge. In the last two decades in the developed and many of the developing countries, the management of infertility has become a major lucrative medical growth industry.

Denial of adequate care for the infertile couple could be argued as the denial of basic human rights. Infertility is not only a health issue but it is also a social issue. In many communities women who have not borne children suffer psychological violence, domestic assault, and social deprivation. Access to health is recognized as basic to all humans as is respect, dignity and security. Yet, the poor do not have access to care.

In the current context of the global development agenda it is unlikely that the care of the infertile will attract direct funding priorities which will allow most to access the latest interventions available. This then leads to the need for other strategies. It is true that there are direct and indirect benefits in reducing poverty, improving nutrition and ensuring that everyone has access to primary education. These endeavors and better infant and child health must also benefit in the longer term. But what can be done more immediately?

Perhaps the most pertinent for those involved in delivering reproductive health care is to identify infertility care as an important component of the entire reproductive health care package. Unplanned pregnancies, unsafe abortions, sexually transmitted infections are all largely preventable. All these have subsequent potential for infertility.

Yet their prevalence continues to increase in many settings. The attitude to reproductive health continues to encourage double standards in those contexts which can least afford them. The lip service to gender equality and the lack of free access to contraception and safe abortion is a sad reflection on society as a whole. The health professional and professional bodies especially in Women's Health have a leadership and advocacy role in meeting this challenge.

The management of the infertile couple in resource poor settings requires several strategic interventions. Firstly, education of the population both about the myths and beliefs that creates the social stigma and violates human rights in almost every society. This campaign does not require sophisticated technology. It requires recognition that infertility exists and where it can not be prevented or corrected it must be managed affording couples dignity and acceptance. Secondly, more effort needs to go into managing unplanned pregnancies, providing safe abortions, and access to contraception. Sexually transmitted infections can be prevented and better managed in all settings. Thirdly, the management of the infertile couple needs to be given a higher priority in health care. This does not mean deploying resources from other pressing health priorities. However, it does mean that we use the available resources efficiently and to maximum benefit. Access to care for all is a shared global responsibility. International nongovernmental organizations must be lobbied to become more involved in the care of the infertile couple. Traditionally only doctors deal with infertility. Other cadre especially nurses need to be involved as do village health workers. At every level, there must be an emphasis on contextually appropriate training. Managing infertility requires the same clinical strategies which are basic to the provision of good health care. A good history and examination will often minimize the need for sophisticated investigations. Management strategies which empower, provide options by adequate counseling are as important as the latest ART. Our colleagues who have an interest in the management of infertility in economically well resourced settings should be persuaded to develop more simple effective approaches to ovulation induction, managing poor semen quality and dealing with tubal patency problems. Training of reproductive health workers in this area has not received the emphasis needed. As knowledge and technology advances, there is hope that management processes in infertility care will become simpler and therefore more accessible.

In the meantime, international professional bodies such as FIGO, AOFOG and SAFOG should consider developing strategies to promote appropriate research to make infertility services more accessible to couples living in the poorer countries. Sharing of resources to remove human suffering must be placed higher on the global development agenda.

BIBLIOGRAPHY

1. Abdallah S, Daar, Zara Merali. Infertility and social suffering: the case of ART in developing countries, December 2007.
2. Low priority level for infertility services within the public health sector:a Brazilian case study. Human Reprod 2010;25(2):430-5.
3. Oxford Journals Medicine Human Reproduction Update 2008;14(6):605-21.
4. Reproductive Health Outlook (RHO). Overview and lessons learned. Infertility www.rho.org/html/ infertility overview.html

Chapter 3

Need for Assisted Reproductive Technology in Low-resource Settings

Rohana Haththotuwa, Upul Senarath

INTRODUCTION

Infertility is a global issue, but the magnitude of the problem and the negative consequences experienced by the women are higher in low-resource settings or developing countries than in the developed countries. The consequences of childlessness create problems related to health and wellbeing of individuals, couples and the society as a whole. This problem of infertility and childlessness is one of the most important and underappreciated reproductive health problems in low-income countries.[1] Though many of the causes that lead to subfertility in these countries can be successfully addressed, less priority has been given to this issue by the respective governments in their health programs. Therefore, it is important that efforts are made to develop a sustainable program for the prevention, evaluation and treatment of the infertility in developing countries. This Chapter aims to highlight the need for assisted reproductive technology (ART) in low-resource settings.

PREVALENCE OF INFERTILITY IN LOW-RESOURCE SETTINGS

The exact prevalence of infertility in low-resource settings is unknown due to a lack of valid data. Global estimates of infertility range between 8 and 12 percent of couples with women of childbearing age.[2] Worldwide more than 80 million couples suffer from infertility and the majority of this population are residents of developing countries with low resources.[3] The problem of infertility in resource-poor countries is underestimated and neglected to a large extent. The prevalence is higher in resource-poor countries, particularly in the sub-Saharan Africa than in the developed countries. The prevalence of infertility among married couples during their reproductive age in the United Kingdom is 8 to 10 percent,[4] and the national average for prevalence in sub-Saharan countries ranged from 12.5 to 16 percent.[5] An 'infertility belt' has been previously described by Inhorn et al[6] involving areas of central and southern Africa, with the highest rate of 32 percent in Namibia. In a recent publication, Pennings et al[7] has pointed out that the rates in sub-Saharan Africa can go up to 30 percent or more, mainly due to infection-related causes which can be preventable.

Magnitude of the problem is also high in the South Asian region, with 8 to 10 million couples in India being estimated to be childless. Further, according to the Delhi IVF Research Center, one in six couples in India suffer from infertility.[8]

Comparison of the measures of infertility between countries has certain limitations due to inconsistency in the definition, lack of household survey data or prevalence studies and poor quality of data. It has been argued that most studies from developing countries have underestimated actual prevalence rates. Despite these limitations, there is worldwide consensus that prevalence of infertility is remarkably higher in the low-resource settings than in the developed countries.[9]

FERTILITY PREFERENCE AND FACTORS INFLUENCING PREFERENCES

The value of having children is high in developing countries due to sociocultural, economic reasons and it is considered as a foundation for a successful married life. Motherhood is often the only way for women to enhance their status within the family and community. Having children is considered as the norm in many societies in the developing countries. Therefore, childlessness creates many problems for the couples especially the women because they are generally blamed for infertility even though the problem may not be in them but in the men.[10]

There are geographical differences in attitudes on fertility, based on sociocultural, religious and political health contexts. In India, for example, motherhood is considered noble, and children, especially boys give the woman status as well as psychological and emotional security within the family.[11]

Consequences of Childlessness

As pointed out by Zandvoort et al[12] in many developing countries, female identity, social status and security depends on their ability to produce children. Failure to comply with this norm is known to have serious consequences which can have a large influence on woman's quality of life. Some of the reported psychological problems women have to face include grief, anxiety, depression, worthlessness and jealousy.

There are more social problems such as family disputes, domestic violence and divorce.[12] Childlessness may result in marital disputes which may have serious consequences.[13-16] According to the 47-country DHS survey, 14 percent of women who have never had a child was found to be divorced or separated possibly due to infertility. Childless women who are divorced are 13 percent more likely to have remarriage than women with children.[17] Furthermore, in societies where polygamy is allowed, men may prefer to take a second wife instead of divorcing or separating. For example, in Kenya, Jordan, Nepal, and Yemen, men whose first wife is childless are 15 to 20 percent more likely to have a second wife.[17] Sometimes, infertile women are forced to prostitution for survival.

In developing countries, poor families depend on their children to bring an income to the family. Childlessness will have severe difficulties in achieving old age security, especially for elderly women.[14] Many of the developing countries do not have social security systems, so people especially in the old age are predominantly dependent on their children to look after their financial and social support.[18] Couple who do not have children will be insecure in old age and this problem will be worse if woman is divorced or left by the husband because of infertility. Infertile women may be discriminated by certain societies and are perceived as a sign of evil. This has led to social stigmatization and exclusion of these women from the opportunities and privileges they deserve.

A recent study has revealed that female infertility is closely associated with psychological distress. A case-control study conducted in Colombo, Sri Lanka has found that the prevalence of psychological distress in infertile women was significantly higher than that in fertile women. Further the study has revealed that Psychological distress among infertile women was associated with poorer education, being previously/currently investigated/ treated, placing higher importance on having children, and having poor marital communication.[19] This highlights the need for addressing the issue of infertility as well as its psychosocial consequences.

It is not only the women, but men also may be severely affected by the stigma of infertility, for example fear of being considered as impotent. However, the men are not usually blamed for the problem of infertility causing women to persistently seek and undergo investigations and treatment. Male infertility too has psychological consequences, and effects on marriage, community relations, etc.

Infertile couples may resort to ineffective medications and interventions possibly by unqualified practitioners. Also they may spend most of their meager earnings for religious rituals with the belief that they would conceive with the help of unseen forces, and that it would help them to dispel the evils which are preventing them from conceiving.

The negative consequences of childlessness are more prevalent in developing countries compared to developed countries. Ombelet et al[18] has summarized psychological and social consequences of infertility in developing countries at six different levels. Figure 3.1 illustrates these consequences in different levels ranging from the psychological consequences such as fear, guilt, and self-blame to the most severe level of lost dignity and death.

Often, at the first level, subfertile women feel a sense of worthlessness and a greater width and depth of distress when compared with Western Societies. At the level 2, the couple is affected by the marital stress, depression and helplessness leading to marital instability, mild marital or social violence. At the level 3, women without children are more prone to be victims of domestic violence. Marital or social violence may end up in divorce, extramarital affairs by the husband and risk of STDs, etc. Further, at this level the social isolation of women will include accusation of 'witch craft', ostracism, exclusion from community functions and from contact with children, subject to ridicule etc. At the level 4, the social status is lost with

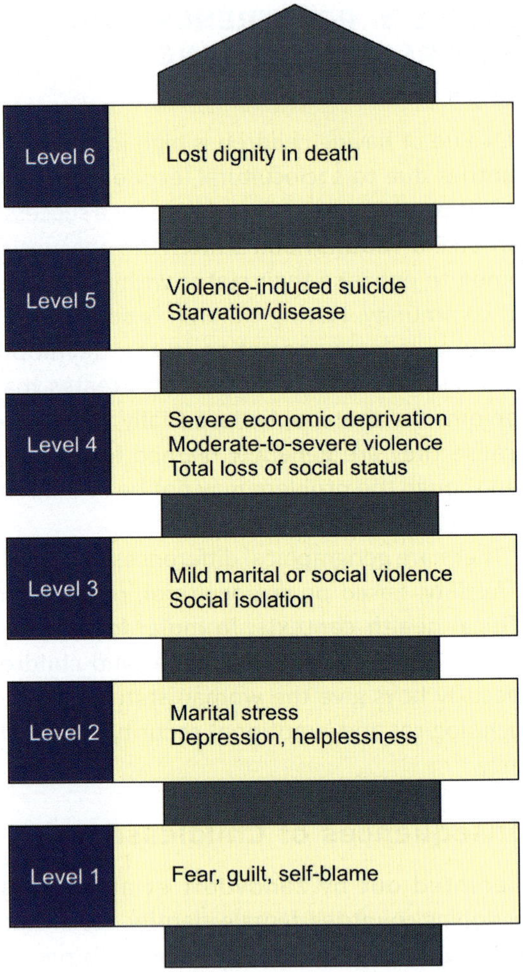

Fig. 3.1: Consequences of infertility in developing countries

[Reproduced with permission from Oxford University Press, from the article Ombelet W, Cooke I, Dyer S, Serour G, Devroey P. Infertility and the provision of infertility medical services in developing countries. Human Reproduction Update, 2008:14(6):605-21(18)]

severe economic deprivation and moderate to severe violence. In developed countries, the consequences of infertility rarely extend beyond level 2, and in developing countries they may manifest at higher levels in a greater frequency. In the subsequent levels, subfertile women face severe economic deprivation, total loss of social status, violence-induced suicide ending up in lost dignity and death.

NEED FOR ART IN LOW-RESOURCE SETTINGS

Individuals have a right to reproduce and freedom to decide when and how often. United Nations' Declaration of Human Rights Article 16:1, states that 'Men and women of full age, without any limitation due to race, nationality or religion have the right to marry and found a family'. An analysis of main ethical arguments for and against provision of infertility treatment in resources poor countries has been performed by the European Society of Human Reproduction and Embryology recently.[7] According to this analysis, the infertility treatment should be part of an integrated reproductive care program including family planning and motherhood care. Education, empowerment of women and economic prosperity are the most effective solutions to most problems related infertility. The review has also justified investments in low-cost interventions in the resource-poor countries.

Health is described as total physical, social and mental wellbeing of an individual and not a mere absence of disease. So it is vital that advanced methods of infertility treatment is available for women in low resource settings to prevent them suffering from the numerous severe consequences of childlessness which will affect their mental and social wellbeing.

One of the leading causes of infertility in developing countries is bilateral tubal occlusion due to sexually transmitted diseases and pregnancy-related infections such as unsafe abortions and postpartum pelvic infections.[18] Sexually transmitted infections caused by *Chlamydia trachomatis* and *Neisseria gonorrhoeae* are most commonly involved in causing the tubal occlusions. Tuberculosis is a major cause of infertility in the Indian subcontinent.[9] Prevalence of genital tuberculosis in tubal factor infertility was 49 percent in women requesting assisted reproduction.[20]

Unsafe abortions done under unhygienic conditions and carried out by untrained personnel is also a leading cause of tubal occlusion. An estimated 21.6 million unsafe abortions took place in 2008 and almost all, amounting to 21.2 million, took place in developing countries.[21]

Another common cause in developing countries is the postpartum pelvic infections due to inadequate care during and after childbirth.

ART should be available to treat these women with tubal occlusion; otherwise these women will be deprived of the opportunity of having a baby. When these advanced technologies are not available in societies where fertility is given a very high value, it can lead to women undergoing various unproven treatments to conceive, which may result in further damage to their reproductive potential.[9]

A review by Obmelet et al[18] recommends that simplification of diagnostic and ART procedures, minimizing complication rate of interventions, providing training courses for health care providers, and incorporating infertility treatment into sexual and reproductive healthcare programs may successfully address the problem of infertility in developing countries. As concluded by this review, the following arguments would make a compelling case for the need of services and programs for ART in low-resource countries:[18]

- Infertility is a disease and needs medical treatment
- Main cause of infertility in developing countries is tubal occlusion
- Negative consequences of childlessness are more severe in low-resource settings
- ART should be available for all, rich or poor
- Adoption is not an option in most developing countries due to sociocultural, religious reasons
- There is a possibility of simplifying diagnostic procedures, clinical procedures, and laboratory procedures.

There is a drastic inequality in the socio-economic status in many resource poor countries. This disparity has led to a situation where a considerably a high fraction of the population will not have access to the infertility management services which are mainly available in the private sector. Usually the infertility management services are not included in the governments' healthcare services available to the public.

BARRIERS FOR ART PROGRAMS

Though the problem of infertility and the need for effective management services have been discussed for many years, not much progress has been made. Hence, it is important to find out the barriers for the ART programs in low-resource settings.

Low Priority

In many low-resource settings, provision of maternal and child care, immunization, family planning services and prevention and control of infections including sexually transmitted infections are the high priorities within the reproductive health programs. Most developing countries have a constricted health budget and financed mainly by the government with support from non-governmental organizations (NGOs). Investments on infertility management is not a common practice due to the low priority of this issue.

Overpopulation

There is a misconception that in developing countries where the objective is to reduce the population growth, the treatment of infertility can lead to overpopulation. According to the projections by the United Nations, the world population is expected to increase from 6.5 billion inhabitants in 2005 to reach 9.1 billion in 2050. In 113 out of 148 developing countries, the average fertility rate has already declined to a level of 2.58 per woman and is expected to decline below the replacement level fertility of 2.1 by 2050. Therefore, it has been argued that in the developing countries, the continuing population rise will be the result of population aging and not because of high fertility rates.[22]

It should also be noted that with the limited success in the ART programs, the contribution made by the ART to population growth is minimal.

High Cost

In Vitro Fertilization-related procedures are regarded as expensive and moderately effective. The direct and indirect costs of conventional ART procedures (IVF, ICSI) are extremely high and therefore only a small proportion of infertile couples in low-resource countries can afford it. *In vitro* fertilization costs are approximately 50 percent higher than the gross national income per capita of most developing countries including China, India, Indonesia, Malaysia and Pakistan.[23] In Nigeria, when one IVF cycle costs USD 2000 to 2700 per month the minimum wage is 52 to 60 USD per month.[24] The poor countries have to incur costs for ART with limited success. However, it must be remembered how it could affect the individual's quality of life, particularly those who are poor.

Therefore, investment on infertility should not be given a low priority, and the development of accessible and affordable assisted reproductive programs will be necessary.

Other barriers for effective implementation of an ART service include limited medical and paramedical staff trained in these procedures, low level of facilities, etc. Limited number of specialized and trained professionals in these technologies to provide the services is also a major factor that prevents introducing ART services in low-resource countries.

SUGGESTED PROCEDURES TO IMPROVE THE MANAGEMENT OF INFERTILITY IN LOW-RESOURCE SETTINGS

Considering the facts and review of scientific literature, the following needs have been recognized in the resource-poor settings. As these would be covered in detail in the subsequent Chapter in this book, only an outline will be made in this Chapter.

Infertility Treatment should be a Part of an Integrated Reproductive Care Program

Though prevention and treatment of infertility is an essential component of the reproductive health program, less attention has been paid to it in the health programs in many developing countries. A high priority has been given on maternal care, infant and child care, family planning and STI control. There is a need to integrate, services to treatment of infertility to the existing reproductive healthcare program of the country.

Establishing an effective referral system in the primary and secondary levels of care should be considered. Primary healthcare providers could be trained in screening patients by simple investigations and in counseling and proving simple advice and making appropriate referral.

Investments for Prevention of Infertility

As sexually transmitted infections (STI), unsafe abortions and postpartum infections are among the main known causes of infertility in developing countries, the governments should invest more on prevention and appropriate treatment for STI, family planning, prevention of unsafe abortions and providing post-abortion care, and prevention of pregnancy-related sepsis, etc.[18]

Public Education

There is hardly any public education in low-resources countries on areas of fertility, infertility, prevention, treatment options and successfulness and what to look for when choosing a provider. This has caused the people to be misled and has led them to resort to unscientific methods of native treatment which can further harm their fertility. Also lack of education will promote misbelieves and make them resort to such methods. Giving them false hopes will not only waste their time but also make them more infertile with age.

Mass media and health education strategies can be used for this purpose. Media can be used as an effective means of educating the public. Fertility awareness programs are relatively low-cost and effective, and it is important to highlight about the importance of male factor in infertility management. Further, counseling on fertility awareness can be provided by the front healthcare providers with adequate training of these health-care providers.

Empowering Women

Educating females will enhance women's autonomy and practice of preventive strategies against infertility. Also women will be able to seek care for infertility and demand for less costly methods, with minimal investigations. The psychosocial consequences of not having children will also be reduced when women are empowered and their status will be high irrespective of the motherhood status.

Simplifying Diagnostic Procedures

Simplified diagnostic procedures would be both feasible and cost-effective in resource-poor settings. The effectiveness and costs of these techniques should be evaluated in different settings in developing countries. The details of these are discussed in a subsequent Chapter of this book.

Simplified Treatment and Non-IVF Assisted Reproduction

There is a great need for simplified and low cost treatment procedures including less costly medication, effective use of procedures such as intrauterine insemination for male infertility, endoscopic procedure, etc.

Simplified Assisted Reproduction

Even after more than 30 years of *in vitro* fertilization (IVF), and more than 15 years of intra-cytoplasmic sperm injection (ICSI), still only a small part of the world population benefits from these technologies.[22] The IVF procedures and expensive and require sophisticated technology and highly competent human resource. Therefore, more research evidence is needed to identify low-cost and simple IVF procedures that can be scaled-up in resource poor settings. Medication used for ovarian stimulation such as gonadotropins, FSH, GnRH agonists and GnRH antagonists are very costly, thus the supply of such drugs will not be sustainable through government health programs. An alternative would be to use mild ovarian stimulation with low-dose regimen or using inexpensive drugs such as clomiphene citrate. Several studies have found satisfactory results with the use of clomiphene citrate regimen in the IVF.[18]

The high-cost laboratory procedures used for IVF programs hampers the establishment of state-of-art laboratories by the governments in resource poor settings.

RESEARCH ON ART

The key research question to be answered should focus on effective low-cost interventions in IVF procedure that can be scaled-up through the wider government health system. On one hand, research should be conducted to invent new low-cost technologies and on the other hand research should be conducted to explore the feasibility and acceptability of such strategies within the existing health system. Research evidence on strategies to adapt advanced technology to local conditions would also be helpful. So far a handful of research is available, and it is recommended that more research on this area should be included in the reproductive health research programs both in developed and developing countries.

Monitoring ART Services

Effective monitoring system is necessary for the benefit of the patients and the care providers and to ensure a successful ART program in a country. All the centers that provide ART services should be registered and should follow a set of minimal standards. A coordinated information system should be established to compile information on resources, procedures and outcomes on regular basis.

Economic Prosperity, Bridging the Economic Disparities

In the long-run, countries should aim at achieving the economic development and bridging the gap between rich and poor with the country. This is far more difficult to achieve in short term, so a more practical solution would be to address the needs in the health system which are feasible within the existing socio-economic and political context.

FUNDING FOR ART IN DEVELOPING COUNTRIES

Allocation for health in government budget is low in many developing countries. Even within this allocation, a major part is spent on treatment of illness and supporting necessary infrastructure and human resources. Governments in low-income countries are not in a position to fund for high-cost ART services such as IVF. Main challenge behind the professional groups is to develop low cost ART procedures and to make the governments understand that treatment of infertility is a health priority and influence them to allocate more funds for prevention and treatment of infertility.

Support from the development assistant partners is utmost important in this regard. The WHO has recognized the importance of ART programs in developing countries, and at present, infertility prevention is the main objective of WHO's infertility-related reproductive health program. At a meeting on 'Medical, Ethical and Social Aspects of Assisted Reproduction' in 2001, WHO called for the integration of infertility into existing sexual and reproductive healthcare programs and for highlighting the value of ART in developing countries,[24] and it is time to recognize more international NGOs to support IVF programs. Since the private sector plays a major role in advanced ART, government's responsibility would be to facilitate them while incorporating ART to the national reproductive/maternal and child health programs.

CONCLUSION

In conclusion, infertility is a public health issue, deserving greater attention in the reproductive health programs in the low-resource settings. Having access to all the methods of treatment is a woman's right. Infertility in developing countries has not been addressed adequately though it has caused serious consequences to the concerned couples and women in particular. Simplified of diagnostic and ART procedures, minimizing complication rate of interventions, providing training courses for healthcare providers, and incorporating infertility treatment into sexual and reproductive healthcare programs may successfully address the problem of infertility in developing countries. Governments should work with healthcare professionals and international development assistant partners to incorporate ART services to the existing reproductive health programs so that it could be reached by all.

REFERENCES

1. Bergstrom S. Reproductive failure as a health priority in the Third World: a review. East Afr Med J 1992;69:174-80.
2. World Health Organization. Infertility: a tabulation of available data on prevalence of primary and secondary infertility. 1991.WHO: Geneva. Programme on Maternal and Child Health and Family Planning, Division of Family Health 1991.
3. Fathalla MF. Current challenges in assisted reproduction. In: Vayena E, Rowe PJ, Griffin PD (Eds): Current Practices and Controversies in Assisted Reproduction, 2002. WHO, Geneva, Switzerland, pp. 3-13.
4. NICE. Fertility: assessment ad treatment for people with fertility problems 2004 [www.nice.org.uk].
5. Larsen V. Primary and secondary infertility in sub-Saharan Africa. Int J Epidemiol 2000:29:285-91.
6. Inhorn MC. Global infertility and the globalization of new reproductive technologies: illustrations from Egypt. Soc Sci Med 2003; 56:1837-51.
7. Pennings G, Wert G De, Shenfield F, Cohen J, Tarlatzis B, Devroey P. Providing infertility treatment in resource-poor countries. Human Reproduction 2011;24(5):1008-11.
8. Dutta S, Guha R. A clinic-anatomical study on the etiological factors pertaining to primary infertility in females using some investigative procedures. J Anat Soc India 2007; 56:14-17.

9. Sharama S, Mittal S, Aggarwal P. Management of infertility in low resource countries. BJOG 2009;116 (Suppl 1):77-83.
10. Ballan FV, Gerrits T. Quality of infertility care in poor-resource areas and introduction of new reproductive technologies. Human Reproduction 2011;16(2):215-9.
11. Riessman CR. Stigma and everyday resistance practices: childless women in South India. GendSoc 2000;14:111-35.
12. Zandvoort HV, Koning KD, Gerrits T. Viewpoint: Medical infertility care in low income countries: the case for concern in policy and practice. Tropical Medicine and International Health 2001;6(7):563-9.
13. Boerma JT, Mgalla Z (Eds). Women and Infertility in Sub-Saharan Africa: A Multi-Disciplinary Perspective. Amsterdam: Royal Tropical Institute, KIT Publishers; 2001.
14. Inhorn MC, van Balen F (Eds). Infertility around the Globe: New Thinking on Childlessness, Gender, and Reproductive Technologies. Berkeley: University of California Press; 2003.
15. Inhorn MC. Reproductive Disruptions: Gender, Technology, and Biopolitics in the New Millennium. New York: Berghahn Books; 2007.
16. Van Balen F, Gerrits T. Quality of infertility care in poor-resource areas and the introduction of new reproductive technologies. Hum Reprod 2001;16(2): 215-9.
17. Inhorn MC. Right to assisted reproductive technology: Overcoming infertility in low-resource countries. International Journal of Gynecology and Obstetrics 2009;106:172-4.
18. Ombelet W, Cooke I, Dyer S, Serour G, Devroey P. Infertility and the provision of infertility medical services in developing countries. Human Reproduction Update, 2008;14(6):605-21.
19. Lansakara N, Wickramasinghe AR, Seneviratne HR. Feeling the blues of infertility in a South Asian context: psychological well-being and associated factors among Sri Lankan women with primary infertility. Women Health 2011; 51(4):383-99.
20. Singh N, Sumana G, Mittal S. Genital tuberculosis: a leading cause of infertility in women seeking assisted conception in North India. Arch GynaecolObstet, 2008; 278-325-7.
21. World Health Organization. Unsafe abortion. Global and regional estimates of the incidence of unsafe abortion and associated mortality in 2008 (6th Edition). 2011: WHO: Geneva.
22. Ombelet W, Campo R. Affordable IVF for developing countries. Reprod Biomed Online, 2007;15:257-65.
23. Vayena E, Peterson HB, Adamson, D, Nygren KG. Assisted reproductive technologies in developing countries: are we caring yet? Fertility and Sterility 2009; 92 (2): 413-6.
24. Vayena E, Rowe PJ, Griffin PD (Eds). Current Practices and Controversies in Assisted Reproduction. Report of a Meeting. Geneva, Switzerland: World Health Organization, 2002;383-8.

Chapter

4

Meeting the Challenges in Low-resource Settings

Bhola Rijal, Rajesh Chaudhary, Sabina Pradhan

INTRODUCTION

Reproductive health has been described as a state of complete social, physical, mental wellbeing and not merely absence of disease, in all matter relating to reproductive system and its function and process. Reproductive health therefore implies an individual's right to reproduce and the freedom to decide when and how often to do so.[1] One of the essential component of reproductive health is the prevention and management of infertility. As per United Nation Declaration on human rights, Article 16:1, men and women have the right to access to sexual and reproductive health services of their choice, which are safe, effective, affordable and acceptable.[2] The 1994 international conference on the population and development (ICPD) has already recommended that the infertility care should be included on the agenda of healthcare planners worldwide, and has acknowledged it as basic elements of reproductive healthcare. WHO, through their different conferences, have declared infertility as a major public health issue and have recommended that infertility management should be incorporated into the national health policy with priorities.[2] The reason why WHO is emphasizing more on infertility care is because of its global magnitude and impact. It is estimated that 60 to 80 million couple are affected worldwide, the majority being residents in developing countries.[3,4] The impact of infertility is immense at all level of society and is not just merely limited to physical disease.[5,6] Its dimension has invaded psychological, marital, socio-cultural, and economical aspect of life. Though WHO has declared infertility as a public health issue, it has received less attention in developing world. Moreover, the implementation of numerous commitments and declarations made by the governments of developing countries and WHO at world conferences at different times of history has been neglected. The health policy makers of these countries usually forward fallacious justification for this neglection: sociodemographic reason (fear of overpopulation), technical and economical constrains due to high cost of IVF and scarcity of resources. Clearly, these rationales are not based on any scientific evidence. The health policies of these countries have reasonably focused on safe motherhood. Unfortunately, their perception on safe motherhood has been restricted to family planning, antenatal care and delivery services, but not the infertility care. They should understand that motherhood is not just about caring for pregnancy but it also implies facilitating women to achieve pregnancy if there is any difficulty.

Unless there is an expansion of existing health policy that includes the issue of infertility, solving infertility problem is still far fetched goal to achieve. The existing health policies of developing countries, impose a major challenge in today's modern date towards solutions of infertility. A favorable health policy addressing the issue of infertility management and incorporating the problem as a public health issue would definitely help in making ART affordable and accessible to common people. In addition, ART is in itself an expensive and technically demanding procedure that makes it inaccessible to many infertile couple as well as health system of low resources countries. Development of low cost ART and promotion of education, training, and research can help ART to become an affordable procedure.[7]

We argue that affordable ART can only be provided if we address the challenges posed by the existing health policies, technical complexities and high cost associated with ART, and lacking trained ART professionals. In this article, we explore the present context of these challenges, and suggest possible recommendations to address the challenges so that ART can be offered to common people who are in need.

BURDEN

Reliable quantification of the problem in low resources countries in term of prevalence is difficult due to poor registration system and lack of well-performed studies. Information on the magnitude of problem and its epidemiology are certainly required while formulating a strategic plan to tackle the disease.

A recent overview of population-based surveillance estimated the current international prevalence of infertility to be 9 percent on an average, with a range of 3.5 to 16.7 percent.[4] For Asia and Latin America, WHO study showed that the prevalence of infertility is between 8 to 12 percent for couples of reproductive age.[8] Different studies suggest that infertility in African countries is widely prevalent ranging from 12.5 to 32 percent.[9–11] The huge burden of infertility is mainly attributed to infection related causes as indicated by available data.[12] The tubal factor in infertility is reported to be as high as 85 percent in sub-Saharan Africa compared with 33 percent of infertile women worldwide.[13,14] Infections also contribute to majority of cases of male infertility.[7,15] The high incidence of tubal disease can be explained by a high rate of unprotected sex at early age, unsafe abortions, and postpartum pelvic infections.[16,17]

What does an infertility really mean for individual couple, the society and for the health service as well? In many countries where children are highly valued female identity, social status and security depend on their ability to produce children. Infertility is known to have serious consequences at all levels of the society. Childlessness often leads to considerable psychological impact on the couple. There is a high risk of assault to the couple particularly the female, which may lead to isolation and abandonment, neglect, economic hardship, domestic violence, marital disruption and even suicide.[5] The impact of infertility problem on health service system is becoming heavier, as larger percentage of couples are seeking medical advice for perceived infertility. A sizeable proportion of time of health care providers, including gynecologist is being spent on the care of infertility and its complication.[18,19]

CONTEXT OF INFERTILITY IN NEPAL

In Nepal, research studies on the field of infertility are sparse. There are no reliable studies or registration system to estimate the magnitude of infertility problem. The situation is so pitiable that the National Demographic Health Survey and Annual Health Report published by the government has no data regarding infertility. Because the global prevalence rate of infertility is between 8 to 12 percent, it can be estimated that approximately 0.6 million couple are likely to be affected in Nepal. However, it seems to be an underestimated data owing to high prevalence of pelvic infections in poor countries.

Bilateral tubal occlusion is the most common cause of infertility in resource poor countries, a condition that is potentially preventable.[13,20] Infertility due to bilateral tubal occlusion is preferably treated by IVF. Therefore, higher prevalence of tubal infertility in developing countries signifies that the need of IVF services is likely to be more than in developed countries. It is estimated that up to 10 percent of all the infertile couples will ultimately require some form of ART, and 5 percent will need IVF.[21] On this basis, some 30000 couples will need IVF treatment for parenthood in Nepal.

ART service in Nepal was first introduced in 1994. By 2010 AD, there were three clinics, all of which are present in Kathmandu and are from private sectors. There has not been any reporting or the surveillance of the quality of the ART services. It increases the risk of exploitation and potentially damaging practice on the infertile couples.[22,23] Moreover, lack of favorable health policies, untrained ART professionals, very few but expensive ART centers have created a huge unmet demand of ART service. Most of the developing countries have similar picture where ART services are either unavailable or very expensive.

THE CHALLENGES IN PROVIDING AFFORDABLE ART: THE PRESENT SCENARIO IN LOW-RESOURCE COUNTRIES

Even after 30 years of the introduction of IVF technology, IVF remains inaccessable to the bulk of population. This is because the problem is mostly underestimated or neglected by health policy makers and medical professionals of developing worlds. Moreover, the cost associated with IVF not only makes it inaccessable to common people but also had contributed in the non-interest of policy makers towards infertility management.

Common misconceptions surrounding the issues of infertility in low resource countries are deeply rooted in the thinking of many, and it has contributed hugely to non-prioritization of infertility management in their public health policy. Two key arguments: over population and limited resources are frequently used to challenge the introduction of ARTs in public sector.[24] The havoc of first argument had compelled policy makers to concentrate more on fertility control, and it leaves no room for other initiatives such as infertility diagnosis and treatment. The existing health policy is not interested in infertility management with fear of over population. If infertile couples do not have access to ART because they should contribute to over population, why to use modern technologies in developing countries, as this would too have overpopulation effect. Medical technology is employed to prevent human suffering, including that of infertility problem. Moreover, the United Nations has reported that the mean fertility rate of most of the developing countries has already dropped as low as 2.58 per woman, and it is expected to decline to 1.92 by mid century (http://esa.un.org/unpp/). Therefore, the problem of over population in low resources countries cannot be used as a reason to disguise the problem of millions of infertile couples.

The limited resources argument suggests that developing countries should not allocate resources for expensive technology that can benefit only a few.[11,25] It has been recommended that public health policy should invest in preventive program and leave the establishment of new ART center to the private sector since it is unlikely to be cost-effective in the public sector.[26] However, as Sen A had rightly mentioned, it is usually the mismanagement of funding in the government sectors rather than resource scarce that has led to the inability to finance on this program by the government.[27] It should be noted that the impact of infertility on individuals are so immense that investment on the treatment program can be totally justified on humanitarian background. Government should not cite scarce resources as the justification for not funding ART and rejecting all the advances and development in ART. Other widespread misbelieves that can be considered as major obstacles in implementing ART in health system are:

i. IVF is too costly and technologically complicated procedure that is not feasible for low resources countries. In fact, few studies have shown that it is feasible to implement the affordable IVF program in these countries if the health budgetary funds are properly managed, IVF technology is simplified, and suitable protocol for infertility treatment specific to the socio-economic context of that country is developed.[28–30]
ii. It is solely a personal problem and is not a life-threatening condition. This belief rudely neglects the devastating impact of infertility on human life and society.
iii. IVF programmes are more suitable for developed countries. Indeed, the consequences of infertility are more severe in developing countries than in developed ones, and so its management should be kept at higher priority in these countries than it does in developed countries.

These misconceptions are widely upheld by the health policy makers and donor agencies, and needs clarification on the scientific ground. Unless and until these misconceptions are clarified, political commitment and raise of fund from international organization for the infertility management is not possible. Therefore, it is the responsibility of the medical practitioners, the researchers, the professional medical organizations, and the drug companies to develop low cost IVF technology, and to convince donors and policy makers to invest on simplified ART program. Health policy of low resource countries are currently devoted to maternal health and fertility control. Though these two are important public health issues to be dealt with, government should also address other issues simultaneously that is related to motherhood, i.e. infertility. However, exclusion of infertility management from health policies of most countries indicates that the lawmakers and policy makers clearly lack knowledge on infertility problem and its impact on society. It seems that the existing policy is not driven by public demand but on donors' demand.

Another major challenge is the lack of basic and system research on the issue of infertility. In the absence of well-conducted research, the measurement of problem and the development of simplified ART/IVF program are not possible. WHO has been at the forefront of conducting epidemiological studies in infertility in low resource countries and producing recommendations.[2,13,31] The 2002 document 'Medical, Ethical and Social aspect of assisted conception' not only suggested a focus on preventive strategies but also recommended the collection and interpretation of population based data.[2] Similarly, researches aiming at simplifying ART procedures that provide safe, effective, acceptable, and affordable treatment for infertility are urgently warranted. Unless cost of ART procedures including IVF are significantly reduced, it is difficult job to get attention of policy makers and to increase the utilization of ART which is currently less than one percent in developing countries.

Inequity in the distribution of ART service between developed and developing countries are another big challenge. It is estimated that developed countries fulfill approximately 20 percent of their demand whereas developing countries hardly reach one percent of their demand.[32] Unless socio-economic status of developing countries is improved, this gap is difficult to bridge. Even within the same countries in developing world, the ART services are mainly situated in the major cities. This inequity can be attributed to lack of development of skilled teams and high cost ART procedures.

Given the magnitude of infertility problem, this hi-tech assisted reproductive technique is expected to find a booming market in developing countries. It has found a multibillion-dollar industry worldwide in which clinicians, medical researchers, and corporate house including pharmaceutical companies have their stakes.[33] This sector is unregulated with low standardization of quality and cost.[34,35] Thus, there is an increased risk of exploitation of infertility patients, who are vulnerable to expand anything that would provide them a chance for parenthood. Furthermore, lack of surveillance and reporting of ART services have made the process of 'informed choice on treatment' a difficult task for the couples. Obviously, it is difficult to make well-informed decision when the options given are complicated and information provided is biased or incomplete.[36] Therefore, to prevent the infertile couples from exploitations and potentially damaging practices as well as wastage of available resources, these booming ART markets need to be organized. Introducing laws and regulation in this profitable sector will be a big forthcoming challenge for governments as it is expected to meet with resistance from the stakeholders. Unfortunately, governments have kept their eyes closed on this important issue.[23]

TOWARDS SOLUTION: A PLEA FOR AFFORDABLE ART FOR ALL

Considering the impact of infertility causing immense human suffering, it is time to move beyond inaction, and to implement the effective and accessible infertility management including ART services in low resources countries. The importance of education and prevention is highly placed in reducing the prevalence of infertility as well as decreasing the need of ART. However, still 10 percent of infertile couple would ultimately need ART. Thus, treatment by ART becomes imperative for them and it cannot be denied because of any fallacious assumptions. However, unless the financial cost of IVF is reduced significantly, it is difficult to campaign for ART program in health system at political level. So maximum effort should be on introducing simplified diagnostic procedure in infertility workup, simplified new assistance reproductive technology and providing training courses including fellowship program for gynecologist. Recent reports appear optimistic about feasibility of low cost ART that are suitable for low resource setting.

How low the price of ART can drop will become clearer over time? In some centers of India, one IVF cycle costs $2000. This amount is still high in poor countries where the minimum wage is $50-60 per month. The cost of IVF can further be made affordable by adopting more innovative approaches: such as, introducing the concept of public private partnership and insurance coverage on this issue, drawing attention of NGOs for funding on research and treatment, motivating government to regularize the services and to waive off import duties on the procurement of equipment and supplies.

Simplifying Technology

The use of public funds on ART program will remain controversial until the cost of ART is reduced considerably. Therefore, before urging the government and NGOs for public sector investment on infertility management, new assisted reproductive technology that are more cheap and safe should be implemented.

a. **Simplified diagnostic procedure**: Currently, the infertile couples have to travel to major cities for the diagnosis of infertility. Ombelet et al have therefore proposed the concept of extending the existing primary healthcare (PHC) to "specialized primary healthcare facility" where the women can get basic diagnostic procedures.[37] If the doctors posted in PHC levels are given comprehensive training on using a microscope and ultrasound equipment, then semen analysis, HSG or hysterosonography can be routinely done in these center which will identify the majority of men's and women's infertility. These techniques are simple, reliable, and comparatively inexpensive. Training courses on how to interpret semen analysis were already successfully organized in sub-Saharan Africa.[38] Even office minihysteroscopy in its simplified version can be done without major costs and side effects, provided there has been appropriate training to the gynecologists.[39,40]
b. **IUI as first line treatment**: In many instances, non-tubal related infertility causes are successfully managed with IUI, and thus it should be promoted as a first line treatment of infertility of non-tubal origin.[41,42] IUI is a simple inexpensive procedure and can be established in low set up infrastructure. Moreover, it can be successfully conducted by paramedics, and requires comparatively less training. This implies that IUI can be set up in many centers across the low resources countries. In addition, cost-effective studies have shown that three IUIs using clomiphene citrate were as successful, but much cheaper than one IVF/ICSI cycle.[43–45] However, if three or more cycles of IUI are failed, IVF can be recommended for the couple.[37]
c. **Simplified and affordable IVF:** The development of low cost but safe and effective IVF technology is mandatory if the governments and non-profit organizations are to be convinced to invest on the infertility treatment program. IVF procedures need modification for affordable and safe IVF treatment for all. Currently practiced protocols of ovarian stimulation and culture of embryos are very much expensive that makes IVF out of reach for treatment. Few studies have worked on this regard and have proposed modification on costly steps of IVF. Unfortunately, the suggested models have never been applied in the market.
   - Concerning oocyte retrieval process, gonadotropins and/or follicle stimulating hormones, GnRH analogues are too expensive, and they carry a high risk of ovarian hyperstimulation syndrome. Unfortunately natural cycle IVF has a high cancellation rates because of premature LH rise and premature ovulation.[46] Mild ovarian stimulation should, therefore, be considered as a potential option in low-resource countries.[47] It has an added advantage of substantially reduced multiple pregnancy rates and overall costs. Among many, the most promising option for mild ovarian stimulation is the use of low-dose clomiphene citrate regimen with acceptable results, minimal side effects, and very low complication rate.[48] In case of clomiphene citrate resistance, the use of letrozole or low dose stimulation regimen with gonadotropins or recombinant FSH could be recommended. Similarly monitoring of the follicular size and the timing of hCG administration can easily be done by simple ultrasound equipment thereby avoiding the need of expensive endocrine investigations.[49,50]

- The cost associated with laboratory procedures imposes another challenge. However, studies have shown that the cost associated with the fertilization technique and culture of embryos can be reduced significantly. Instead of using an expensive laminar flowhood for the handling of gametes and embryos, 'humidicrib' plant box can be used with modification.[28,30] This approach will reduce the price nearly by one tenth. Similarly, for the purpose of incubation and culture of embryos, we can borrow the technique that was already in use in veterinary IVF for more than last ten years.[51] In this technique, a plastic bag containing the petri-dish with the embryos is dropped into the warm bath that can efficiently culture the embryos and thus avoid the need for expensive incubator.

Furthermore, Ranoux et al[52] in 1987 and Taymor et al[53] in 1992 described a promising technique that is more suitable for low resources countries, in which the process was done intravaginal or intrauterine fertilization and culture of embryos. A tube filled with 3 ml of cultural medium containing 1-5 oocyte with 10000-20000 washed spermatozoa per milliliter was hermetically closed and was placed in the vagina. It was then held by a diaphragm for 44-50 hours. Though this was a safe and simple method of culture with comparable success rate with conventional IVF, it did not receive wide attention.[54] Probably the introduction of such a simplified and low cost IVF technology in the market of developed countries could not have served the economic purpose of stakeholders. During late 1980s, IVF was new technique and was the only hope for western rich infertile couple who were ready to pay any price for taking baby home. With such a high unmet demand due to expensive IVF, it is high time to re-introduce this simple and low cost effective reproductive technology in the IVF clinics of developing countries, and developed countries as well.

Recently in 2009, Blockeel et al conducted a pilot study that was designed to explore the safety and feasibility of a novel *in utero* encapsulation technology.[55] This study showed that *in utero* culture system (IUCS) supports normal fertilization, embryo development, and normal chromosomal segregation. Fertilization and embryo development were comparable in the *in vitro* and IUCS arms, with a tendency towards better embryo quality in the IUCS. It also demonstrates the possibility of obtaining pregnancies after transient presence of silicone device in the uterus. In this technology, the microinjected oocytes were loaded into the capsule in a dish filled with HEPES-buffered medium kept at 37°C under microscopic control. The capsule was inserted into a catheter and transferred to the uterus. After *in vivo* culture for 18 hours, the IUCS was removed from the uterine cavity and immediately placed into HEPES-buffered medium at 37°C. The silicone capsule was opened at both ends, and the zygotes were recovered. Zygotes were individually placed into 25 µl droplets of cleavage medium under oil. Fertilization obtained *in vivo* was evaluated by the appearance of two pronuclei at 20 hours after injection, and all zygotes were further cultured *in vitro*. In this technique, no special incubation is needed, and the embryos thus obtained are transferred in the uterus after 24 hours of insemination, with the same catheter. These interesting observations, however, need to be confirmed in a large RCT.

Education and Training

The implementation of affordable and accessible ART will require many well-trained doctors and paramedicals. So training course on ART should be sponsored by state, and should be provided to those professionals who are motivated to work for the cause of infertile couples. Sponsoring these training courses to motivated medical personnel could discourage them from profit seeking practices in the private sector.[10] Following training, implementation of quality control, regular audit, and system of accreditation and registration should be done in order to maintain appropriate standards of care.

Surveillance and Reporting for Affordable ART of Quality

Vayena E et al had identified the surveillance and reporting of outcomes of ART treatments as a pre-requisite for ART services in any country.[56] Surveillance and reporting system would ensure safe and efficient infertility service in ART centers. It would also help patients for treatment options, professionals for clinical policy adjustments and state for regulation and resource allocation. The reporting of ART results are at the stage of infancy in developing countries. Many countries have no reporting system at all. This demonstrates that how unregulated ART services are in developing countries. ART professionals and centers should voluntarily initiate to report the quality and result of ART service. Otherwise, it is duty of government to make sure, thorough regulatory bodies, that their citizens get the right information, and protect the infertile couple from exploitations and potentially damaging practice.

Affordable IVF through Private Public Partnership

While governments of low resource countries are not interested in establishing public ART centers, mainly due to limited resource availability, the concept of cooperative public private partnership (PPP) in the infertility care could be the best option and could raise hope of successful implementation of affordable ART. This approach also seems to be more realistic in developing countries.[25] These partnerships can bring technical expertise, research work, equipment, and supplies to low-resource settings. In addition, PPP can help influence the establishment of standards, regulations, and policies to safeguard the health of couples undergoing treatment.[5]

Role of Government

ART programs in developing countries can only be made accessible and affordable if they are supported by government's health policy. Policy makers should give attention to infertility and needs of infertile patient. First, they should acknowledge it as a public health issue as recommended by WHO meeting on 'Medical, Ethical and Social Aspects of Assisted Reproduction', Geneva, 2001. Additionally the government should offer the treatment of infertility through "specialized primary healthcare facility". They should also support for continuous research work and ART training program. Where public funding is insufficient for public sector ART program, government should facilitate alternative sources of funding. Moreover, the government should consider introducing the health insurance policy. While developing countries generally lack adequate, efficient, and low cost ART services at public level, the government should encourage the growth of private sectors through subsidies, and waiving of import duties to improve the procurement of equipment and supplies. At the same time, it should regulate the private sector through regulatory bodies to monitor misuse and prevent them to deliver low quality low success IVF treatment.

CONCLUSION

Infertility remains a central issue in the lives of 60 to 80 million couples worldwide, majority of them resides in developing countries. The consequences of infertility are devastating. The higher prevalence of infection related tubal infertility in low resources countries implies that the need of IVF treatment is going to be more in these countries than in the developed ones. Unfortunately, the available ART services in low recource countries just meet one percent of the need. The huge unmet demand for infertility treatment is mainly attributed to costly and technically demanding ART procedures, as well as existing health policies neglecting the infertility treatment totally.

Studies have shown that a cost-effective and feasible ART program can be successfully implemented in low-resource countries. Keystones in the successful implementation include simplification of the diagnostic and ART procedures, organizing training courses, incorporating infertility treatment into existing reproductive health program, cooperation between public and private sectors, and appropriate reporting and surveillance of ART activities. With economical constrains, governments could still involve in assisted reproduction by encouraging the growth of the private sector through subsidies, incentives and waiving of import duties. Additionally, they have added responsibility to ensure safe and effective ART services through feasible regulatory mechanism.

ACKNOWLEDGMENTS

The authors would like to thank Prof Dr Pushpa Chaudhary for her comments on the draft. We would also like to thank Dr Angel Magar for his contribution in reference section, and resident Dr Nikita Dhakal for her help during computing the draft.

REFERENCES

1. WHO Department of Reproductive Health and Research. Reproductive health strategy to accelerate progress towards the attainment of international development goals and targets. Geneva: World Health Organization, 2004.
2. Vayena E, Rowe PJ, Griffin PD. Current Practices and Controversies in Assisted Reproduction. Report of a Meeting. Geneva, Switzerland: World Health Organization; 2002. pp.383-5.
3. Fathalla MF. Reproductive health: a global overview. Early Hum Dev 1992;29:35-42.
4. Boivin J, Bunting L, Collins JA, Nygren KG. International estimates of infertility prevalence and treatment-seeking: potential need and demand for infertility medical care. Hum Reprod 2007;22:1506-12.
5. Daar AS, Merali Z. Infertility and social suffering: the case of ART in developing countries. In: Vayena E, Rowe PJ, Griffin PD (Eds). Current Practices and Controversies in Assisted Reproduction. Geneva, Switzerland: World Health Organization; 2002. pp. 15-21.
6. Araoye MO. Epidemiology of Infertility: social problems of the infertile couple. West Afr J Med 2003;22:190-6.
7. Ombelet W, Cooke I, Dyer S, Serour G, Devroey P. Infertility and the provision of infertility medical services in developing countries. Hum Reprod Update 2008;14(6):605-21.
8. World Health Organization. Infertility: A tabulation of available data on prevalence of primary and secondary infertility. Geneva: WHO; 1991. WHO/MCH/91.9.
9. Larsen V. Primary and secondary infertility in Sub-Saharan Africa. Int J Epidemiol 2000;29:285-91.
10. Inhorn MC. Global infertility and globalisation of new reproductive technologies: illustrations from Egypt. Soc Sci Med 2003;56:1837-51.
11. Okonofua FE. The case against new reproductive technologies in developing countries. Br J Obstet Gynaecol 1996;103:957-62.
12. Barten J. Screening for infertility in Indonesia: results of examination of 863 infertile couples. Andrologia 1978;10(5):405-12.
13. World Health Organization. Infections, pregnancies, and infertility: perspectives on prevention. Fertil Steril 1987;47(6):964-8.
14. Cates W, Farley TM, Rowe PJ. Worldwide patterns of infertility: is Africa different? Lancet 1985;2(8455):596–8.
15. Gerais AS, Rushwan H. Infertility in Africa. Popul Sci 1992;12:25-46.
16. Grimes DA, Benson J, Singh S, Romero M, Ganatra B, Okonofua FE, et al. Unsafe abortion: the preventable pandemic. Lancet 2006;368(9550):1908-19.
17. Okumu CV, Kamau RK, Rogo KO. Past reproductive and sexual characteristics of women with tubal

infertility at Kenyatta National Hospital. East Afr Med J 1990;67(12):864-72.
18. Katz SS, Katz SH. An evaluation of traditional therapy for barrenness. Medical Anthropology 1987;(1): 395-405.
19. Sundby J, Mboge R, Sonko S. Infertility in the Gambia: frequency and health care seeking. Soc Sci Med 1998;46:891-9.
20. Nachtigall RD. International disparities in access to infertility services. Fertil Steril 2006;85:871-5.
21. Sharma S, Mittal S, Aggarwal P. Management of infertility in low resource countries. Br J Obstet Gynaecol 2009;116(1):77-83.
22. Van Balen F, Gerrits T. Quality of infertility care in poor resource areas and the introduction of new reproductive technologies. Hum Reprod 2001;16:215-9.
23. van Zandvoort H, Koning K, Gerrits T. Medical infertility care in low income countries: the case of concern in policy and practice. Trop Med Int Health 2001;6:563-9.
24. Akande EO. Affordable assisted reproductive technologies in developing countries: pros and cons. ESHRE Monogr 2008:1:12-4.
25. Sheth SS, Malpani AN. Inappropriate use of new technology: impact on women's health. Int J Gynecol Obstet 1997;58:159-65.
26. Oknofua FE. New reproductive technologies and infertility treatment in Africa. Afr J Reprod Health 2003;7:7-11.
27. Sen A. Freedoms and needs. The New Republic 1994;17:31-2.
28. Pilcher H. Fertility on a shoestring. Nature 2006;442:975-7.
29. Huyser C. Affordable ART services in Africa: synthesis and adaptation of laboratory services. ESHRE Monogr 2008. pp.77-84.
30. Hovatta O, Cooke I. Cost-effective approaches to in vitro fertilization: means to improve access. Int J Gynaecol Obstet 2006;94:287-91.
31. WHO Department of Reproductive Health and Research. Accelerating Progress towards the Attainment of International Reproductive Health Goals and Framework for implementing the WHO Global Reproductive Health Strategy. Geneva, Switzerland: WHO Department of Reproductive Health and Research, 2006.
32. Collins J. An international survey of the health economics of IVF and ICSI. Hum Reprod Update 2002;8:265-77.
33. Heitman E. Social and ethical aspects of in vitro fertilization. International Journal of Technology Assessment in Health Care 1999;15:22-35.
34. Brugha R, Zwi A. Improving the quality of private sector delivery of public health services: challenges and strategies. Health Policy and Planning 1998;13:107-20.
35. Sengupta A, Nundy S. The private health sector in India. British Medical Journal 2005;331:1157-8.
36. Unisa S. Childlessness in Andhra Pradesh, India: treatment seeking and consequences. Reprod Health Matters 1999;7:54-64.
37. Ombelet W, Campo R, Frydman R, Huyser C, Nargund G, Sallam H, et al. The Arusha project: accessible infertility care in developing countries—a reasonable option? ESHRE Monogr 2010. pp.107-15.
38. Franken DR, Smith M, Menkveld R, Kruger TF, Sekadde-Kigondu C, Mbizvo M, et al. The development of a continuous quality control programme for strict sperm morphology among sub-Saharan African laboratories. Hum Reprod 2000;15(3):667-71.
39. Campo R, Molinas CR, Rombauts L, Mestdagh G, Lauwers M, Braekmans P, et al. Prospective multicentre randomized controlled trial to evaluate factors influencing the success rate of office diagnostic hysteroscopy. Hum Reprod 2005;20(1): 258-63.
40. Ombelet W, Campo R. Affordable IVF for developing countries. Reprod Biomed Online 2007;15:257-65.
41. Ombelet W, Deblaere K, Bosmans E, Cox A, Jacobs P, Janssen M, et al. Semen quality and intrauterine insemination. Reprod Biomed Online 2003;7:485-92.
42. Verhulst SM, Cohlen BJ, Hughes E, Te Velde E, Heinmen MJ. Intrauterine insemination for unexplained subfertility. Cochrane Database Syst Rev 2006;4:CD001838.
43. Philips Z, Barraza-Llorens M, Posnett J. Evaluation of the relative cost-effectiveness of treatments for infertility in the UK. Hum Reprod 2000;15:95-106.
44. Peterson CM, Hatasaka HH, Jones KP, et al. Ovulation induction with gonadotropins and intrauterine insemination compared with in vitro fertilization and no therapy: a prospective, nonrandomized, cohort study and meta-analysis. Fertil Steril 1994;62:535-44.
45. Goverde AJ, McDonnell J, Vermeiden JP, et al. Intrauterine insemination or in-vitro fertilisation in idiopathic subfertility and male subfertility: a randomised trial and cost-effectiveness analysis. Lancet 2000;355:13-8.

46. Pelinck MJ, Hoek A, Simons AH, Heineman MJ. Efficacy of natural cycle IVF: a review of the literature. Hum Reprod Update 2002;8:129-39.
47. Philips SJ, Kadoch IJ. Natural cycle IVF: a question of semantics? Reprod Biomed Online 2007;15(3): 255-6.
48. Daya S, Gunby J, Hughes EG, Collins JA, Sagle MA, Young EV. Natural cycles for in-vitro fertilization: cost-effectiveness analysis and factors influencing outcome. Hum Reprod 1995;10(7):1719-24.
49. Steinkampf MP, Kretzer PA, McElroy E, et al. A simplified approach to in vitro fertilization. J Reprod Med 1992;37:99-104.
50. Rojanasakul A, Choktanasiri W, Suchartwatanachai C, Srisombut C, Chinsomboon S, Chatasingh S. 'Simplified IVF': program for developing countries. J Med Assoc Thai 1994;77:12-8.
51. Vajta G, Holm P, Greve T, Callesen H. The submarine incubation system, a new tool for in vitro embryo culture: a technique report. Theriogenology 1997;48:1379-85.
52. Ranoux C, Dubuisson JB, Foulot H, Aubriot FX. Intravaginal culture and embryo transfer. A new method for the fertilization of human oocytes. Rev Fr Gynecol Obstet 1987;82:741-4.
53. Taymor ML, Ranoux CJ, Gross GI. Natural oocyte retrieval with intravaginal fertilization: a simplified approach to in vitro fertilization. Obstet Gynecol 1992;80:888-91.
54. Ranoux C, Aubriot FX, Dubuisson JB, Cardone V, Foulot H, Poirot C, et al. A new in vitro fertilization technique: intravaginal culture. Fertil Steril 1988;49:654-7.
55. Blockeel C, Mock P, Verheyen G, et al. An in vivo culture system for human embryos using an encapsulation technology: a pilot study. Hum Reprod 2009;24(4):790-6.
56. Vayena E, Peterson HB, Adamson D, Nygren KG. Assisted reproductive technologies in developing countries: are we caring yet? Fertil Steril 2009; 92(2):413-6.

Chapter 5

Establishing an ART Unit in a Low-resource Setting

Haroon Latif Khan

Reproductive health implies good health of the woman to fulfill her desire to reproduce whenever she wishes. This is part of the human rights declaration of the United Nations. Reproduction is the basic desire of all human beings but a large number of married couples fail to conceive and reproduce. Hence every country should have a strategy to prevent causes of infertility and plans to investigate and treat all the couples. In spite of the prevalence of the problem in low resource setting, the facility for such a care is not available.

Infertility is failure to conceive after unprotected coitus for two years. In recent years, the duration of living together has been reduced from two years to one year.[1]

National Institute for Clinical Excellence (NICE) recommends two years in its guidelines. According to this definition in United Kingdom at least 8 to 10 percent couples are infertile.[2]

The incidence in some African countries is 15 to 22 percent (Botswana, Zimbabwe, Lesotho) but the incidence in Egypt is 8 to 13 percent. Okonofua suggests the incidence in Nigeria is 20 to 30 percent.[3]

According to Delhi IVF Fertility Research centre, the incidence in India is one out of six couples. A survey conducted in three Indian states found out overall prevalence out of 7000 couples was 24 percent in low income group and 31 percent in higher income group. The incidence of secondary infertility is higher in low resource countries. In India, primary infertility is more common in younger age groups and secondary infertility increase with age.[4]

Boivin in a survey in 25 countries found out similarity in incidence 5 to 15 percent. He also found out remarkable similarity in the prevalence of sexually transmitted infection (STI).

In recent years, the incidence of STI has fallen from 30 to 40 percent in 1960 and 1970 to the low level of six percent in recent years.[5]

Infertile couples need medical advice and help. Unfortunately due to prevailing unhygienic conditions, lack of public education and awareness this problem is more prevalent in the low economic groups.

Infertility carries with it additional social, financial and family problems which make the life of the couple extremely unhappy and emotionally stressful, moreover the quacks and charlatans exploit such couples financially and add to their misery. In addition, they not only leave them financially poorer but add additional medical problems by their wrong treatment.

The ratio between patient and doctor in low economic countries is very poor. Trained medical practitioners are overwhelmed by the life-threatening medical diseases therefore they neither have time nor the expertise to handle cold cases such as infertility.

Management of infertility in low resource setting does not always require high tech equipment. The preliminary workup of a couple is possible even in the poorest and financially deprived couples. Management at grass root level requires minimal assistance from the laboratory and radiology.

In 2001, World Health Organization (WHO) recommended that infertility be treated as a global problem which called for innovative approaches in treatment, such as low cost ART.[6]

European Society of Human Reproduction and Embryology (ESHRE) created task force which has been active in creating forums for debate on the strategic and technical issues increasing access to assisted reproductive technique (ART). The low cost IVF foundation was established in 2007.[1] The foundation's specific goals are to establish low cost ART centers at selected sites, training clinicians and scientists.[7-9]

The International Society for Mild Approaches in Assisted Reproductive Techniques (ISMAAR) was established in 2007 with the objective of encouraging medical community to develop and use simpler treatment protocols.[10]

The focus has shifted to determine adaptation of ART to developing countries and make it a low cost treatment suitable to the local economic environment.[11,12]

In Nigeria, one IVF cycle costs $2000 to $2700. The minimum wage is $52 to 60 per month. How can this gap be reduced to make it possible for all Nigerians to use ART when needed?[13,14]

ETIOLOGY

Causes of infertility are multiple. They could be due to some abnormality in male partner or female partner or remain unexplained. In the male partner it could be defective or no production of the spermatozoa (oligospermia or azoospermia) or impotency or any other sexual dysfunction. Similarly in the female partner, it could be related to ovulation or fallopian tubes.

These could be either due to genetic, hormonal or immunological factors. There could be an infective cause. The infection could be acquired by STI or iatrogenic. In India and Pakistan, tuberculosis (TB) is still a common cause of genital tract infection which may lead tubal obstruction. In a study, it was found that there was a history of TB in 68 percent of women who complained of infertility, amenorrhea or oligomenorrhea.[15]

In Africa nearly 85 percent of women had infertility due to infection[16] which is double of rest of the world.

The type and mode of infection varies from country to country, depending upon the health care system and social factors.[17] Iatrogenic causes are responsible in 5 percent in Europe and 15.5 percent in Africa.[16]

In sub-Sahara region, the STI are responsible for more than 70 percent cases of pelvic infection. Most of these infections are caused by Chlamydia and Gonorrhea.[18] They also cause male infertility. In addition other causes are postabortal or postpartum infections. HIV-infected persons are also at a higher risk of infertility either due to damage to the tubes or altered spermatogenesis.

A WHO report of 2006 estimated that in 1995 nearly 26 million legal and 20 million illegal abortions were performed worldwide.[21] In developing countries, nearly 97 percent were unsafe abortions. These interventions can have serious consequences leading to tubal blockage and infertility in 20 to 30 percent cases. Unhygienic obstetrical practices also contribute to secondary infertility, which is why secondary infertility is more common in later age groups.[19-21]

Local cultural practices also may causes infertility. In Africa genital mutilation is still commonly practiced. A WHO report of 2005 shows 100 to 140 million young girls had undergone genital mutilation.[22] This procedure may lead to sepsis, scarring leading to dyspareunia and infertility. Early marriage, polygamy, lack of health care access may be other factors responsible for disparity in the incidence of infertility in rural and urban areas.[23]

In Pakistan and India due to higher priority for fertility, the patients approach local midwives for treatment under social pressure and end up with iatrogenic cause of infertility.[24]

INVESTIGATIONS

NICE guidelines are that certain basic principles should be followed. Minimal time should be spent before embarking upon investigations and treatment.

This includes evaluation of the couple by history, physical examination of both partners and use of evidence-based investigations. It is important that a clinical diagnosis is made without delay and appropriate treatment is provided.[17,25]

Detailed and accurate history is obtained from the partners, especially about social habits and coitus. Past history of an intervention or infection is enquired. Special enquiry is made about local endemic infections. A past history of STI, urinary tract infection (UTI), induced abortion and postpartum infection are most important in relation to secondary infertility.

Preliminary Workup

In low economic setting clinical evaluation is the most important component. A detailed history and physical examination to find out the cause of infertility is the most important step to pin point the cause and subsequently management of the couple (Flow chart 5.1).

Generally speaking, it is the wife who approaches the medical facility for any investigation and treatment. A detailed history and physical examination will establish any possible cause and further line of investigations. If on clinical grounds all is well then it can be reassuring for the wife and she can impress upon her husband the need for his check-up.

After clinical evaluation, investigations for both partners can be planned.

- Clinical Assessment
  - History
  - Physical examination
- Semen analysis (abstinence 2–8 days)
- Tests for patency of the fallopian tubes (HSG or laparoscopy) CD 8–10
- Ovulation Tests (CD 21 progesterone).

  All these can be completed within one month.

  If one wishes to reduce the cost of workup in low economic group of patients, all these factors can be worked out with minimal expense.

A simple semen analysis and cycle day 21 progesterone test will cost less than $5 and similarly for tubal patency tests a hysterosalpingogram (HSG) will cost $20 to 30. Hence, the total cost of the work-up is reduced to less than $50. It gives reassurance and provides sense of direction for the treatment of the couple.

HYSTEROSALPINGOGRAPHY

Hysterosalpingography (HSG) is a useful low cost tool to establish pathology of uterine cavity and fallopian tubes. It can be performed in an outdoor setting, without the need of an operation theater or anesthesia. Common side effects include pain, drug reaction and risk of infection.

Sonohysterography

This is a similar procedure to HSG but performed under ultrasound (U/S) guidance. Somehow

Flow chart 5.1: Infertility workup map

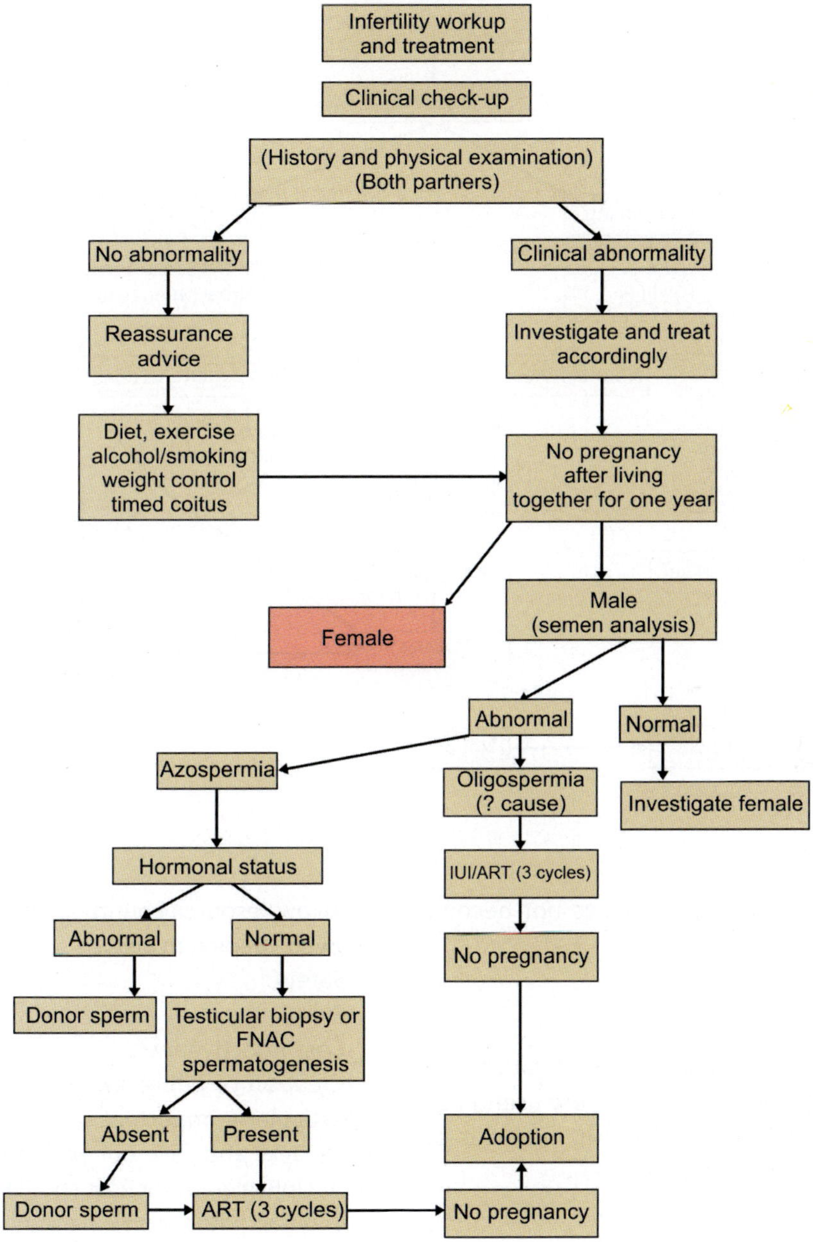

Contd...

Contd...

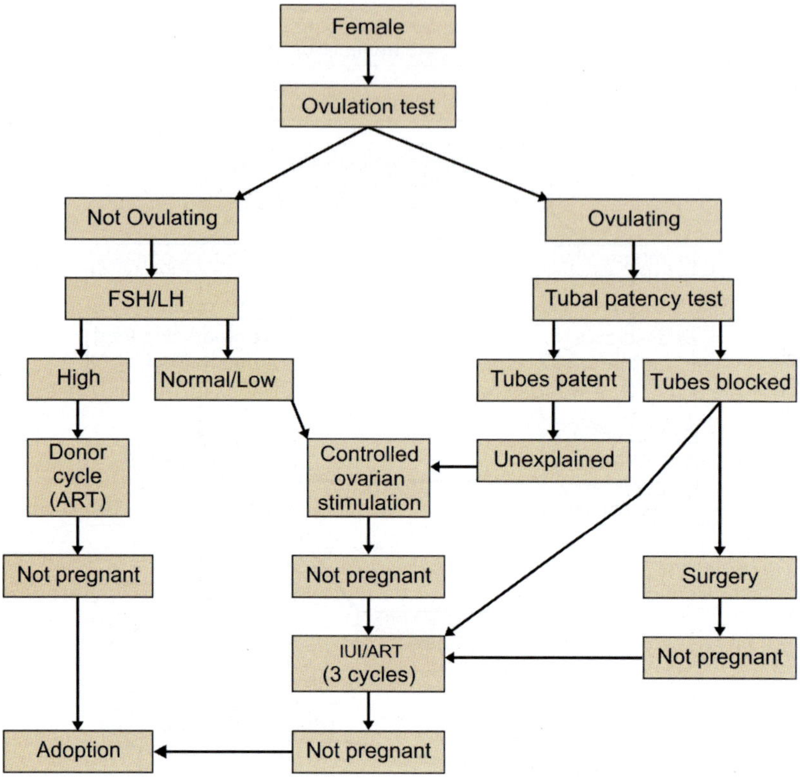

because of its less reliability it has not become popular even in low-cost setting.

Laparoscopy

Laparoscopy is a second line of investigation. It is invasive and expensive but it is a very useful tool for investigations after HSG.[24] It may not be indicated in all infertile couples.

Treatment

NICE and Royal College of Obstetricions and Gynecologists (RCOG) (London) have produced guidelines for the treatment of infertility.[25]

In low resource countries, these guidelines are followed keeping in view:

- Safety
- Simplicity
- Cost effectiveness.

Creation of public awareness about infertility is particularly important to eliminate charlatans and quacks and save our patients from maltreatment. Unhygienic practices should be excluded and early contact with the physicians should be promoted.

Healthy dietary habits should be encouraged and bad habits of alcohol and smoking discouraged. Counseling about public health issues should be part of media campaign.

Once a specific diagnosis is established, it should be treated according to the international guidelines (NICE/RCOG).

Controlled Ovarian Stimulation (COS)

In a low cost set-up, the commonly used protocols and drugs for ART are:

- Natural cycle
- Clomiphene citrate (CC) only
- Aromatase inhibitors (Letrozole) only
- Clomiphene citrate (CC) + Human menopausal gonadotropin (HMG)
- Purified follicle stimulating hormone (FSH) only
- Letrozole + Purified FSH
- Gonadotropin-releasing hormone (GnRH) agonists + Gonadotropins (Short protocol)
- Small doses of gonadotropins with antagonists or analogs (Mild protocol).

Natural Cycle

Louise Brown was conceived by natural cycle and tracking of ovarian follicle by estimation of estradiol levels. This method involves no ovarian stimulating drugs but practically it is extremely inconvenient for the ART team for tracking luteinizing hormone (LH) surge and planning ovum pickup (OPU). LH surge may be at an odd hour. Secondly, it means procurement of only one to two eggs which reduce the chances of fertilization and subsequent embryo transfer (ET).

It carries the benefit of no OHSS or hyperstimulation. The risk of cancellation of the cycle remains high and overall success rate is low (7.5–19% per cycle).[26,27,43,44] Generally it is an unpopular method even in the lowest income group.

Clomiphene Citrate

This is the least expensive method of ovarian stimulation. When combined with injection human chorionic gonadotropin (hCG) it is useful in ART. This salt has been in use for ovarian stimulation for nearly five decades. It was the most popular method for ovarian stimulation in 1980s.[18] In spite of its antiestrogenic side effects, it is still the most commonly prescribed drug for ovarian stimulation protocol.

The problem with this stimulation regimen is premature LH surge. Such surge can be prevented by injection of GnRH antagonists but these injections are expensive which makes the stimulation cost very high.

CC achieves 20 percent ovulation and with timed coitus up to 25 percent pregnancy rates.[18,28]

The risks are OHSS and multiple pregnancies when combined with gonadotropins.

The success rate improves further when combined with intrauterine insemination (IUI) but this requires monitoring and infrastructure of andrology laboratory which increases the cost of treatment. For some low socioeconomic groups it may be too expensive.[29]

Aromatase Inhibitors

Transient inhibition of aromatase activity in early menstrual cycle is achieved by giving aromatase inhibitor (Letrozole). It results in stimulation of folliculogenesis in the ovaries. This folliculogenesis is similar to clomiphene citrate.

Letrozole is particularly useful in polycystic ovarian (PCO) patients. The ovulation and pregnancy rates are higher than clomiphene citrate.[38]

The indications for use and results are comparable with CC. The usual dose of 2.5 mg is given orally from CD 3–7 or CD 5–9. If required in the next cycle dose is increased up to 7.5 mg/day. The results in terms of endometrial thickness, estradiol levels and ovulation are comparable with CC. The cost of letrozole is higher than CC (almost 3–4 times). This makes CC as first choice for ovulation induction. In special cases like PCO letrozole may be used in low income groups. Letrozole may also be used if CC fails to stimulate ovaries.[39,40]

Intrauterine Insemination

Intrauterine insemination (IUI) is a popular method of treatment of subfertility. In this treatment, processed semen of the male partner is inseminated into the uterus using a specialized catheter. The insemination is timed with the ovulation time of the female partner. It may be performed in a natural cycle or with controlled ovarian stimulation.

Common indications include mild-to-moderate cases of oligospermia, infrequent ovulation, PCO, sexual dysfunction (male and female) and unexplained infertility.

IUI if performed with proper expertise can do wonders in low socioeconomic groups.

Low Cost IUI Facility

IUI is a fairly basic treatment which does not require expensive equipment and highly expert personal like other ART procedures. It can easily be performed in rural settings and basic health units.

A low cost set-up for IUI treatment facility includes:

- Ultrasound with transvaginal sonography probe
- Andrology laboratory:
  - Laboratory size 6′× 6′
  - Trinocular microscope
  - Laminar flow hood
  - Centrifuge machine
- Disposables:
  - IUI catheter
  - Other (Test tubes, pipettes, etc.)
- Culture medium
- Personnel:
  - Clinician
  - Trained laboratory technician (Andrologist).

Surgery for Tubal Blockage

The results of surgical correction depend upon the causes of blockage and techniques used for operative procedures.

Surgery after bilateral tubal ligation (BTL) with clips produces best results especially when microsurgical techniques are used. The success rate maybe up to 50 percent in such cases.[29,31]

In low income countries generally blockage is due to pelvic inflammatory disease and microscopic surgery is not available.

In such situations surgery when performed laparoscopically or open laparotomy carries lesser chances of success as compared to ART.[29,31]

Assisted Reproductive Technique

These days assisted reproductive technique (ART) is the gold standard of infertility treatment. It is worked out that nearly 10 percent of all infertile couples will need ART treatment.[29]

When translated into national figures population of one million needs one ART set-up. In most of the low income groups such help is available only in rich urban localities. The overall cost makes it prohibitively expensive for low income rural groups.

The lower rate of take home baby makes it even more expensive.[32]

On the other hand, the way infertile women are exposed to psychological, physical trauma and even physical violence at any cost ART is the need of poor population.[33,34]

ART is not on the priority list of national health budget hence in low income countries it is available only in the private sector. Because of initial investment and cost of drugs and overhead expenses the cost of ART treatment is beyond the reach of most needy couples.

In light of this, we should work out the ways of minimizing the cost of ART and make alternative treatments available in teaching hospitals so that most of the infertile couples can be helped.

The doctors and other staff dealing with infertility should impress upon the political leaders and planners of health in the low income countries that infertility affects not only the couples emotionally and socially it carries ramifications at work, home and in the society. To make amends in this aspect, ART should be made available to infertile couples at low cost public sector hospitals. ICPD recommendations should be cited to support the case of infertile couples and create political will in the society.[35]

The political governments should be impressed upon that ART as a treatment of infertility should the part of the national health plan.

WHO has recommended improvement in maternal and child health program.[36]

The side effects of infertility are such that its treatment should become priority in the budget for health care and it should be attempted that ART and all treatments of infertility should be available to all members of the society irrespective of its cost.

On the other hand, we should plan and try to reduce the cost of ART especially in low income countries.

HOW TO REDUCE THE COST OF ART?

The high cost of ART is due to:

- Infrastructure:
  - Exclusive facility
  - Laboratory equipment
  - Ovarian monitoring equipment (TVS/doppler), etc.
- Ovarian stimulation drugs
- Disposables for ART
- Culture medium
- Overhead expenses
  - Utilities
  - Salaries of staff
    - Embryologist
    - Clinician (Endocrinologist, sonologist)
    - Counselor.

Facility (Fig. 5.1)

Adequate premises should be marked for infertility workup and ART program. At least minimal physical and personnel requirements should be provided.

Personnel

- Clinician (gynecologist)
- Counselor
- Sonologist
- Embryologist
- ART nurse.

Laboratory Equipment

The cost of setting up an ART program can be minimized by providing minimal equipment. To establish an ART unit in a low resource setting following is the bare minimum requirement:

- Stereozoom microscope
- CO_2 Incubator
- Laminar flow hood
- ART disposables (OPU needles, dishes, pipettes and embryo transfer catheters)
- Culture medium [homemade (reduces the cost)/commercial].

Use of autoclaving for the pipettes and other glassware, where permissible, will reduce the cost tremendously.

Follicular Tracking

Ultrasound machine with TVS probe is most important for any ART program. It is most useful for follicular tracking and OPU. Low cost set-up does not need Doppler, 3D or other advanced ultrasonographic machines.

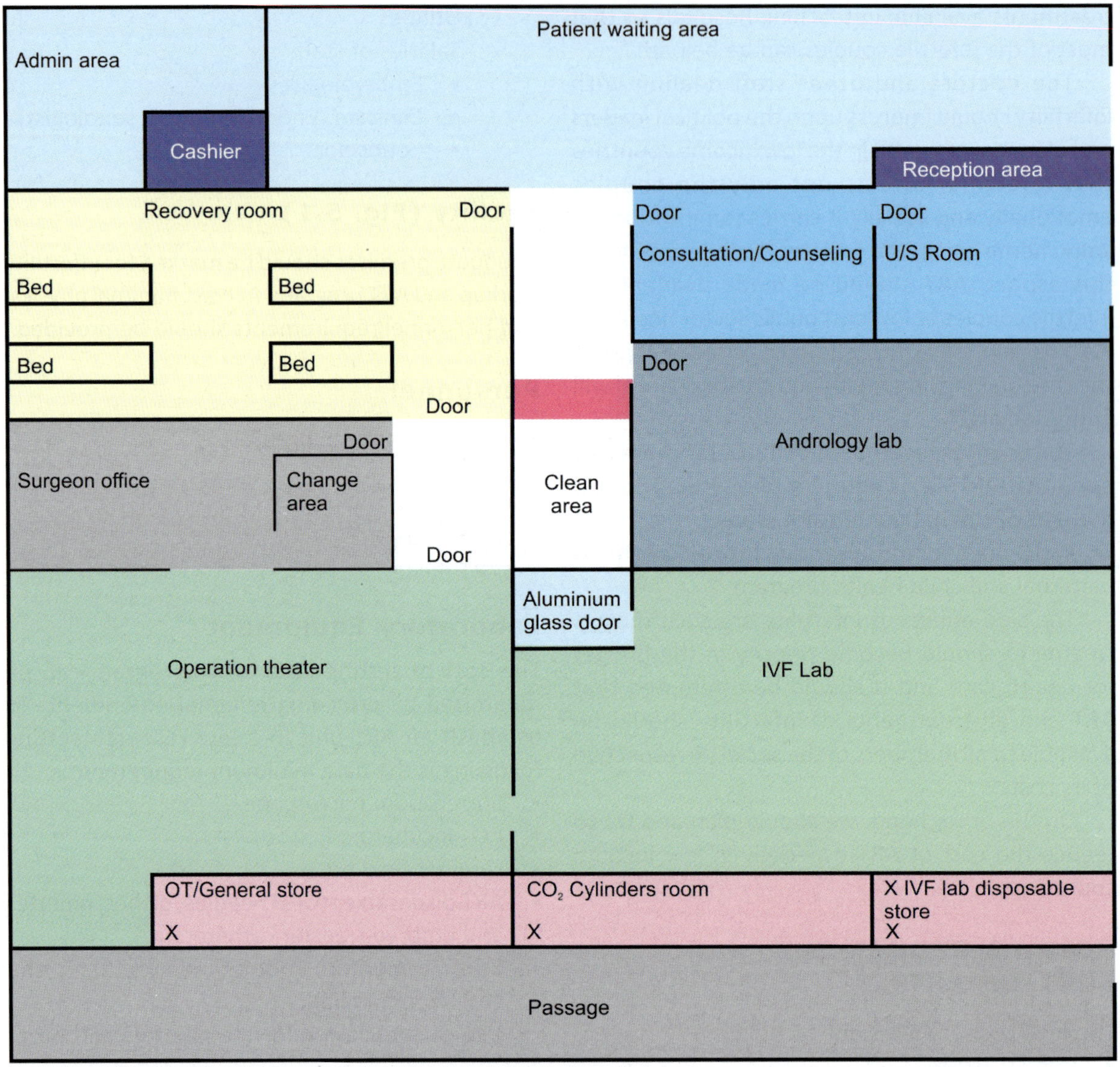

Fig. 5.1: IVF lab

Training

The most difficult component of setting up ART program is nonavailability of trained embryologists and other members of the ART team. Training slots all over the world are limited and their training fees are rocketing high hence their salaries commensurate with the expense of their training fees. A good ART program needs a good embryologist who are expensive to engage and not easily available.

In a low cost set-up, it makes extremely difficult to engage well-trained but low paid staff. Such a center should have a close liaison with a central ART set-up and seek rotation and advice from the central/parent department regularly. Working in isolation carries the risk of trouble shooting not being available to identify and rectify problems. All laboratories, every now and then, develop these technical issues.

In a low cost set-up one can minimize the number of staff but cannot compromise on the quality of expertise. Success of any program depends heavily on the performance of the embryology laboratory.

Cost of Disposables/Culture Medium

In addition to the cost of setting up ART laboratory the running cost of a program is substantially high due to the use of expensive disposables and short shelf-life of culture medium. Disposables are generally for use only once.

If the manufacturers could come out with reuseable disposables after autoclaving, which will be the greatest service to ART programs. At present the only choice is to keep their use to the minimum but remember that there is no cutting of corners in ART programs; any such measure may lead to immediate drop in results.

Similarly latest culture media are very expensive and have short shelf-life. Minimizing its use and maintaining optimal results require expertise and skills of the embryologist, which in a low cost setting is scarcely available.

Nevertheless, the cost can be brought down by paying attention to these aspects in a low cost program.

Treatment in Batches

In those clinics which are not very busy use of visiting embryologist is recommended. Collecting a batch of patients by synchronizing their last menstrual dates can save expenses on the constant availability of expert embryologist, use of culture medium and laboratory staff salaries.

Satellite Clinics

Another method of reducing the cost of ART is to set-up satellite clinics in low economic areas in affiliation with tertiary state of the ART clinics. These satellite clinics could perform basic infertility workup, controlled ovarian stimulation, follicular monitoring with timely referral to the main clinic.

These clinics may perform IUI procedure provided they have proper expertise and equipment for andrology.

Intravaginal Culture (INVOCEL)

In 1986, Renoux C[41,42,45] described insertion of a small commercially available tube containing oocytes and prepared spermatozoa into the vagina of the patient for incubation. This method used vaginal temperature as a natural incubator and reduced the use of laboratory incubation. In this procedure after 72 hours of vaginal incubation, the tube is retrieved and the embryos are examined under a microscope for fertilization and cleavage. Two embryos are transferred by ET method into the uterus.

This short cut reduces the cost of incubator and is promoted as an effective technique for low cost ART.

IN VITRO MATURATION OF OOCYTES

In vitro maturation of oocytes (IVM), no hormonal stimulation is required and multiple oocytes can be procured without the use of ovarian stimulation. Therefore, the cost of stimulation drugs is excluded.

The laboratory techniques required are much more demanding than those from the treatment stimulated cycles.

This technique is particularly useful for PCOD patients who stand higher risk of OHSS with ovarian stimulated cycles.[37]

Ovarian Hyperstimulation Syndrome (OHSS)

OHSS is one of the major complications, of controlled ovarian stimulation (COS). Its incidence ranges 5 to 6 percent.[23,24]

OHSS patients require intensive care because the patient can become seriously ill and rarely it is life-threatening.

In a case of natural cycle there is no such risk. Low dose stimulation when used to keep the cost down the risk of this high cost complication is also reduced or ruled out.

In a low cost setting avoiding OHSS is an important component of reducing the overall cost of ART treatment.

By use of gonadotropins, especially recombinants, more embryos are procured with higher pregnancy rates and lower cancellation rates but with a higher risk of OHSS.[9]

CC and letrozole with injection hCG may be used more frequently for ART in low-cost setting.

Single Embryo Transfer

Transfer of multiple embryos (>2) gives higher chances of multiple pregnancies. Routine transfer of two or more embryos results in higher rates of twin pregnancies, up to 24 percent.[9,46-48]

The rate of twins, triplets and even higher number carries the more risk of preterm births. Preterm babies carry risk of developing neurological deficit and other anomalies.

They require intensive neonatal care, the cost of which may go prohibitive. The cost effectiveness of three embryo transfers is more but long-term economics with single embryo transfer (SET) is better.

Multiple pregnancies add astronomic cost to the total expenditure of ART. Hence most of the countries are making laws promoting SET (Finland Sweden, Belgium).[9]

Lesser stimulation with CC + hMG or low dose gonadotropins would mean lesser number of embryos and SET will be possible. In a low cost setting such a benefit in reducing the overall cost will be most welcome. Such an approach may increase the cancellation of the cycles and lower the pregnancy rates but it will be cost beneficial to the patient. Hence SET should be the norm for two attempts at least.

CONCLUSION

Exploring low cost ART suitable to third world countries should be aim of the future research. Such ART should be incorporated in the national health care program.

The widespread perception that infertility is the problem only in the developed countries is wrong. Prevention of the causes of infertility should be part of health care in the country but complete workup and treatment including ART should be available to the infertile couples.

More constructive approach is needed to find out the ways of low cost ART for developing nations. This is a challenge we have to face and find solutions for the future approaches.

In spite of best efforts universal availability of ART is unlikely but we should continue to explore means of reducing the cost of ART but maintain the quality of care which is the hallmark of success in ART.

To make ART accessible to most of the population of a developing country we need to address the following:

- Evaluate national infertility needs
- Present position of infertility in the country
- Incorporate ART in the health care program
- Transfer of knowledge and technology of low cost ART and lay down low cost protocols
- Develop rules and regulations for ART in the country (Regulatory Authority)

- Surveillance and reporting of ART program
- Maintain ethics and standards of care.

REFERENCES

1. Cates W, Farley TMM, Row PJ. Worldwide patterns of infertility: is Africa different? Lancet 1985;2:596-8.
2. NICE: Fertility: assessment and treatment for people with fertility problems, 2004 (www.nice.org.uk) ref. CG11.
3. Jindal UN, Gupta AN. Social problems of infertile women in India. Int J Fertil 1989;34:0-33.
4. Talwar PP, Goel OP, Murali IN. Prevalence of infertility in different population groups in India and its determinants. ICMR, 1986 (www.icmr.nic.in).
5. Boivin J, Bunting L, Collins JA, Nygren KG. International estimates of infertility prevalence and treatment seeking: potential need and demands for infertility medical care. Hum Reprod 2007;22:1506-12.
6. Jindal UN, Gupta AN. Social Problems of infertile women in India. Int J Fertil 1989;34:0-33.
7. The Low Cost Foundation. Available at: http://www.lowcost-ivf.org Last accessed 3 March, 2008.
8. Huyser C. Affordable ART services in Africa: Synthesis and adaptation of laboratory services. ESHRE Monogr 2008. pp. 77-84.
9. Hovatta O, Cooke I. Cost-effective approaches to in vitro fertilization: means to improve access. Int J Gynaecol Obstet 2006;94:287-91.
10. Nargund G, Frydman R. Towards a more physiological approach to IVF. Reprod Biomed Online 2007;14:550-2.
11. Oknofua FE. Nes reproductive technologies and infertility treatment in Africa. Afr J Reprod Health 2003;7:7-11.
12. Ombelet W, Campo R. Affordable IVF for developing countries. Reprod Biomed Online 2007;15:257-65.
13. Vayena E, Rowe P, Griffin PD (Eds). Current practices and controversies in assisted reproduction: Report of a World Health Organization meeting. Geneva: World Health Organization, 2002.
14. Habbema JD. Is affordable and cost-effective assisted reproductive technology in low-income countries possible? What should we know to answer the question? ESHRE Monogr 2008. pp. 21-4.
15. Cates W, Farley TMM, Row PJ. Worldwide patterns of infertility: is Africa different? Lancet 1985;2:596-8.
16. Aboulghair MA. The importance of fertility treatment in the developing world. BJOG 2005;112:1174-6.
17. RHO archives. 2002 (www.sho.org/html/infertility) Accssed 2 March 2009.
18. Ombelet W, Cooke I, Dyer S, Serour G, Devroey P. Infertility and the province of infertility medical services in developing countries. Hum reprod Update 2008;14:605-21.
19. Leke RJ, Oduma JA, Bassol-Mayagoitia S, Bacha AM, Grigor KM. Regional and geographical variations in infertility; effects on environmental, cultural and socioeconomic facts. Environ Health Prospect 1993;10173-80.
20. Stanton C, Blanc AK, Croft T, Choi Y. Skilled care at birth in the developing world: progress to date and strategies for expanding coverage. J Biosoc Sci 2007; 39:109-20.
21. WHO. Unsafe abortion: global and regional estimates of the incidence of unsafe abortion and associated mortality in 2000, 4th edn. Geneva, Switzerland: WHO, 2004.
22. WHO. Female genital mutilation. 2005 Fact sheet No. 241 (www.WHO.int/mediacenter/fs241/en/index.html).
23. Dickens BM, Cook RJ. Reproductive health and public health ethics. Int J Gynaecol Obstet 2007;99:75-9.
24. Ombelet W, Campo R. Affordable IVF for developing countries. Reprod Biomed Online 2007;15:257-65 (www.Rbmonline.com/article/2820) Accessed 2 March 2009.
25 WHO. Infections, pregnancies and infertility: perspectives on prevention. Fertil Steril 1987;47: 944-9.
26. Cooke ID, Lenton EA. Folliculogenesis: the natural way. Aust NZ J Obstet Gynaecol 1994;34:268-71.
27. Pelinck MJ, Hock A, Simons AH, Heineman MJ. Efficacy of natural cycle IVF: a review of literature. Hum Reprod Update 2002;8129-39.
28. Inhorn MC, Buss KA. Infertility care in poor resource areas and the introduction of new reproductive technologies. Hum reprod 2001;16:215-9.
29. Fathalla MF, Sinding SW, Rosenfield A, Fathalla MMF. Sexual and reproductive health for all: call for action. Lancet 2006;368:2095-100.
30. Cheap IVF needed editorial Nature Publishing Group. Nature 2006;442:958.
31. Okonofua FE, Essen UI, Nimalaraj T. Hysterosalpingography versus laparoscopy in tubal infertility: comparison based on findings at laparotomy. Int J Gynaecol Obstet 1989;28:143-7.
32. Macklin R. Reproductive technologies in developing countries Bioethics 1995;9276-81.

33. Dyer SJ, Abrahams N, Mokoena NE, Lomard CJ, Van der, Spuy ZM. Psychological distress among women suffering form couple infertility in South Africa: a quantitative assessment. Hum Reprod 2005;20:1938-43.
34. Daar AS, Merali Z. Infertility and social suffering: the case of ART in developing countries. In: Vayena E, rowe P, David Griffin P, editors: Current Practices and Controversies in "Assisted Reproduction" Geneva: WHO, 2004. pp. 15-21.
35. Programme for Action – Declaration, Paragraph 7.6 United Nations International Conference on Population and Development (ICPD) 5-13th September 1994, Cairo, Egypt.
36. WHO (2002) In: Vayena E, Rowe P, David Griffin P (Eds). Introduction Current Practices and controversies in Assisted Reproduction "Medical, Ethical and Social Aspects of Assisted Reproduction" Geneva: WHO 15-17.
37. Grochowski D, Wolczynski S, Kuczynski W, Kulikowski M, Szamatowicz M. The results of an in vitro fertilization program: two regimens of superovulation. Gynecol Endocrinol 1995;9:59-62.
38. Mosammat Rashida Begum, et al. Comparison of efficacy of aromatase inhibitor and clomiphene citrate in induction of ovulation in polycystic ovarian syndrome; Fertility and Sterility 2009;92(3):853-87.
39. Fozan HA, Khadouri MA, Tan SL, Tulandi T. A randomized trial of letrozole versus clomiphene citrate in women undergoing superovulation. Fertil Steril 2004;82:1561-3.
40. Fisher SA, Reid RL, Vugt DA, Casper RF. A randomized double-blind comparison of the effects of clomiphene citrate and the aromatase inhibitor letrozole on ovulatory function in normal women. Fertil Steril 2002;78:280-5.
41. Taymor ML, Ranoux CJ, Gross GL. Natural oocyte retrieval with intravaginal fertilization: a simplified approach to in vitro fertilization. Obstet Gynecol 1992;80:888-91.
42. RanouxC, Dubuisson JB, Foulot H, Aubriot FX. Intravaginal culture and embryo transfer: a new method for the fertilization of human oocytes. Rev FR Gynecol Obstet 1987;82:741-4.
43. Child TJ, Abdul-Jalil AK, Gulkeli B, Tan SL. In vitro maturation and fertilization of oocytes form unstimulated normal ovaries, polcystic ovaries, and women with polycystic ovary syndrome. Fertill Steril 2001;76:936-42.
44. Soderstroom-Anttila V, Makinsen S, Tuuri T, Suikkari AM. Favourable pregnancy results with insemination of in vitro matured oocytes from unstimulated patients. Hum Reprod 2005;20:1534-40.
45. Sterzik K, Rosenbusch B, Sasse V, Wolf A, Beier HM, Lauritzen C. A new variation of in vitro fertilization: intravaginal culture of human oocytes and cleavage stages. Hum Reprod (4suppl 8):83-6.
46. Vilska S, Tiitinen A, Hyden-Granskog C, Hovatta O. Elective transfer of one embryo results in an acceptable pregnancy rate and eliminates the risk of multiple birth. Hum Reprod 1999;14:2392-5.
47. Martikainen H, Tiitinen A, et al. Finnish ET study group. One versus two embryo transfer after IVF and ICSI: a randomized study. Hum Reprod 2001;16:1900-2003.
48. Bergh C. Single embryo transfer: a mini-review. Hum Reprod 2005;20:323-237 (electronic publication 2005 Jan 21).

Chapter 6

The Laboratory Minimum Acceptable Standards

Manish Banker, Bharat Joshi

INTRODUCTION

Assisted reproductive techniques (ARTs) are increasingly used as a part of infertility management. Success of an ART program depends on various aspects: patient recruitment, counseling, optimal ovarian stimulation, egg collection and embryo transfer and embryology, etc. Establishing, equipping and maintaining a good laboratory form a very crucial integral part of the ART set-up.

MINIMAL PERSONNEL REQUIREMENTS OF AN ART CLINIC

The ART team consists of all or some of the following persons—medical director, clinician, sonologist, andrologist, embryologists, anesthesiologist, scientists, counselor, medical secretary, nurses and cleaning staff. The success of an IVF set-up is directly proportional to the degree of coordination and positive interactions between the members of this team. Total posts in an IVF Laboratory should be Director, Supervisor, Senior and junior Embryologist and Laboratory Technicians.

Laboratory Staff Requirement

Laboratory Director

The laboratory should be directed by an appropriately qualified and experienced responsible person with postgraduate qualifications and expertise in the field of embryology and biological or medical sciences according to national rules.

The responsibilities of the laboratory director include:

a. Ensuring that laboratory facilities are appropriate and safe by systematically controlling their functioning and programming with periodical maintenance.
b. Ensuring that written procedure manuals for all procedures exist and are carried out appropriately by the laboratory staff in compliance with a quality system.
c. To periodically review and update procedure manuals, and ensure that only the updated version of the manual is available in the laboratory.
d. To ensure that appropriate numbers of staff are in place, having the required experience to undertake the workload of the laboratory in relation to the techniques offered.
e. To ensure that all new staff are given a comprehensive orientation and introduction program. Beginners should follow a training scheme under the assistance and supervision of experienced embryologists and of the laboratory Director.

f. To organize and control laboratory staff training and ensure that the staff receive continual scientific and medical education.
g. Evaluation and analysis of data and having regular exchange of information and discussion with the clinical colleagues.

Clinical Embryologist

Must be knowledgeable in mammalian embryology and all other related biological field and must also be familiar with ART procedures. Should be either a medical graduate or postgraduate in life sciences. A complete supervision by a qualified and experienced embryologist is mandatory for the duration of up to six months to one year or first 100 cases depending upon workload and skill requirement.

a. The chief responsibilities of an embryologist are to perform all ART procedures as laid down in compliance with a quality system.
b. Embryologist should not preferably be loaded with responsibilities of general patient care, counseling, administration and marketing to avoid distraction.
c. Perform routine checks and maintaining detailed logs of changes and incidents.
d. Computerized data management, evaluation and analysis.

Total number may vary according to the actual workload,[1] as shown in Table 6.1.

Table 6.1: ART cycles and embryologist required

No. of ART cycles	*No. of embryologist required*
1–150	2
151–300	3
301–600	4
>600	1 additional per 200 cycles

(Fertility sterility, 2008;90:S165-8, Practice committee, revised minimum standards)

MINIMAL PHYSICAL REQUIREMENTS OF AN ART CLINIC

The location of an ART set-up involves several considerations like population of the area to decide on patients flow, their staying arrangements through egg collection to embryo transfer, their easy accessibility to the clinic, etc. neighborhood, i.e. polluting industries, vicinity to the airport to receive supplies.

Considering the data published worldwide it is now clear that of all possible methods including transport IVF, part-time clinics, and clinics with egg transport after collection to other center, one with fully integrated laboratory with clinical areas is likely to give best possible results.

A well-designed ART clinic should have minimum rooms for designated procedures which can be divided as nonsterile and a strictly sterile area as shown in Table 6.2.

The semen processing laboratory can be accommodated in a semisterile area. Entry to the main culture area should be made through double door interlock.

Table 6.2: Laboratory area requirement with dimensions

Nonsterile area	*Sterile area*
Waiting room	Ovum pick-up theater
Consulting room	Embryo transfer room
Examination-sonography room	Culture laboratory
Semen collection room	Cryopreservation room
Intrauterine insemination (IUI) room	
Sterilization room	
Postoperative ward	
Library, Data record room	
Store room	
Utility room	
Air-conditioning and power supply room	

Knowledgeable structure engineer and architect are of prime importance in designing or upgrading such a unit. Proper coordination of medical team, laboratory director, designers and air-conditioning team is key to establish an ideal set-up.

In modern laboratories air quality can be controlled to an extent but before selecting site for designing laboratory and clinical area thorough consideration should be given to exterior environment as ongoing construction work in surroundings, high-level of certain industrial gases and pollutants and also during construction or renovation many paints, chemicals and adhesives used may have significant negative impact on overall results of a program. So, these changes should be carefully monitored and program can be accordingly planned. In cases of pollutants generated outside or in neighborhood could be isolated by physical barriers or by creating negative pressure in the area between laboratory and renovation site. Many physical and chemical filtration systems are available with acceptable standards especially for set-ups where outside air directly cannot be used based on the analysis. The system installed must be capable of supplying filtered air with a temperature ranging 20 to 25°C with relative humidity less than 40 percent.

Laboratory Design

The construction of the laboratory should ensure aseptic and optimal handling of gametes, zygotes and embryos during all phases of the treatment. Laboratory walls and ceilings should have minimum penetrations. A solid ceiling with sealed light fittings and lockable, seal and sweep doors are preferred. Door width should be planned in such a way that allows easy movement of heavy and large sized equipment. Attention should be given to the ergonomics of the operator: bench height, adjustable chairs, microscope eye height, anti-slippery floors, efficient use of space and surfaces, sufficient air-conditioning with controlled humidity and temperature, all contributing to a working environment that minimizes distraction and fatigue. Rooms for changing clothes should be located close to the laboratory, having hand washing facilities. Access to the laboratory should be limited to authorized personnel only. Pass-box for all materials and disposables coming into the laboratory are recommended. Separate office space should be provided for administrative work, such as record keeping and data entry.

Semen collection rooms should be well planned and be adjacent to semen processing lab where collected sample can be immediately and easily handed over to laboratory personnel with a specially designed signaling method.

Central air-conditioning system with its outlet in various rooms should also be installed preferably with HEPA filters. DOP leak testing for checking the filter efficiency is to be carried out at each servicing. Minimum acceptable number of Particles per Cubic Meter by Micrometer Size for LAF (class -100) and IVF laboratory (class -10,000) is given in Table 6.3.[2]

Frequency of required and optional tests for class 100 and class 10,000 is given in Table 6.4.[3]

Table 6.3: Acceptable number of particles per cubic meter by micrometer size

CLASS	*0.1 μm*	*0.2 μm*	*0.3 μm*	*0.5 μm*	*1 μm*	*5 μm*	*Remarks*
100	100	24	10	4	-	-	for LAF
10,000	10,000	2,370	1,020	352	83		for IVF lab

(ISO 14644-1, *Cleanrooms and associated controlled environments Part 1: Classification of airborne particulates, Revised 1999)*

Table 6.4: Schedule of required and optional tests to demonstrate continuing compliance

Schedule of required tests to demonstrate continuing compliance	
Test parameter	*Maximum time interval*
Particle count test	6 months
Air pressure difference	12 months
Airflow	12 months
Schedule of optional tests to demonstrate continuing compliance	
Test parameter	*Maximum time interval*
Installed filter leakage	24 months
Containment leakage	24 months
Recovery	24 months
Airflow visualization	24 months

(ISO 14644-2, *Cleanrooms and associated controlled environments Part 2: Testing and monitoring to prove continued compliance with ISO 14644-1*; Revised, 1999)

Laboratory Equipment

Inside	*Outside*
Incubators	AF unit, AC
Microscopes	Gas cylinders
Laminar air flow	UPS
Micromanipulators	Generator

Cryofreezer, Containers

In an ideal set-up appropriate placement of incubators, laminar flow units and micromanipulator stations will minimize the distances that material need to transfer. In ideal conditions, all procedure modules should be arranged in such a way that embryologist can complete one procedure without moving more than three meters in any one direction, "lesser the footprints—better the results". Great care should be taken in designing to minimize collisions especially in busy units. Cryopreservation and storage facilities should preferably be partitioned but always just adjacent to the main laboratory. Same stands for the andrology laboratory being a separate unit altogether, with space for microscope, centrifuge, incubator and freezing. Separate place for ample storage capacity is part of good laboratory design as too many store cases and cupboards added later on may disturb the environment.

The laboratory equipment must be adequate for laboratory work and easy to clean and to disinfect. Critical equipment, including incubators and frozen gamete, zygote and embryo storage facilities, should be appropriately alarmed and monitored. An uninterrupted power supply and automatic emergency generator backup in the event of power failure should be in place. Instead of each instrument having its own voltage stabilizer, a centralized voltage stabilization unit is the better option. Records of ordinary and extraordinary maintenance on all the equipment must be documented and retained. Devices for the maintenance of temperature of media, gametes, zygotes and embryos during each phase of the procedure, when they are out of the incubators, should be in place (i.e. warm stages, heating blocks). Regular checks of functional parameters for devices used to maintain temperature and CO_2 should be performed using calibrated thermometers and extra methods of CO_2 analysis and/or pH measurement. Record of these measurements, as well as those shown by the digital displays of each device, must be retained. The instruction manual for every instrument should be available in the laboratory. Written instructions should be available to all members of the staff for actions to be taken in the case of equipment failure.

While selecting equipment, emphasis is given to the available space, ease of operation, ease of cleaning and more importantly to the after sales services available for their smooth functioning. Considering the events of sudden malfunction, extra crucial equipments such as incubators and cryopreservation systems may be considered in spare though it may add to the overall cost. Many a times supplier may provide the backup in cases of such emergencies which may turn out to be cost effective. It is also good practice to formerly tie up with other such unit in cases of such adverse event for equipment backup.

CO_2 Incubator

A minimum number of two incubators are recommended. Good practice is to keep approximately four cases per normal sized incubator. Gas cylinders should be placed outside or in a separate room with an automatic backup system. Incubators should be frequently cleaned and sterilized.

Conventional CO_2 incubators with 5 or 6 percent CO_2 in air and Bench top incubators with premixed 5 or 6 percent CO_2, 5 percent O_2, rest N_2 are available. Use of medical grade gases is recommended. A 0.22 micron filter should be attached at gas input if not inbuilt. Incubator should have an emergency power backup and remote alarm system for power failure and for high and low levels of both CO_2 and temperature. One CO_2 Incubator should be totally devoted for sperm preparation for IUI, IVF or ICSI procedures. Only the processed sperm sample at the time of insemination should enter the embryology laboratory. If workload demands, an additional incubator can be introduced which would serve as a standby unit. Or, one incubator can be used as working unit where eggs after pick-up and insemination are kept, whereas the other unit (culture unit) can hold embryos after fertilization till transfer.

Laminar Air Flow

Integrated vertical laminar air flow (LAF) workstations are available providing the hood with filtered air (0.3 micron) thus decreasing the chances of microbial contamination. A germicidal (UV) lamp is also provided. While ordering for LAF the table should be constructed in a way to fix stereozoom microscope on the table. This is so that the working levels of microscope stage and LAF table are same for easy handling of Petri dishes. Microscope stage and about 70 percent part of the table are provided with heating coils to maintain a constant temperature of 37°C.

Microscope

Besides the phase contrast microscope for sperm analysis and a stereozoom microscope for egg and embryo handling, a high quality inverted microscope equipped with differential interface contrast (DIC) or Hoffman modulation contrast optics is highly desirable for micromanipulation procedures. Attachment to CCTV camera provides simultaneous visualization of procedures for training, assessment and record.

Additionally, laser system, spindle viewing and attachment for morphologically selected sperm before ICSI can also be added. Spares for breakdown like fuse and lamps should be readily made available in the laboratory.

Cryostorage

Use of eye and face protection, and of cryogloves when cryogenic materials are handled is recommended. While designing the place for nitrogen containers in cases of power failure or other emergency their easy exit should be planned. Liquid nitrogen low level alarms and remote notification capabilities are useful add ons. Liquid nitrogen container should be placed just adjacent to the laboratory in a room with outside access so at the time of their change or usage laboratory environment is least disturbed. Proper patient identification and location of stored semen and embryos should be documented and annually audited.

MINIMAL QUALITY CONTROL PARAMETERS

A quality assurance system that incorporates the principle that "an ounce of prevention is better than a pound of attempted cure" can eliminate or reduce hours, days or even weeks of frustration associated with failure. In an IVF set-up, with multifaceted procedures a systematic approach to quality control relies on careful and logical organization, accurate record maintenance, regular analysis and communication, routine testing, verification of regular data analysis and common sense. Although many genetic, environmental and intrinsic factors influence the outcome of IVF procedures, basic laboratory sanitation and QC measures are relatively simple but often overlooked factors that have a real impact on success. The QC parameters includes, maintaining and calibrating equipment on a periodical basis (daily/weekly/monthly/yearly). The following indicators for clinical and laboratory performance should be regularly reviewed, analyzed and discussed:

I

Parameters	*In relation to/ compared to*	*Acceptable range*
No. of follicles	No. of eggs collected	>90%
No. of eggs	Mature eggs	Around 90%
Mature eggs (inseminated/ injected)	Normal fertilization	60–80%
	Abnormal fertilization	10–15%
	Degeneration	10–15%
Normal fertilization	Cleavage rate	90%
Cleaved	Usable	80%
No. of embryos transferred	ET days—(2 or 3)	Max. 3
Fresh embryo transfer cycle	Cumulative pregnancy	30%
Frozen embryo transfer cycle	Cumulative pregnancy	20%
ART cycles	Freezable cycles	50%
Embryos thawed	Survival rate	75%
Semen thawed	Survival rate	50%

Following parameters should also be considered as important and should fall in the acceptable range.[4]

II

Parameters	*Vs*	*Acceptable range*[4]
Stimulation cycles	OHSS	0.2–8%
Total pregnancy	Multiple gestation	20–30%
Total pregnancy	Spontaneous abortion	20–35%
Total pregnancy	Ectopic pregnancy	Up to 8%

[as per National Guidelines for Accredition, Supervision and Regulation of ART Clinics in India, ICMR, National Academy of Medical Sciences (India), 2005]

Growth potential of the unutilized embryos is good indicator of laboratory culture conditions. All batches of media should be subjected to sperm survival test before routine use.

The basic science underlying these factors should be well understood. These are hydrogen ion concentration, osmolality, humidity and temperature.

Hydrogen Ion Concentration (pH)

Human oocytes have been reported to be able to grow in media with a pH as low as 7.2 and as high as 7.6, however a pH of 7.4 yield the optimum growth rates.

Osmolality

Like pH, osmolality can vary over a range from 280 to 300 mOsmol/kg for successful human IVF.

Temperature

Most IVF procedures for eutherian mammals are performed at 37°C. Early embryos are often adversely affected by elevated temperatures but seldom harmed by temperatures that are slightly lower. Layering with mineral oil equilibrated with culture media serves as cushion for eliminating abrupt changes in pH, smolality and temperature.

Light

Deleterious effects of long-term exposure to light radiation (wavelength and duration of exposure) on the developmental stage have been noticed. Filters are used on microscope light source to reduce effects of spectrum below 500 mm. Fluorescent light source which emits ultraviolet waves can be replaced by yellow light (560 to 580 nm). Efficiency in performing procedures is highly desirable to counter these effects.

MISCELLANEOUS

Identification

At each stage, patient identification on each and ever disposable material should be clearly done. At the time of insemination and embryo transfer sperm and embryos respectively should be identified by two persons before use.

Record Keeping

Perfect record of each patient: (1) clinical file—with informed consents from both the partners for all the procedures performed for them (2) Embryology sheet showing each oocyte till the time of their use. Daily quality control records are to be maintained. Entries should be made when a new batch of media or supplies are introduced. Where computerized records are routinely used a backup hard copy should be retained. List of daily activities and due dates of LN_2 refilling, cleaning of incubators, calibration of instrument, etc. should be displayed.

During the journey from gametes to the preimplantation embryo formation several factors play a critical and decisive role. Following precautionary measures should be practiced:

a. Use of nontoxic (nonpowdered) gloves, head cover and masks where appropriate.
b. Aseptic handling of culture media.
c. Use of mechanical pipetting devices.
d. Food, drinks, cigarettes and cigars are strictly forbidden.
e. The use of make-up and strong perfumes should be limited.
f. Each and every surface of the whole laboratory is periodically to be cleaned first with mild surface disinfectant, sterile water and final wiped with 70 percent alcohol, whereas the immediate working area for routine work should be wiped with 70 percent alcohol at the end of each day.

Data Analysis

Data form the laboratory should be regularly analyzed to determine that minimum satisfactory standards are achieved in the following parameters:

- Satisfactory percentage of mature oocytes are collected in the pick-up
- Oocyte survival rates following microinjection of sperm
- Fertilization and cleavage rates
- Embryo growth and their quality
- Proportion of surplus embryos cryopreserved
- Post-thaw survival of frozen embryos
- Pregnancy/implantation rates for each procedure.

The term "satisfactory" can be defined as the results compared with the national standards and published literature.

The success in ART procedures and its reproducibility depend highly on integrated, high efficiency laboratory activities which consistently provide acceptable results. Close coordination and frequent interaction between the team members to discuss the best possible strategy for each patient's protocol help achieve this goal.

Corrective actions to be taken to restore the expected efficiency level after some disruption or lean phase in results. This may involve trouble-shooting to correct malfunctioning of equipment, re-evaluating protocols or even retraining personnel.

REFERENCES

1. Practice committee, revised minimum standards, Fertility sterility, 2008;90:S165-8.
2. Classification of airborne particulates, ISO14644-1. Clean rooms and associated controlled environments Part 1: Revised 1999.
3. Clean rooms and associated controlled environments ISO14644-2, Part 2: Testing and monitoring to prove continued compliance with ISO14644-1; Revised, 1999.
4. National Guidlines for Accredition, Supervision and Regulation of ART Clinics in India, ICMR, National Academy of Medical Sciences (India), 2005.

Chapter

7

Counseling of the Infertile Couples

Kamini A Rao

The psychological and sociological implications of infertility on infertile couples are well recognized. Every step they take in the pathway to achieve their dream of having a baby can add to their emotional turmoil and financial and physical strains. The problem of infertility becomes a problem within the relationship of the partners.

Stress, as such, is unlikely to result in infertility but individual coping mechanism, the extent of support, level of optimism and resilience are important confounding factors. Infertility, its investigations and treatment can cause significant stress. Added to this is social and family pressure. Couples are continually reminded of their inability and sense of failure every month when the woman menstruates.

There are individual reactions to infertility such as depression and anxiety (psychological aspects) and there are social implications such as the stigma and taboo associated with infertility (social aspects).

Gender specific reactions to infertility and assisted reproductive technology (ART)—men and women react differently and manage this crisis in different ways. Women tend to show their emotional reactions more visibly than men and they perceive the inability to conceive as the most upsetting life event. Also, their social life alters as female friends become mothers and infertile women tend to lose contact with such friends or isolate themselves.

Men, generally, are more reserved about displaying emotions and are less affected by treatment, both physically and emotionally. However, they indicate high levels of stress when male factor infertility is diagnosed.

Regarding management strategies, men tend to benefit from information and often prefer a pragmatic and aim oriented approach whereas women find it helpful to share their emotional reactions.

Women may also experience an identity crisis as there is a conflict between their ideal sense of self as a woman who can become a mother and their real self as being infertile. The manifold diagnostic and treatment procedures require couples to adapt their identity not just once, but several times and in stages.

FUNDAMENTAL ISSUES IN COUNSELING

Counseling can be formally defined as an interpersonal process, based on a theoretical framework which is used to bring about change in a skilled and systematic way.

During the last two decades, great advances have been made in the field of ART. Treatments such as

IVF and ICSI have given new hope to many infertile patients. In addition to necessary medical, and surgical procedures, one should also focus on the patients psychosocial and emotional needs by:

- Understanding childlessness
- Giving information about the relevant medical aspects.
- Implications counselling
- Support counseling and/or
- Therapeutic counseling.

Caring for the emotional needs of the patient demands continuity and is not a single event.

Implications Counseling

This is meant to enable the couples to understand the implications of the proposed treatment for themselves, their family and for the children born as a result. This may be of particular relevance for couples seeking treatment with donor eggs, donor sperm, donor embryos or surrogacy.

Genetic counseling should be offered when there is an increased risk of passing on an inherited disease to the offspring.

Psychological counseling should be offered for partners suffering from psychosexual problems such as impotence and vaginismus.

Support Counseling

This is intended to give emotional support and information from the start of the treatment. The family doctor, infertility specialist and support group may help the couples.

Support groups consist of couples who are going through or have experienced infertility and its treatment; their support and guidance can often prove invaluable. Group sessions can be a liberating and empowering experience. At these meetings, patients are encouraged to speak up about their situation, feelings of isolation being to disappear when couples having similar problems come in contact with each other.

Therapeutic Counseling

This focuses on:

- Individual problems and (family) history
- The acceptance of the situation
- The meaning and impact of infertility
- Work on alternative life and self concepts for the future
- The development of coping strategies and strategies to minimize distress
- Problem and conflict solving, and/or
- Specific issues such as sexual, marital and other interpersonal problems.

The basic aim of counseling is to ensure that the patient understands the implications of their treatment choice, the patient receives adequate information and emotions support, and that they can cope in a healthy way with the consequences of treatment. Counseling can contribute significantly to improving the psychological and social health, and minimize drop out rates.

Mandatory counseling ensures that all patients have access to a professional service with the opportunity to discuss their own personal circumstances and issues. However, the fact that the service is mandatory may mean that patients are unwilling to discuss any issue openly and/or that they feel suspicious about the true purpose of the session (i.e. support or screening?).

Voluntary counseling may also give rise to worries concerning screening but since the patient is the one to initiate counseling, there is usually a greater willingness to overcome these fears. However, it must be ensured that information concerning counseling is easily and clearly available.

Counseling is of particular importance at time of stress such as frustration of the desire for a child, or social and family pressure, or the treatment received with its limited success rate. Anxiety is tremendous whilst waiting the results of treatment couples are often torn between hope and fear of failure.

THE COUNSELOR

He can be a part of the medical team treating the couple or be independent. A counselor should be aware of the particular needs of the couple. Counseling must be informed and effective. For patients undergoing infertility treatment, counseling should be available at any time — before, during and after treatment. Counselors should have up-to-date knowledge of infertility and ART. Couples must recognize that infertility treatment may not produce immediate results and with patience, a positive attitude and appropriate treatment, most couples can eventually become parents.

THE BENEFICIARIES

Though counseling is beneficial in most infertile couples undertaking treatment, there are certain special groups of patient who are particularly eligible for this:

- Patients who receive donor eggs, sperms or embryos
- Patients who use surrogacy or adoption
- Patients who experience great distress such as depression
- Patients considered to be at risk such as those with history of psychiatric illness and substance abuse
- Patients with marital disharmony
- Patients who require genetic counseling.

Individuals may also seek counseling to help make decisions regarding the continuation or termination of treatment. Counseling may be used to discuss alternatives to parenthood such as adoption or fostering and/or it may be used to identify ways of living a meaningful and fulfilling life without children.

SPECIAL ISSUE

Pregnancy after infertility treatment couples are anxious about the risk of miscarriage, multiple pregnancy and fetal reduction, fetal abnormality and also the fear of being separated from the baby after it is born. The patient who used donor sperm or embryo also experiences a lot of worries and anxiety about the baby father, there anxiety about the physical characteristics of the baby. Counseling can, with time, help people to adjust and accept the situation and move forward in life with a positive outlook.

Hence, for the infertile couples undertaking treatment, it is recommended to have:

- An ongoing relationship with a qualified counsellor
- The best estimates for pregnancy rates for all forms of treatment available at any point in time
- The option of stopping treatment at any point of time
- Encouragement to seek second opinions throughout treatment
- Time off from treatment
- The opportunity to set arbitrary but relatively firm time limits to stop treatment.

BIBLIOGRAPHY

1. ESHRE. Psychology and Counselling. Hum Reprod on 14, 1384-91.
2. Hammer Burns L, Covington S. Psychology of infertility. In Covington SN, Burns LH (Eds): Infertility counselling. A comprehensive handbook for clinicians New York: Cambridge University Press 2006;pp 1-19.
3. Petra Thorn. Understanding Infertility: Psychological and Social Considerations from a counselling perspective. Intl J Fertil Steril 2009;3:48-51.
4. Verhaak CM, Smeenk JM, van Minnen A, Kremer JA. Longitudinal, prospective study on emotional adjustment before, during and after consecutive fertility treatment cycle. Hum Reprod 2005;20:2253-60.
5. Wright J, Duchesne C, Sabourin S, Bissonnette F, Benoit J, Girard Y. Psychosocial distress and infertility: men and women respond differently. Fertil Steril 1991;55:100-8.

Chapter

8

Transvaginal Sonography in Infertility

Narendra Malhotra, Jaideep Malhotra, Neharika Malhotra, JP Rao, Sakshi Tomar

Transvaginal sonography (TVS) (Figs 8.1 and 8.2) has an important role in the management of infertility. Serial pelvic ultrasound examinations are useful in monitoring patients undergoing ovulation induction using ovulation-inducing drugs. In addition, the correct prediction of timing of ovulation is critical for infertility, therapies such as intrauterine insemination, artificial or therapeutic insemination using donor sperm and the timing of intercourse during ovulation induction therapies.[1]

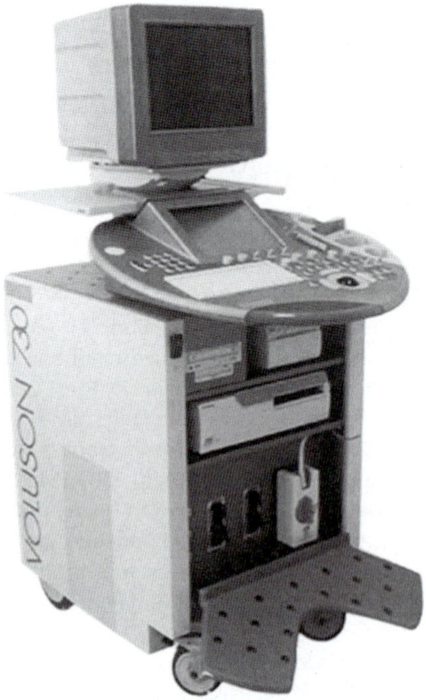

Fig. 8.1: USG machine and probes

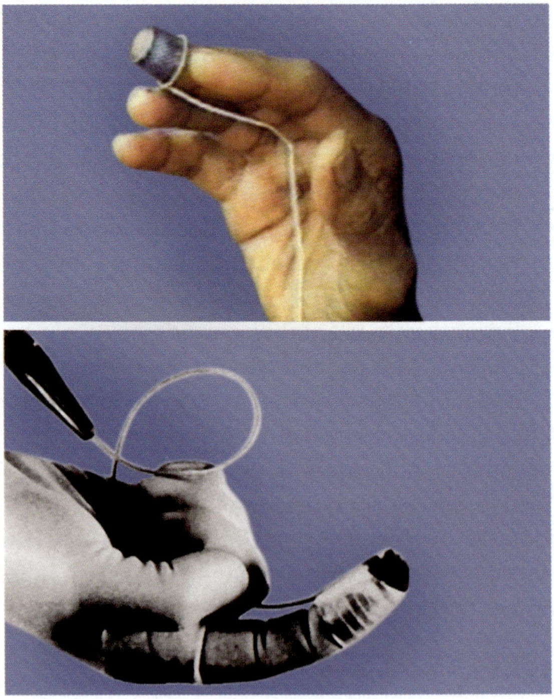

Fig. 8.2: Fingertip probe

CERVIX

Cervix is evaluated for echotexture cervicitis, nabothian cysts, cervical mucus. It is best seen in the AP view with the probe just away. TVS gives a good idea of the cervical factors of infertility (Figs 8.3 to 8.6).

UTERUS

Transvaginal ultrasound examination of the body of the uterus is done to observe detailed view of the myometrium and any anomalies (Figs 8.7 to 8.9).

Endometrium

The endometrial cavity should be visualizable as a separate entity within the uterus in virtually all menstruating patients. It is generally centrally located in the uterus. The cyclic histologic changes and changes in the thickening of the endometrium with hormonal stimulation can be imaged using transvaginal ultrasound during the different phases of the menstrual cycle (Figs 8.10 to 8.12).[1,2]

Sakamoto described the characteristic sonographic image noted during the menstrual cycle in 1985. The proliferative endometrium is characterized by:

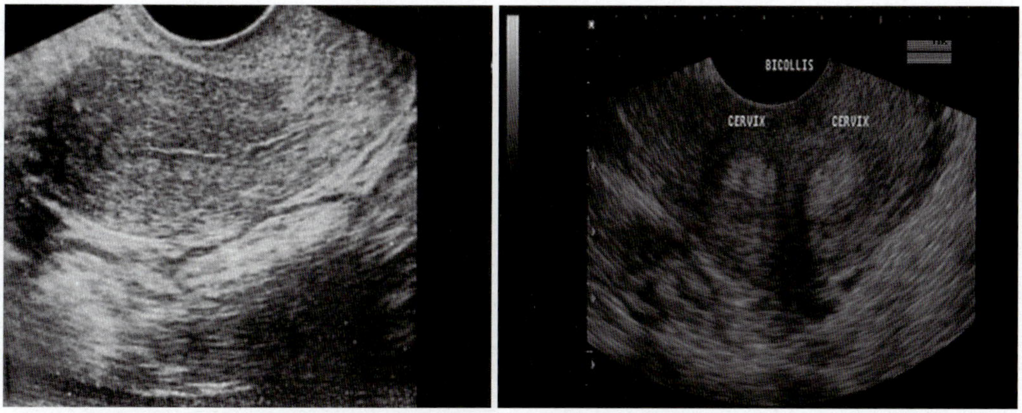

Figs 8.3 and 8.4: Two cervices

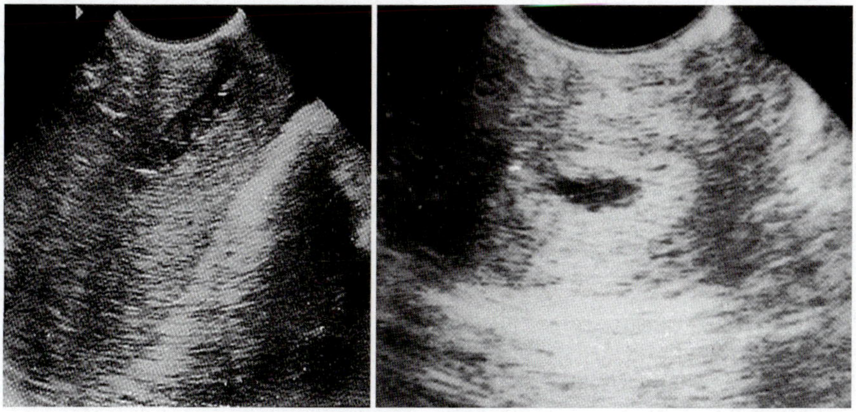

Fig. 8.5: Cervical mucus

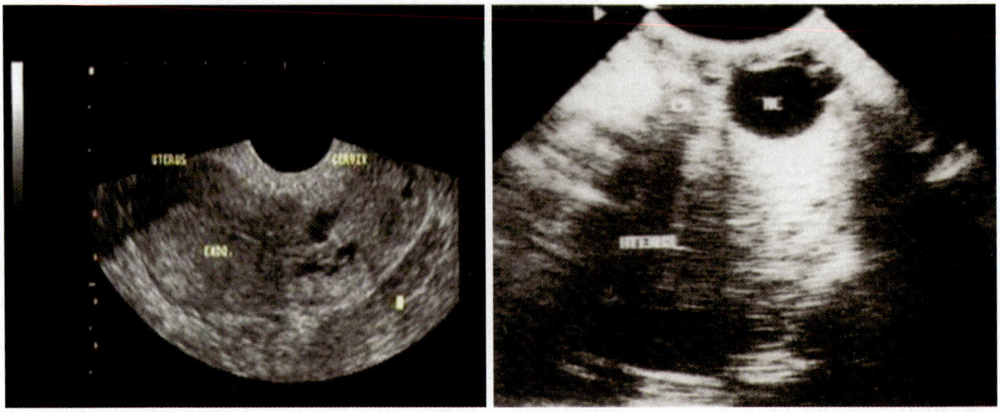

Fig. 8.6: Nabothion cysts

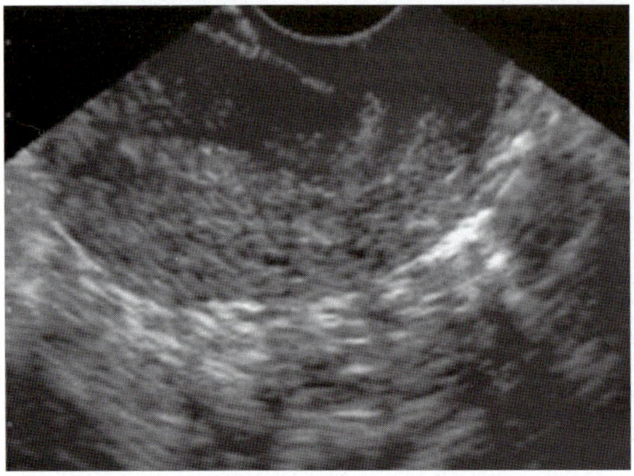

Fig. 8.7: Normal uterus

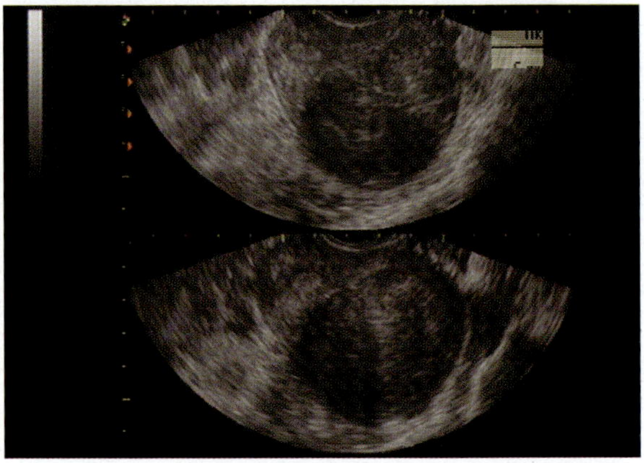

Fig. 8.9: Fibroid causing contour problem

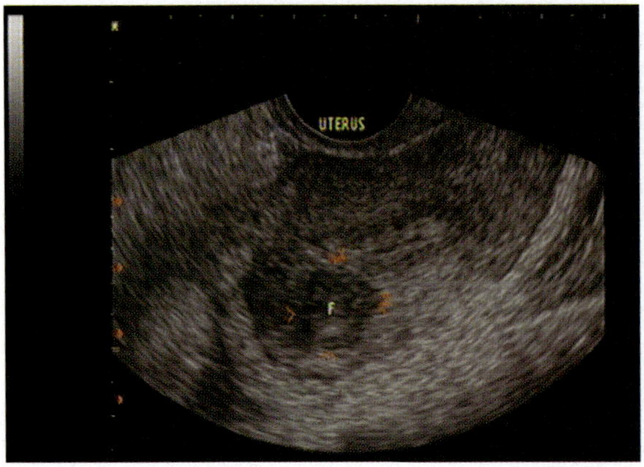

Fig. 8.8: Fibroid uterus

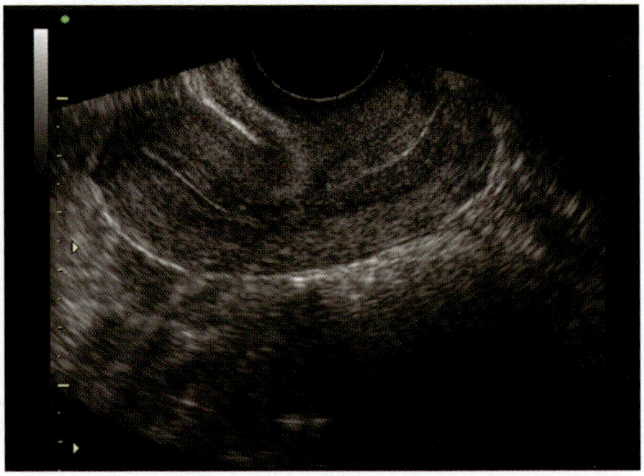

Fig. 8.10: Day 10 endometrium

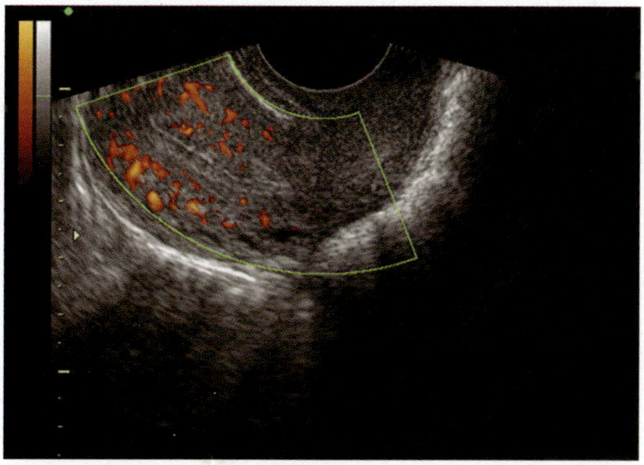

Fig. 8.11: Periovulatory endometrium

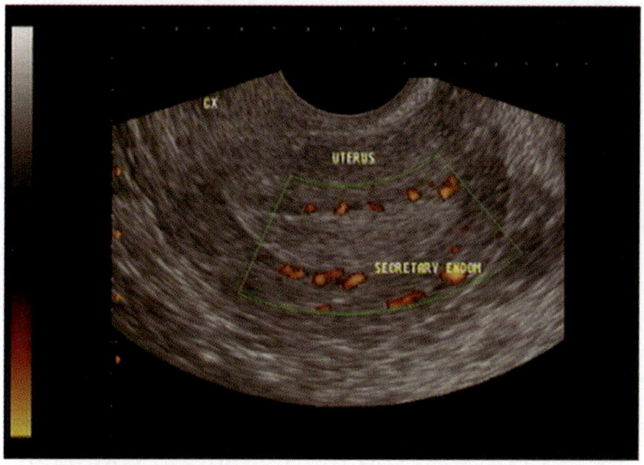

Fig. 8.12: Secretory phase endometrium

- The presence of a well-defined three line sign
- A hypoechogenic functional layer
- A minimal or absent posterior acoustic enhancement.

The three-line sign is formed by the central hyperechoic reflection representing the endometrial cavity and the additional hyperechoic reflection representing the thin developing layer of endometrium. There is also a surrounding hypoechoic halo.

Luteal phase endometrium is: (1) Hyperechoic; (2) Posterior enhancement is present; (3) Three line sign and halo are absent.

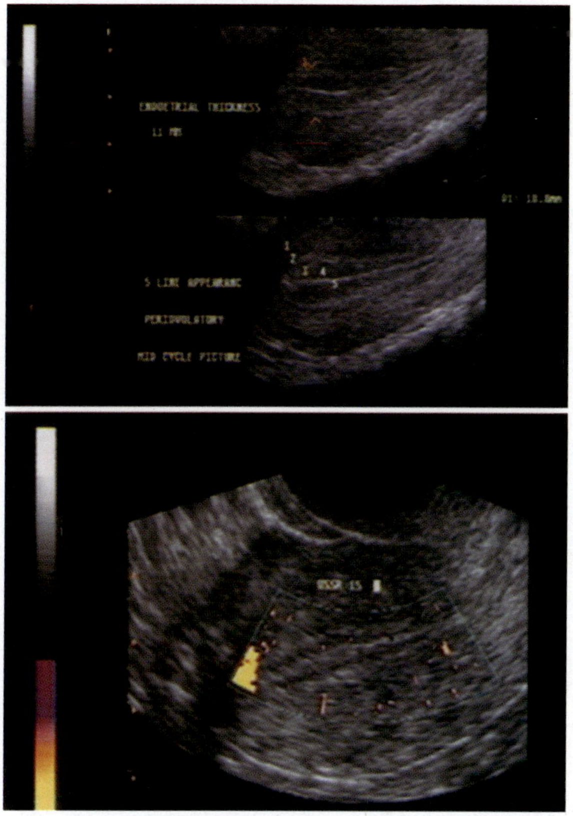

Fig. 8.13: Uterine zones

Uterine Biophysical Profile[3]

During the normal mid-cycle certain sonographic qualities of the uterus are noted:

- Endometrial thickness in greatest AP dimension of 7 mm or greater (full thickness measurement)
- A layered (5 line) appearance to the endometrium (Fig. 8.13)
- Blood flow within zone 3 using color Doppler technique (Fig. 8.14)
- Myometrial contractions causing a wave like motion of the endometrium
- Uterine artery blood flow as measured by PI, less than 3.0
- Homogeneous myometrial echogenicity

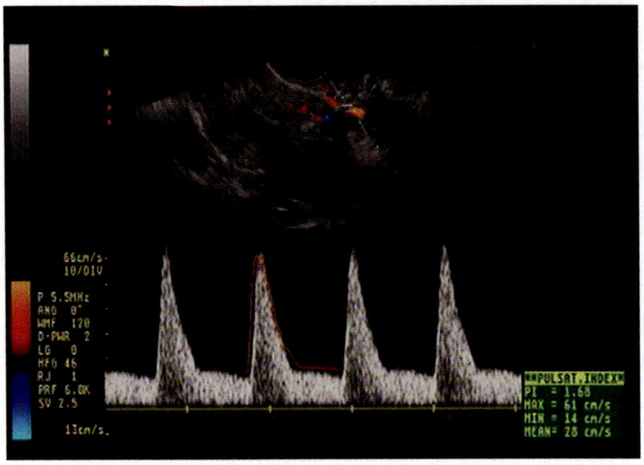

Fig. 8.14: Uterine A

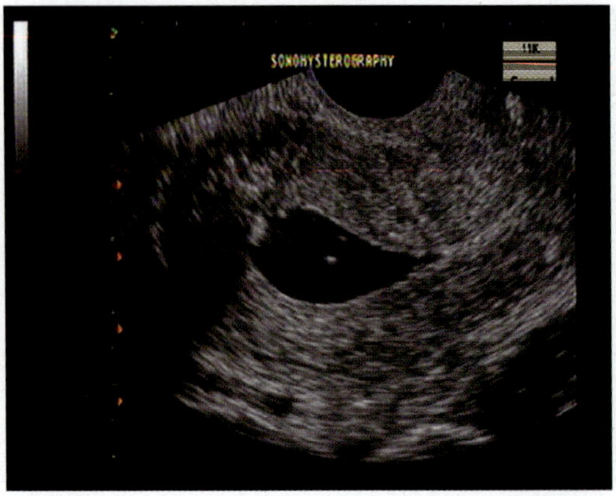

Fig. 8.15: Sonohysterography: Uterine cavity

- Myometrial blood flow seen on gray scale examination (internal to the arcuate vessels).

Uterine Cavity Evaluation

Transvaginal ultrasound with sonohysterography can very accurately delineate the cavity and pick up irregular endometrium, polyps, Asherman syndrome, submucous fibroids, double cavity, septum, unicornuate and T- shaped uterus.

Sonohysterography or contrast sonohysterography (Hyscosy) is done by introducing a No. 8 Foley's catheter or an infant feeding tube into the uterine cavity and injecting a sterile fluid media under ultrasound visualization (Normal saline, hydrotubation fluid or commercially available echocontrast media - ECHOVIST). This offers a very accurate noninvasive method to evaluate cavity and should be routinely done after SSG and also in all infertile cases (Fig. 8.15).

3D ultrasound and 3D reconstruction with echo contrast media is also a very accurate and good method for uterine cavity evaluation.

TUBES

Fallopian tubes are isoechoic and cannot be normally seen on ultrasound unless pathological or fluid surrounds the tubes.

Sonosalpingography also known as 'SION TEST'[6] uses transvaginal sonography to confirm the tubal patency by visualizing the spill of fluid from the fimbrial end of fallopian tubes. This test is not a substitute for hysterosalpingography or laparoscopy but is a noninvasive, cheap outdoor screening procedure in infertility patients.

Method—No. 8 Foley's calheter is put inside the uterus. The bulb is inflated with 2 ml of distilled water. Prior to procedure, the patient is asked to evacuate the bladder and base line vaginal scan is performed. 20 to 60 ml of solution containing diploes, hylase and dexamethasone is taken in 50 ml catheter tip syringe and pushed via Foley's catheter; spill is studied by TVS from the fimbrial end (Fig. 8.16).[7]

OVARY

TVS can accurately inform about follicular development, prediction of ovulation and confirmation of ovulation (Fig. 8.17).

- *Follicular development:* Developing follicles destined to ovulate increase in size 2 to 3 mm/day and reach a maximum diameter of 16 to 33 mm before ovulation. Selection of the dominant follicle is thought to occur by cycle days 5 to 7 but is not apparent sonographically

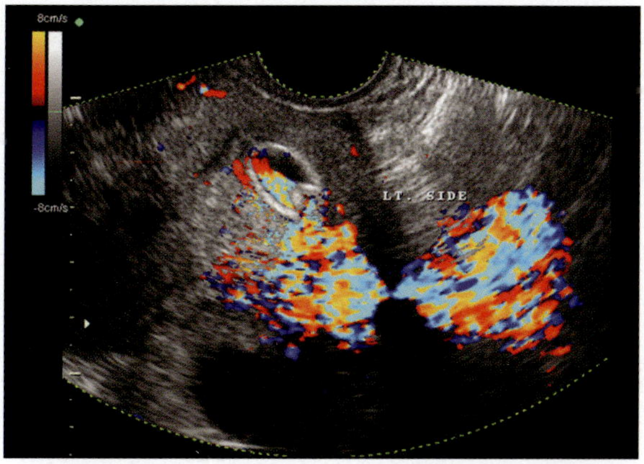

Fig. 8.16: Patent tubes by color flow imaging sonosalpingography

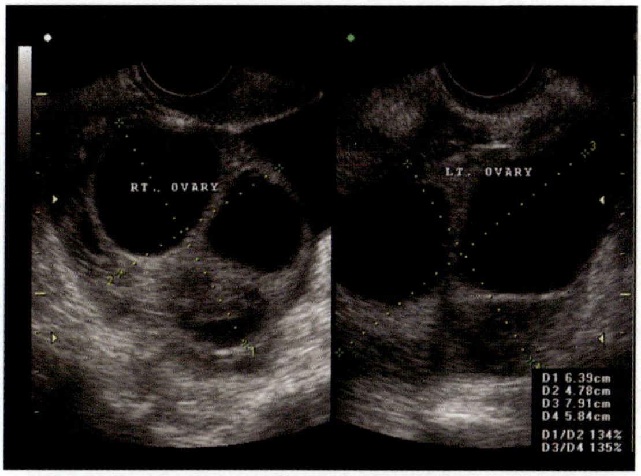

Fig. 8.18: Dominant follicle

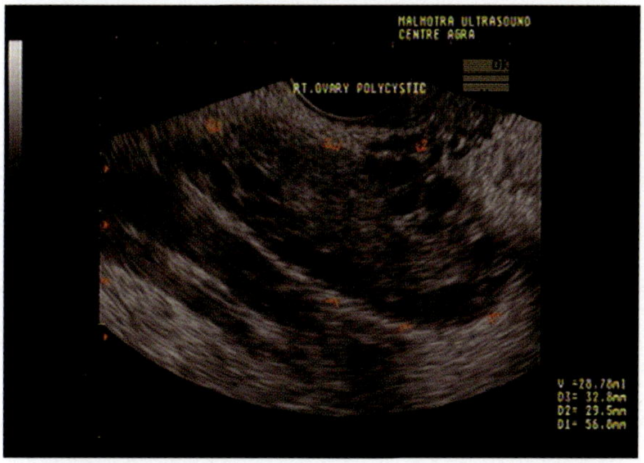

Fig. 8.17: Normal ovary in front of iliac vessels

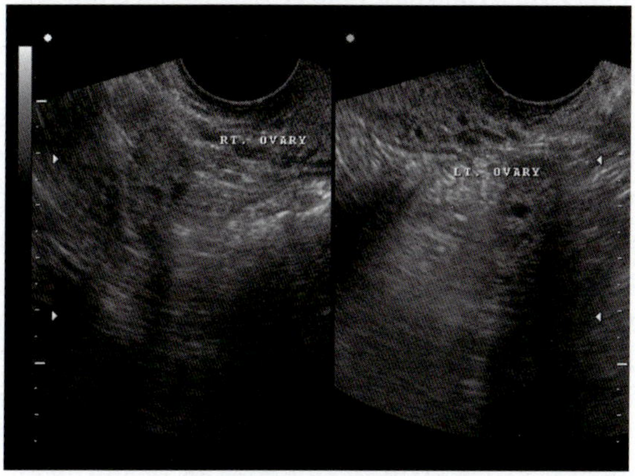

Fig. 8.19: Preantral follicles

until cycle days 8 to 12. Other antral follicles of the developing cohort will generally undergo atresia and will not exceed 14 mm in diameter.

- *Prediction of ovulation:* Potential signs of impending ovulation are:
  - Presence of a dominant follicle (usually >16-18 mm) (Fig. 8.18)
  - Anechoic area, double contour, around the follicle (possible ovulation within 24 hours)
  - Separation and folding of the follicle lining (ovulation within 6 to 10 hours)
  - Thickened proliferative endometrium.
- *Confirmation of ovulation:*
  - Disappearance of the follicle (91% cases)
  - Decrease in follicle size (9% cases)
  - Fluid in culde-sac when not present in a previous scan
  - Development of intrafollicular echoes suggesting the formation of a hemorrhagic corpus luteum.

Ovary in anovulatory cycles: Following may be seen (Fig. 8.19):

- Lack of any follicular development particularly in the hypogonadotropic hypogonadal patient
- Few nonovulatory (less than 11 mm) follicles,
- A cyst
- PCOD—characterized by (Fig. 8.20)
  - Enlarged ovary (>8 cms)

- Multiple small cysts (0.2–0.6)
- Anovulation (lack of follicular development)
- Resting or follicular endometrium.

Today with modern technology it is possible to occurately measure follicles by SONOVAC (Fig. 8.21).

FOLLICULAR MONITORING

Monitoring of follicular growth by ultrasound is now an established practice in most fertility centers. The ability to visualize and monitor follicular growth was first postulated by Kratochavil et al (1972). Hackelor et al (1979)[4] reported a good correlation between follicular diameter and plasma estradiol levels in women in spontaneous menstrual cycles. The follicular diameters must be measured in the transverse and longitudinal planes to get the average diameter. Follicles may be seen in the ovaries as early as day 2 or 3 of the menstrual cycle, measuring 3 to 4 mm in size. The rate of follicular growth is between 1 and 2 mm per day (Hackeloer and Robinson 1978). Thus by day 12, the dominant follicle is around 12 to 16 mm in sizes. Follicular rupture in normal cycle occurs when the mean follicular diameter is between 18 and 28 mm (Hackeloer 1979). In clomiphene stimulated cycles follicular rupture occurs between 18 and 24 mm (O' Herlihy 1980), whereas in HMG stimulated cycle it occurs between 15 and 20 mm (Ylostalo 1979). For timing of accurate ovulation, serial scanning is needed. Follicular collapse, disappearance of follicle and enlargement of follicle with appearance of internal echoes—indicate ovulation.

Oocyte Retrieval

After performing a preliminary scan to assess the number of follicles, position of both the ovaries, intervening bowel loops, adhesion, chocolate cysts, etc. follicles in the ovary are tapped by a sterile disposable ovum pick up needle with attached silicon tubing and suction apparatus (set at 150 mm Hg). At the end of one side, the needle is withdrawn and flushed with culture medium before proceeding to the ovary on the opposite side (Fig. 8.22).

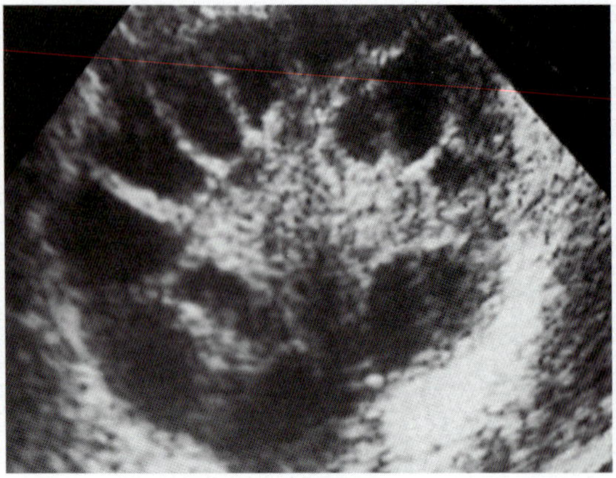

Fig. 8.20: Polycystic ovary

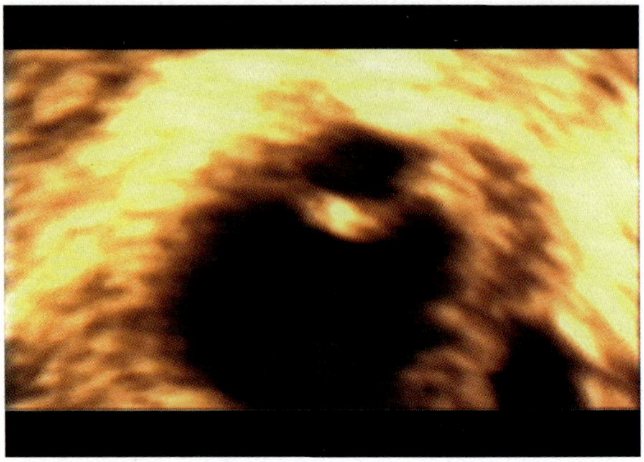

Fig. 8.21: Dominant follicle showing cumulus

ROLE OF COLOR DOPPLER IN INFERTILITY

The advent of transvaginal color Doppler sonology has added a new dimension to the diagnosis and treatment of infertile female. Color Doppler innovation is a unique noninvasive technology to investigate the circulation of organs like uterus and ovaries. Dynamic changes occur almost every day of the menstrual cycle in a reproductively active female.

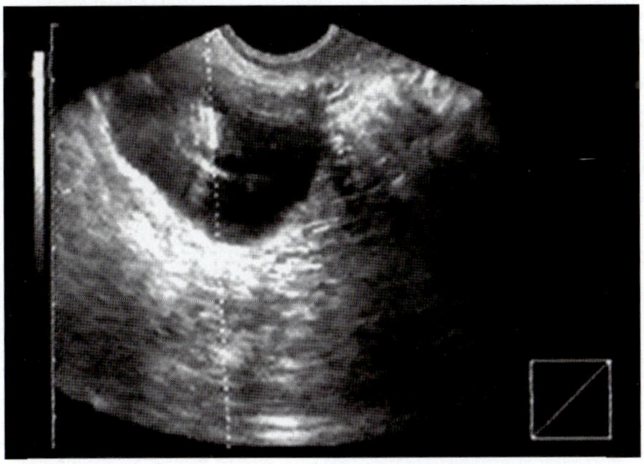

Fig. 8.22: Ovum pick-up

These events are picked-up very well by transvaginal color Doppler and definite conclusions can be drawn regarding the diagnosis, prognosis and treatment of infertile patients. As the, vaginal probe lies close to the organs of interest, various vessels supplying these structures can be studied in detail like the uterine artery, ovarian artery and their branches.

STUDY OF MENSTRUAL CYCLE BY COLOR DOPPLER

It is very important to study the whole of the menstrual cycle by transvaginal color Doppler during the evaluation of infertility. It provides vital information about follicular dynamics like blood flow to the growing follicle, the vascular supply of the endometrium and corpus luteum vascularization which are very important for a successful outcome in terms of pregnancy.

Changes in the Ovary

The ovaries are situated on either side of the uterus and measure about 2.2 to 5.5 cm in length, 1.5 to 2.0 cm in width and 1.5 to 3.0 cm in depth and are recognized by the presence of follicle of different sizes. The blood supply is by ovarian artery via the infundibulopelvic ligament and ovarian branch of the uterine artery. There is anastmosis between the two sources of blood supply. The primary and secondary branches of the ovarian artery grow along with the development of the follicle. Dominant follicle within the ovary can be recognized by transvaginal color Doppler by day 8th or 10th of the cycle by a ring of angiogenesis around it, when compared to the subordinate follicles which do not demonstrate this. These vessels become more abundant and prominent as the follicle grows to about 20 to 24 mm in size.

The phases are described as early follicular (Day 5–7), late follicular (Day 11–13), early luteal (Day 15–17) and late luteal (Day 26–28). In general, the index values are high in the early part of menstrual cycle and fall as ovulation approaches. According to Kurjak et al the RI in the early proliferative phase is 0.54 ± 0.04 and declines the day before ovulation (LH peak) when it is about 0.44±0.04.

This is the best time for administration of surrogate hCG. The increase in peak systolic velocity with a relatively constant is a particularly interesting finding that might herald impending ovulation. It is hoped that information on ovarian perfusion may be used to predict ovulation and to investigate ovulatory dysfunction. The lowest RI values were obtained during the mid-luteal phase (RI 0.42±0.06) with a return to higher vascular resistance (0.50±0.04) during the late luteal phase (Fig. 8.23).

The dominant ovary corpus luteum show a low impedance waveform with a RI of 0.39–0.49, characteristic of blood flow in early pregnancy. The contralateral ovary shows a high impedance flow with a RI of 0.69–1.00 characteristic of nondominant ovary (Kurjak et al). If the ovary having corpus luteum shows high RI (>0.50) it is associated with nonviable outcome.[8]

Uterine Perfusion

The uterine artery give rise to the arcuate arteries which are oriented circumferentially in the outer third of the myometrium. These vessels give rise to the radial arteries, which after crossing the myometrium-

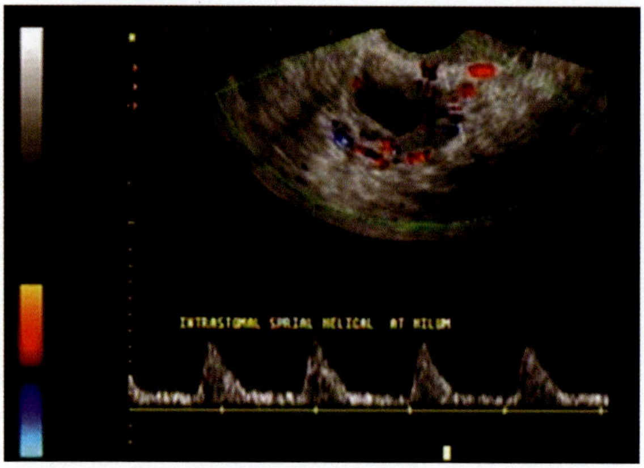

Fig. 8.23: Resistance index (RI) of Ovarian a

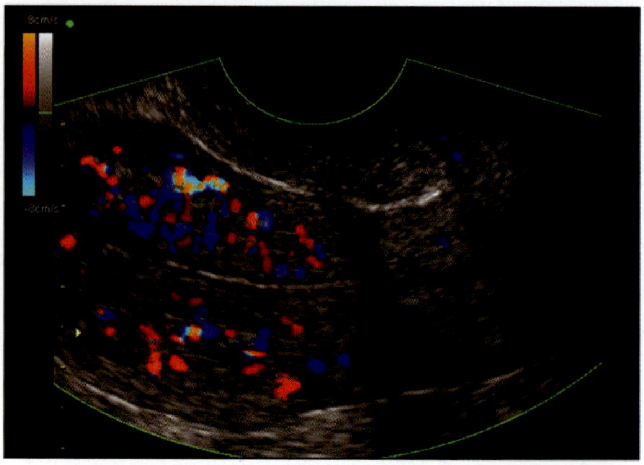

Fig. 8.24: Vascularity of endometrium

endometrium border, further branch and give rise to the basal arteries and the spiral arteries.

The RI in the uterine artery hovers around 0.88 ± 0.04 until day 13 of the 28 day menstrual cycle. Increased uterine artery impedance is seen 3 days after the LH peak (Day 16). This is explained by increased contractility and compression of vessels traversing the uterine wall, which decrease their diameter and consequently cause higher resistance to flow. Lowest blood flow impedance occurs during peak luteal phase (RI = 0.84±0.04) during which implantation is likely to occur. RI of radial vessels is 0.78±0.10.

Blood flow velocity wave form changes in the spiral arteries during normal ovulatory cycles are characteristics of by lower velocity and lower impedance to blood flow than are those observed in the uterine arteries with larger diameter. It seems that features of endometrial blood flow may be used to predict the implantation success rate and to reveal unexplained infertility problems more precisely than evaluation of the main uterine artery alone (Fig. 8.24).[5]

Changes in the Endometrium

Michael Applebaum in his study with transvaginal color Doppler divided the endometrium and periendometrial areas into four zones. In the study conducted by him, no pregnancy was reported in IVF patients unless vascularity was demonstrated in Zone III or with in Zone III or IV prior to transfer.

- Zone I : 2 mm thick area surrounding the hyperechoic outer layer of the endometrium
- Zone II : The hyperechoic outer layer of the endometrium
- Zone III : The hypoechoic inner layer of the endometrium
- Zone IV : The endometrial cavity.

ULTRASOUND TECHNIQUE FOR UTERINE BIOPHYSICAL PROFILE

To perform the uterine biophysical profile (UBP) special care should be taken. The following guidelines are recommended (Apple baum 96):

- To determine the presence of a 5-line appearance, information from both the transabdominal and transvaginal studies may be useful. For example, although a 5-line appearance may be noted transabdominally, it may not always be possible to see it endovaginally due to uterine position (and vice versa). In this case, a 5-line appearance is considered to be present and endometrial vascular penetration may be estimated when performing the endovaginal study.

- Perform the Doppler study slowly: The flow of blood in the endometrium is of low velocity, it may take time for the ultrasound machine to register the presence of blood flow and create the image. If one sweeps through the endometrium too quickly, flow may not be seen. Additionally endometrial blood flow has a mercurial personality—it may appear as if it comes and goes. It may also appear in some areas and not others. Do not observe hastily.
- Endeavor to make the endometrium as specular a reflector as possible. Use the techniques of manual manipulation of the anatomy and probe pressure to achieve this.
- Scan endovaginally both coronally and sagittally. There may be a difference in how well the blood flow is imaged.
- When measuring the endometrium in the A-P dimension, try to obtain the value when no contraction affecting it is present. Contractions may affect this value. Also when possible, obtain the measurement in a standard plan such as when both the endometrial and cervical canals continuous.

Uterine Biophysical Profile[3]

In our experience, certain sonographic qualities of the uterus are noted during the normal midcycle. These include:

- Endometrial thickness in greatest AP dimension of 7 mm or greater (full-thickness measurement)
- A layered (5-line) appearance to the endometrium
- Blood flow within zone III using color Doppler technique
- Myometrial contractions causing a wave like motion of the endometrium
- Uterine artery blood flow, as measured by PI, less than 3.0
- Homogeneous myometrial echogenicity
- Myometrial blood flow seen on gray-scale examination (internal to the arcuate vessels).

The uterine scoring system for reproduction (USSR) comprises evaluation of the following parameters:

- Endometrial thickness (full-thickness measured from the myometrial-endometrial junction to the endometrial-myometrial junction)
- Endometrial layering (i.e. a 5-line appearance)
- Myometrial contractions seen as endometrial motion
- Myometrial echogenicity
- Uterine artery Doppler flow evaluation
- Endometrial blood flow
- Gray-scale myometrial blood flow.

Each parameter is scored as follows:

- Endometrial thickness
  - < 7 mm = 0
  - 7–9 mm = 2
  - 10–14 mm = 3
  - >14 mm = 1
- Endometrial layering
  - No layering = 0
  - Hazy 5-line appearance = 1
  - Distinct 5-line appearance = 3
- Myometrial contractions (seen as wave-like endometrial motion high-speed playback from videotape)
  - < 3 Contractions in 2 minutes (real-time) = 0
  - ≥ 3 Contractions in 2 minutes (real-time) = 3
- Myometrial echogenicity
  - Coarse/inhomogeneous echogenicity = 1
  - Relatively homogeneous echogenicity = 2
- Uterine artery Doppler flow
  - PI—2.99–3.0 = 0
  - PI—2.49 = 1
  - PI < 2 = 2
- Endometrial blood flow within Zone 3
  - Absent = 0
  - Present, but sparse = 2
  - Present multifocally = 5

- Myometrial blood flow internal to the arcuate vessels seen on gray-scale examination
  - Absent = 0
  - Present = 2.

The values assume a technically adequate ultrasound examination with no abnormalities of uterine shape or development, no other gross uterine abnormalities (e.g. significant masses) and a normal ovarian cycle (e.g. without evidence of ovarian-uterine dyscoordination). A male factor component to the infertility is not present.

In our limited experience (Applebaum) with this system thus far, a USSR "perfect score" of 20 has been associated with conception 100% of the time. (The number of patients in which we predicted successful conception cycles based upon the UBP and USSR perfect score was 5. The group included 2 spontaneous cycles (non-IVF, non-IUI), 2 IUI and 1 IVF). Scores of 17-19 (10 patients) have been associated with conception 80% of the time. Scores of 14-16 (10 patients) have a 60% chance, while scores of 13 or less (25 patients) have resulted in no pregnancies.

Absent endometrial flow despite highest values for the other parameters, has always been associated with no conception.

ROLE OF THREE-DIMENSIONAL ULTRASONOGRAPHY

Three-dimensional ultrasonography (3D-USG) is an exiting and rapidly developing field, providing images of the target organ in multiple tomographic sections. In particular, for the first time, the volume of the target organ can be accurately measured, regardless of its shape. Three-dimensional sonography allows physicians to understand and appreciate the complex anatomy of the pelvis with ease.

Future modifications of 3D ultrasound in the field of infertility could include a combination with color Doppler ultrasound to give an index of vascular changes, 3D realtime ultrasonography and direct quantitative computation of the volume of target. It is likely that 3D ultrasound will be accepted in the future as the diagnostic gold standard for the female pelvis (Figs 8.25 to 8.29).[9]

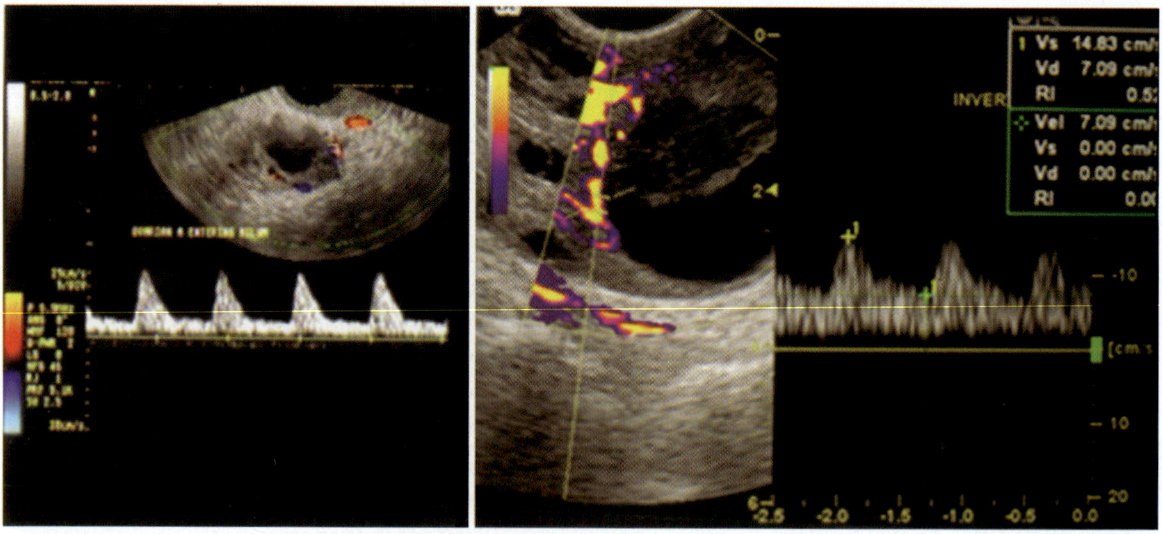

Fig. 8.25: Functioning corpus luteum blood flow

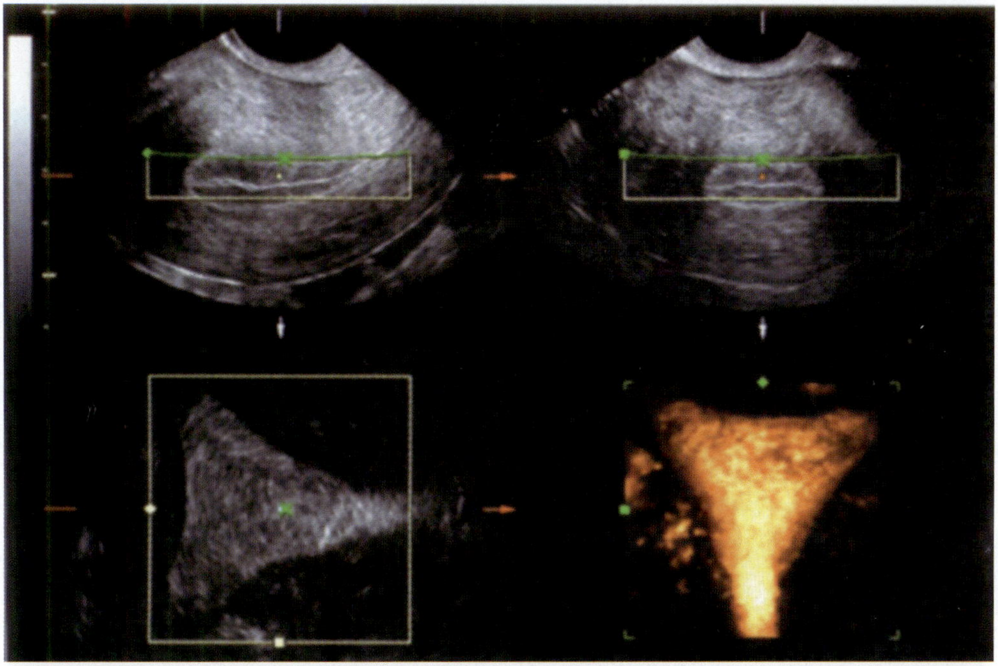

Fig. 8.26: 3D of uterine cavity

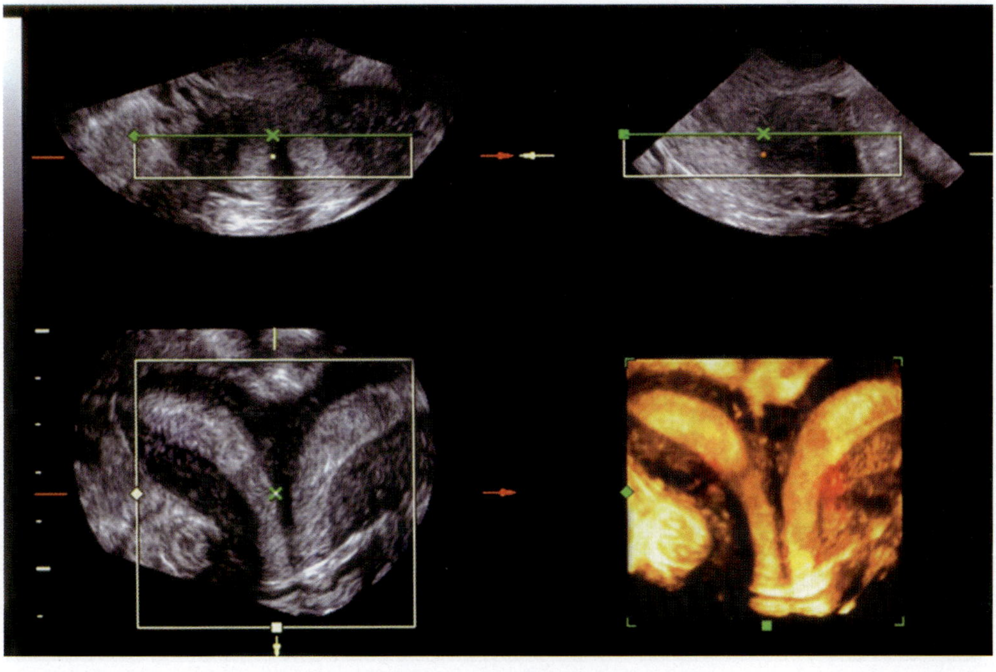

Fig. 8.27: 3D showing bicornuate uterus

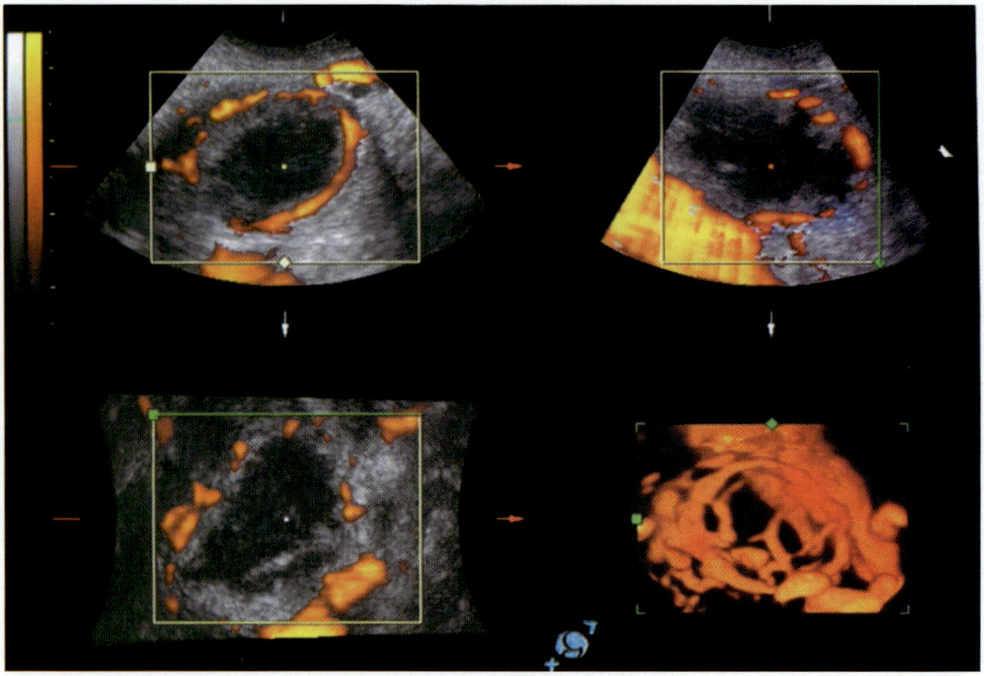

Fig. 8.28: 3D color of corpus luteum

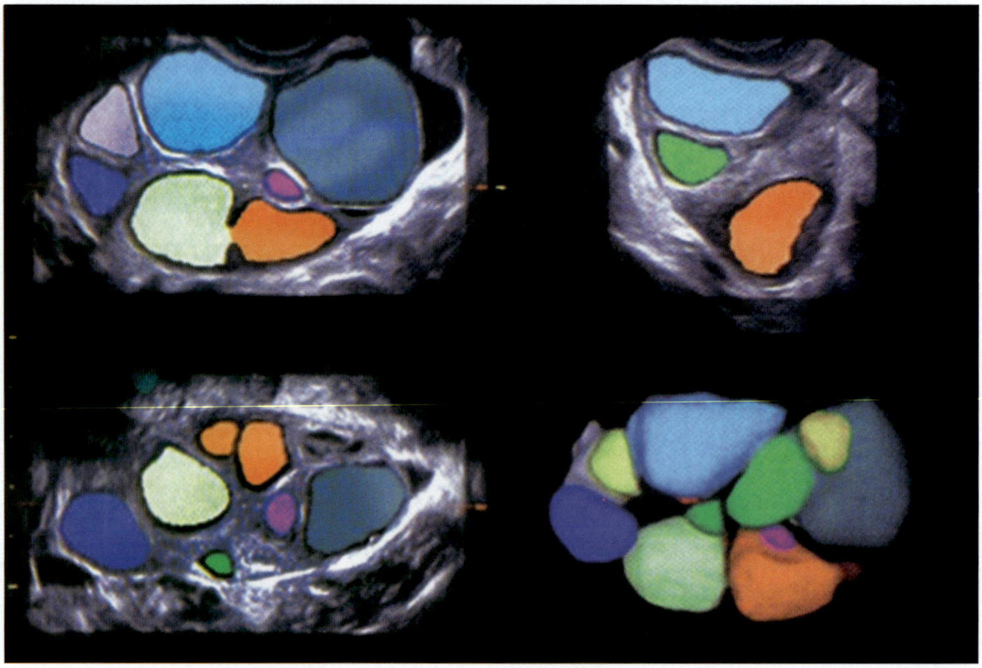

Fig. 8.29: Sonovac of follicles in stimulated ovary

ROLE OF TVS IN INTERVENTIONAL PROCEDURES

With the addition of intervention, today a specific pathological diagnosis is possible as now a needle can be guided into the lesion to take biopsies, fluid for cytology and to even treat simple cysts and localized pyogenic collections and even PCO puncture is being attempted.

The ability to diagnose conditions earlier and better than with transbdominal approach has put vaginosonography in an enviable position for interventional procedures to be carried out on the pelvic organs. Thus, the transvaginal transducer coupled with the biopsy guide, has become of late a crucial weapon in the armamentarium of the interventional ultrasonologist. Whereas with trans abdominal ultrasound, intervention is mainly a free-hand technique; with transvaginal ultrasound it becomes a guided procedure where in the operator can be confident that the needle will follow the path charted out by the software generated biopsy line on the monitor. Also, transvaginal ultrasound guided procedures have the advantage of easy accessibility to the pelvic organs in the needle path.

CONCLUSION

Transvaginal sonography offers a very accurate, easy and reproducible method to evaluate the female pelvis and the female factors of infertility. Addition of color gives us more information about organ perfusion and addition of 3D has opened a new dimension to diagnosis of pelvic pathologies.

To practice infertility without TVS is like walking in dark without a torch.

REFERENCES

1. Matijevic R, Grgic O. Predictive values of ultrasound monitoring of the menstrual cycle. Curr Opin Obstetri Gynecol 2005;17(4):405-10
2. Persadie R. Ultrasonographic assessment of the emdometrial thickness: a review. J Obstet Gynecol Can 2002;24:131-6.
3. Applebaurm M. The uterine biophysical profile (UBP). In endosonography in obstetrics and gynecology. Allahabadia G (Ed) Rotunda Medical Technologies Ltd, Mumbai 1997;343-52.
4. Hackeloer BJ, Fleming R, Robinson HP, et al. Correlation of ultrasonic and endocrinologic assessment of human follicular development. Am J Obstet Gynecol. 1979;35:122.
5. Balakier H, Stronell RD. Color Doppler assessment of folliculogenesis in in vitro fertilization patients. Fertil Steril 1994;62(6):141-6.
6. Gautam Allahabadia fallopian tubes and ultrasonography: FOGSI FOCUS issue No. 7 Oct 93. Recent Advance in of Obstetric and Gyn. Ultrasound.
7. Sharma RP. Fallopian tube patency by ultrasound scan. Obstet Gynecol India 1984;39:700-1.
8. Kurjack A, Kupesic-Urek S, Schulman H, et al. Transvaginal color Doppler in the assesm. of ovarian and uterine blood flow in infertile women. Fertil Steril 1991;56:870-3.
9. Kyei-Mensah A, Zaidi J, Pitlrof R, et al. Transvaginal three dimensional ultrasound. Fertil Steril 1996;65: 371-6.

Chapter 9

Fertility Enhancing Surgeries

Shyam V Desai

Surgical procedures to improve the chances of fertility which are concerning intra-abdominal pathology may be carried out by laparotomy or laparoscopy depending upon the skill and training of the surgeon. In todays age with gynecologists being trained in laparoscopic surgery all over the world, laparoscopic surgery should be the first choice for many a surgical procedure. However, the surgical procedures that involve intrauterine pathologies are best performed by hysteroscopy.

The hysteroscopic surgeries that are commonly performed in an infertile patient are:

- Uterine septum excision
- Adhesiolysis of intrauterine adhesions
- Endometrial polyp excision
- Hysteroscopic submucous myomectomy
- Removal of intrauterine foreign bodies.

UTERINE SEPTUM INCISION

A uterine septum can cause reproductive failure in 25 percent of patients. Early miscarriages are usually the result of the septum due to implantation of the embryo on the septum leading to improper vascularity. The diagnosis is made with a characteristic appearance the dark cornua separated by a central fibrous band A metroplasty seems to be indicated in the following situations—women more than 35 years of age, unexplained infertility resistance to any form of assisted reproduction discovery of the septum at the time of investigations in patients in whom it is assumed that some form of ART is needed and women with a past history of early abortions.

Procedure

The operation can be carried out under general anesthesia using distention of the uterine cavity with 1.5 percent glycine and a resectoscope.

The septum can be incised using a Collins knife or hysteroscopic scissors the septum being divided millimeter by millimeter till both the tubal ostia are seen in the same plane and the fundus being devoid of a arcuate appearance. The division of the septum results in fibromuscular tissue retracting into the uterine wall and the cavity assumes a capacious appearance. The raw area soon heals with endometrium growing over it in the next cycle.

Israel and March[1] after carrying out hysteroscopic septectomy in 91 patients found a significant improvement in the pregnancy outcome.

A uterine septum may also be responsible for early pregnancy loss and may be found in women with a missed abortion. Operative hysteroscopy with its simplicity its reproducibility and low morbidity remains the gold standard treatment of uterine septae.

DeCherney[2] treated 72 patients with a septum hysteroscopically 58 percent of these had a successful outcome.

Birinyi L et al[3] have reported 36 deliveries in their series of 66 cases of metroplasty with normal delivery in 28 cases.

INTRAUTERINE ADHESIONS

Asherman's syndrome was recognized in the causation of amenorrhea and infertility in 1920. It usually follows severe infection such as genital tuberculosis or excessive curettage in a recently pregnant uterus resulting in damage to the basal endometrium. The symptoms of these adhesions are hypomenorrhea or amenorrhea. The adhesions are a recognizable cause of infertility and the diagnosis is made on a hysterosalpingogram or a hysteroscopic examination.

Adhesions may also play a role in habitual abortions by reducing the capacity of the uterine cavity.

The adhesions can be either flimsy or mild and these are easily divided, however, some of them may be thick and then the division becomes more difficult.

Classification

Mild: Filmy adhesions composed of basalis endometrial tissue producing partial or complete uterine cavity occlusion.

Moderate: Fibromuscular thick covered with endometrium that may bleed on division and partially or totally occlude the endometrial cavity.

Severe: Composed of connective tissue only lacking endometrial lining and not likely to bleed on division.

The American Society of Reproductive Medicine has suggested another classification correlating it with menstrual abnormalities. These classifications help in comparing the efficacy of various therapies in the treatment of the problem.

The extent and location of the adhesions would determine the success of the procedure. A skilled endoscopic surgeon would have better success in restoring the uterine cavity to its optimum status as it is important to seek out a proper plane for the dissection allowing pockets of endometrium to grow and cover the fibrotic areas.

Procedure

Adhesiolysis of intrauterine adhesions is carried out under general anesthesia with 1.5 percent glycine as the distending medium and using the scissors or the Collins knife. The Versapoint a bipolar probe can also be used. Dissection should begin at the internal os and once a niche has been created distention should proceed to the fundus and the contour of the uterus should be followed to prevent dissection into the myometrium. Incase one is not confident of the anatomy the dissection can be carried out under laparoscopic guidance. If a monopolar current is being used the cautery setting should be blended with 90 watts cutting and 20 coagulation current. Postoperatively it is usual to administer an estrogen-progesterone combination pill so that the islands of endometrium proliferate and cover the fibrous areas.

The more severe the adhesions worse is the prognosis especially tuberculous infection can impair the results in aspect of return of normal menstruation and pregnancy rates. A secondlook hysteroscopy and/or a hysterosalpingography may be carried out 3 months after the surgery.

In a study by Magos[4] et al, 192 patients with hysteroscopic adhesiolysis 71 (41.4%) became pregnant. Twenty-nine (36.7%) had a spontaneous abortion, 2 had premature deliveries and 45 (23.4%) had a term delivery.

ENDOMETRIAL POLYPS

Endometrial polyps can occur at any age after the menarche and it is not unusual to detect a polyp in an infertile patient. The location may vary from near the internal os to the fundal region and these polyps may range from 1 to 2 cm in size. These polyps should be differentiated from dislodged strips of endometrium. Polyps undulate gently with the distention medium. Large polyps are uncommon but they bring about an inflammatory reaction and act as foreign bodies in the uterine cavity preventing a conception.

Procedure

This is a simple procedure carried out with an operating hysteroscopic channel. Excision in toto can be carried out under hysteroscopic vision using a resectoscope with a loupe electrode and cutting current or it may be vaporized using a Versapoint coagulator.

Grasping the polyp with a grasper and removing the compressible mass through the cervix is also possible in excising the polyp though at times cauterization of the base may be required.

Liberis[5] reported a 86 percent success in hysteroscopic polyp removal.

Hysteroscopic polypectomy is a safe procedure with a low complication rate In a study of 183 patients with a diagnosed polyp the menstrual pattern was normalized in 91.6 percent of patients. The rates of spontaneous pregnancy and delivery at term increased after the procedure and were 61.4 percent and 54.2 percent respectively.

SUBMUCOUS MYOMAS

Submucous location of uterine fibroids can be responsible for symptoms such as dysmenorrhea menorrhagia and intermenstrual bleeding and due to their location they may also result in infertility and early miscarriages. The diagnosis is made on a pelvic USG or MRI and confirmed with a diagnostic hysteroscopy. Fibroids appear as smooth firm pale and rounded masses. They may be sessile or pedunculated the extent of the intramural extension should be known before the procedure so as to prevent perforation of the uterus. The first hysteroscopic myomectomy was reported by Neuwirth and Amin[6] in 1976. Pregnancy rates as high as 66 percent have been reported after hysteroscopic myomectomy.

The methods of hysteroscopic myomectomy are:

1. Under hysteroscopic control scissors can be used to cut the stalk and then morcellate the fibroid.
2. Use the resectoscope to resect the mass piecemeal.
3. Laser vaporizer to dissolve the tumor.
4. Versapoint to vaporize the myoma.

The use of the resectoscope is by far the most widely used method.

Coddington[7] et al (1985) reported that lesions 5 cm or less which protrude 75 percent or more into the uterine cavity and are single can be resected in a single sitting procedure. GnRH analogs may be used to reduce the size of a myoma which is larger and which protrudes less than 50 percent into the cavity.

At times a two sitting procedure is safer for the patient as far as glycine overload is concerned.

Procedure

The fibroid is gradually resected with the use of 1.5 percent. Glycine for distention of the uterine cavity. A standard removal technique involves the use of the resectoscope and wire Loupe electrode cutting current 50 to 90 watts Bleeders are controlled with 50 watt coagulating current.

The extended part of the fibroid into the myometrium has to be removed carefully and the bed of the fibroid may have to be coagulated to prevent excessive bleeding myometrial contractions being adequate to stop the bleeding in most cases.

A 1 cm thickness of the myometrium above the fibroid is desirable for safety.

Prior to an IVF procedure a second look hysteroscopy may be performed to note the endometrial lining.

Donnez et al (1990)[8] have reported out of 134 infertile patients undergoing hysteroscopic myomectomy by resectoscope or Nd: YAG laser have been recorded of these 79 (58.9%) patients conceived. This outcome is similar to that occurring after open myomectomy. The hysteroscopic approach has several advantages over the open method. The operative risk of hysteroscopic myomectomy is 3 percent. Uterine perforation distention system hazards infection and hemorrhage being the most common problems.

Fernandez et al (2001)[9] reported a 27 percent pregnancy rate with 10 percent delivering at term. The symptoms improved in 62 percent of patients the pregnancy rate was 27 percent and there were 10 term deliveries.

REMOVAL OF FOREIGN BODIES

A foreign body in the uterine cavity could be due to remnants of a previous pregnancy such as fetal bones or a part of a IUCD inserted many years ago.

The foreign body could prevent a conception and hence a diagnostic hysteroscopy can be carried out the exact location determined and a curettage performed to remove the mass. Sometimes a hysteroscopic forceps is useful in dislodging the foreign body before curettage.

HYSTEROSCOPIC TUBAL CANNULATION (Figs 9.1 and 9.2)

Tubal cannulation is a procedure carried out for blockage of the fallopian tube at the cornual end. Cornual blockage can be diagnosed on a hysterosalpingography or at the time of an endoscopic evaluation of an infertile patient.

Weidmann et al (1996)[10] classified cornual blocks as follows:

1. Non-nodular
2. Nodular
3. Pseudo-occlusion

DONNEZ AND CASANAS-ROUX CLASSIFICATION OF CORNUAL BLOCKS[11]

1. Pseudo-occlusion—23 percent
2. Fibrosis—33 percent
3. Salpingitis isthmica nodosa—26 percent
4. Chronic salpingitis—1 percent.

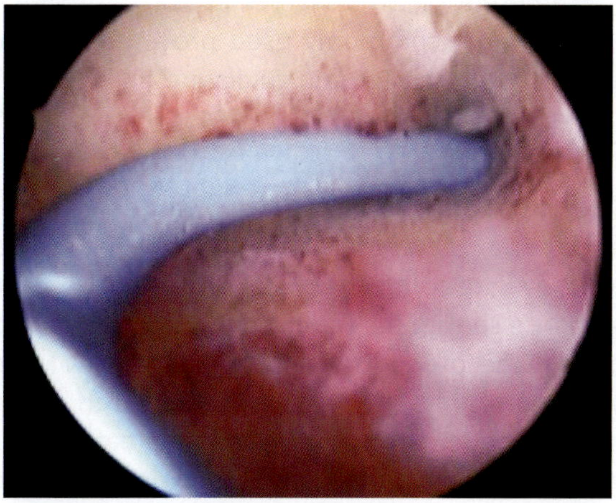

Fig. 9.1: Hysteroscopic tubal cannulation

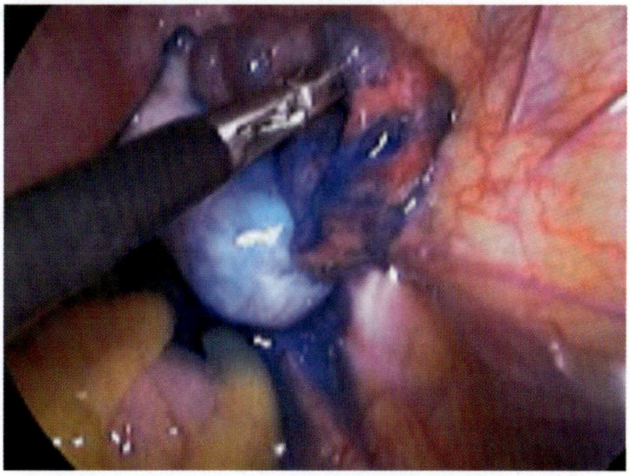

Fig. 9.2: Hysterolaparoscopic cannulation spelt

Novy et al have stated that the blocks which are most likely to respond to tubal cannulations are blocks due to muscular spasm, mucosal agglutination viscous secretions and amorphous debris. It is unlikely that the procedure will benefit patients with salpingitis isthmica nodosa, luminal fibrosis, tuberculosis and leiomyomas in the cornual region.

The procedure is simple and involves the use of a tubal cannulationset. The methods available are:

1. Passage of a flexible guidewire through catheter.
2. Falloposcopic guided cannulation
3. Transcervical balloon cannulation with linear catheters.

The most commonly used procedure is the catheter with the Terumo guidewire.

Procedure

The procedure is carried out under general anesthesia. Hysteroscopically with normal saline as the distending medium with laparoscopic guidance so that the cannulated tube is visualized during the procedure and the patency of the salpinges is seen and documented. The hysteroscope is introduced and the catheter is placed in the ostium. The guide-wire is passed through the catheter so that it bypasses the block and enters the tube. The Novys coaxial system is most ideal as it conforms to the anatomy of the uterotubal junction 1988 Novy.[12]

The procedure also serves to determine whether the block is due to an organic problem or as a result of collection of mucinous plugs and debris which prevent passage of dye or the presence of a spasm of the tube at the time of testing patency.

The problem with establishment of patency in an organically blocked tube is that even though patency is procured the block tends to recur and the purpose of the procedure is not served besides the incidence of a tubal ectopic pregnancy can be expected to increase in a partially blocked tube.

However, if the procedure can ensure patency in a small percentage of patients it would spare them the cost and emotional stress of undergoing an ART procedure.

LAPAROSCOPIC PROCEDURES FOR FERTILITY ENHANCEMENT (Figs 9.3 to 9.7)

The fertility enhancing procedure that are commonly performed laparoscopically are:

- Tubal surgeries
- Adhesiolysis
- Endometriosis surgery
- Laparoscopic myomectomy
- PCOD cauterization
- Bicornuate uterus unification.

TUBAL SURGERIES

Tubal disease is responsible for subfertility in 25 to 30 percent of women and about 10 to 15 percent have proximal tubal disease.

Laparoscopic correction of tubal disease is an important indication for laparoscopic surgery. A

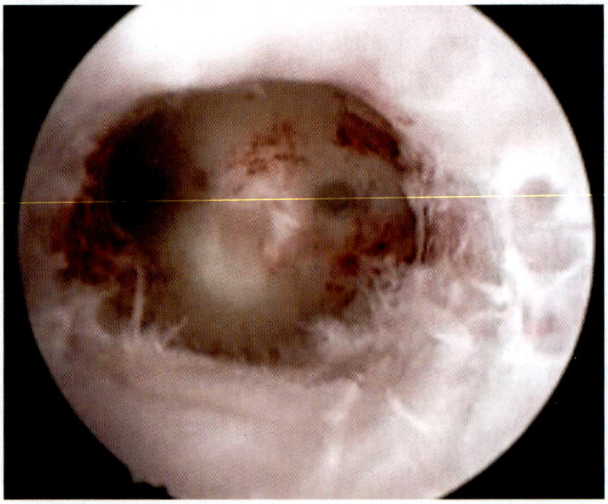

Fig. 9.3: Adhesions left lateral wall

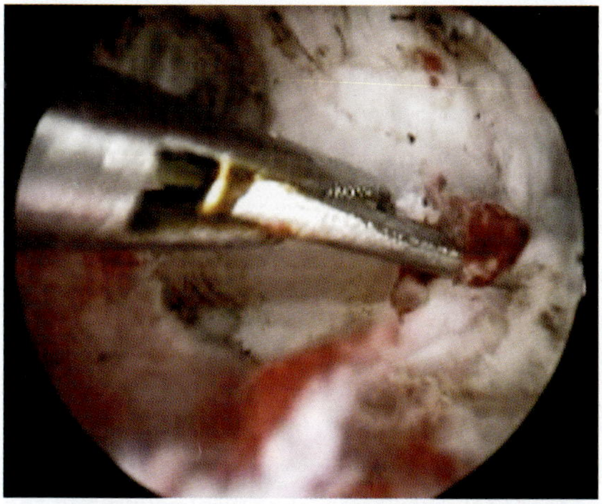

Fig. 9.4: Adhesions cut with scissors

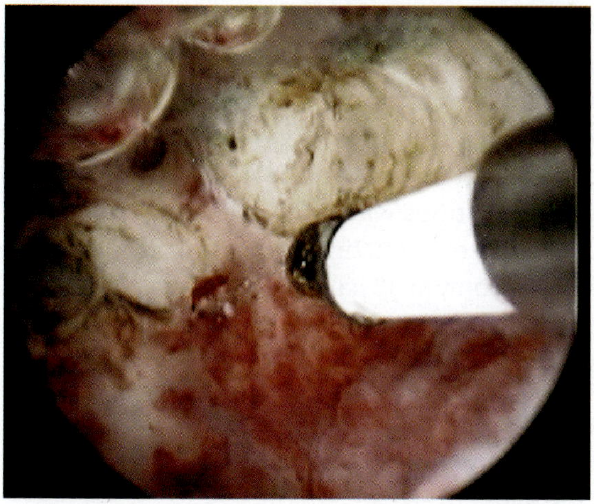

Fig. 9.5: Adhesions cut with versapoint

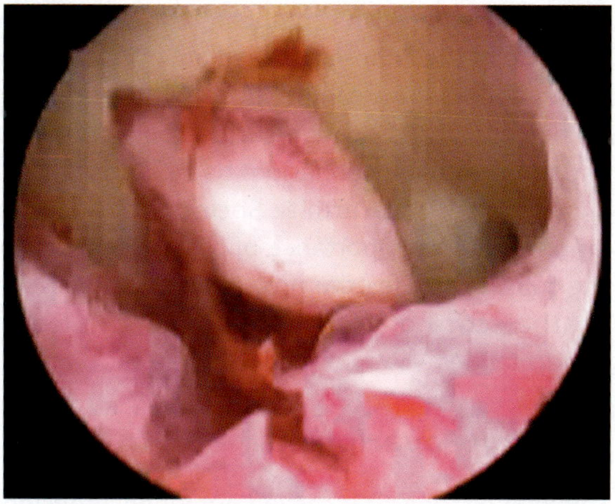

Fig. 9.6: Small polyp

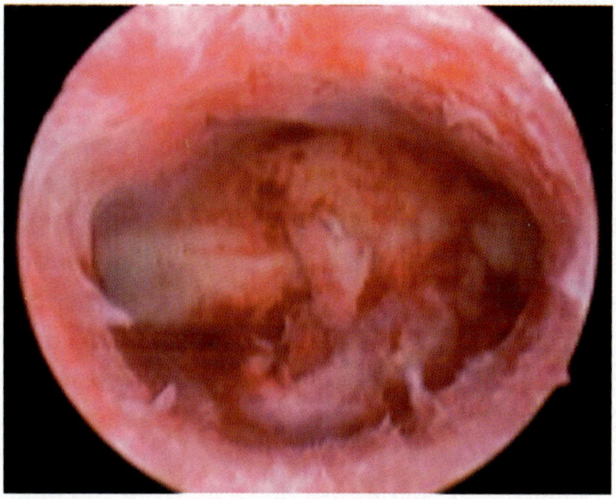

Fig. 9.7: Polyp removed

large number of patients have adhesions developing between the fallopian tubes and the ovaries and between the fallopian tubes and the posterior aspect of the uterus.

The etiology of these adhesions are usually inflammatory following an episode of mild to severe pelvic inflammatory disease or they may result from endometriosis. A patient may also develop adhesions following previous surgery, e.g. laparotomy for appendicectomy.

Laparoscopic procedures that can be carried out also serve to restore the normal anatomy of the pelvic organs so that the process of ovulation and ovum pickup by the fallopian tubes and the transport through the tube into the uterine cavity is made easy.

There are two classifications for grading the adhesions present.

Hulka (1982) described a prognostic classification system based on a 5 years retrospective survey of the outcome of fertility operations. The extent of ovarian involvement and the nature filmy or dense of the adhesion played an important role in the eventual outcome. Those with more than 50 percent of the ovarian surface being involved and those with thick adhesions had a bad prognosis

The American Fertility Society classification emphasizes the importance of the fimbrial end of the tube and bases the prognosis for conception on the score of the adnexa with the lesser abnormalities.

Salpingo-ovariolysis

Salpingo-ovariolysis is carried out when adhesions bind the tubes and ovaries preventing normal functioning of the organs and this results in impaired ovum pickup.

Procedure

The patient is subjected to laparoscopy under general anesthesia with a three or four puncture technique. Dissection begins at the fundal region and the operator works his way downwards excising the adhesions and not merely dividing them. The adhesions are coagulated and divided if they are thick and vascular gradually exposing the pouch of Douglas. The adnexae are then put on a stretch making adhesiolysis easier and the salpinges and ovaries are released from the pelvic sidewall from the bowel and from each other. Irrigation is carried out and all except the smallest bleeding points are coagulated to achieve hemostasis. The success of such an operation depends on the hemostasis of the operating field at the end of surgery.

Gomel V et al (1983)[13] reported that out of 92 patients who underwent salpingo-ovariolysis 54, i.e. 59 percent had at least 1 term pregnancy 5, i.e. 5 percent had an ectopic pregnancy.

Salpingostomy

Salpingostomy is carried out when the fimbrial end is inverted or blocked resulting in the formation of a hydrosalpinx.

Procedure

The patient is under general anesthesia and a laparoscopy is performed with three or four punctures.

The Fallopian tube is separated from the ovary and posterior surface of the uterus by carrying out adhesiolysis. The hydrosalpinx is distended by transcervical instillation of normal saline and the tube is incised on the punctum in a cruciate manner to expose the underlying mucosa. The opening is widened with the insertion of an atraumatic forceps and the fimbriae gradually everted A cuff salpingostomy ensures that the neostoma remains open. This can also be ensured by bipolar coagulating the serosa adjacent to the opening or by taking sutures with 3-0 prolene or vicryl.

Mettler et al (1979)[14] carried out laparoscopic salpingostomy in 38 patients out of which 10 (26%) conceived. The ectopic pregnancy incidence is not reported.

Fimbrioplasty

Fimbrioplasty can be carried out when there is a simple inversion of the fimbriae into the tubal lumen.

Procedure

An atraumatic grasper is introduced into the point where inversion has taken place and opened up in the lumen of the tube. Gradual withdrawal of the forceps will bring about eversion of the fimbriae. It is a delicately carried out procedure and only minimal trauma to the fimbriae should occur.

In todays scenario the extent of tubal disease should be taken into account as far as operative procedures on the Fallopian tubes are concerned. In the milder grade of tubal disease pregnancy rates are in the region of 50 percent but in the more advanced tubal diseases the rates may be as low as 10 to 20 percent. With ART procedures giving 40 to 50 percent success with procedures like ICSI it may be prudent to subject the patient to ART rather than operative laparoscopic surgery.

However, procedures such as tubal cannulation and salpingo-ovariolysis and salpingostomy may have a place in special situations like when ethical or religious objections to ART exist or when financial problems preclude IVF.

SURGERY FOR ENDOMETRIOSIS

The correlation between endometriosis and infertility is well established. Infertility is a presenting symptom in 30 to 50 percent of patients with endometriosis. Besides anatomical abnormalities as a result of endometriotic adhesions impaired folliculogenesis,ovulatory dysfunction and luteal phase defects are some of the reasons given to explain infertility.

Diagnosis of endometriosis is made on pelvic and transvaginal sonography (TVS) but laparoscopy is the gold standard for diagnosing small lesions.

At the time of diagnostic laparoscopy facilities for treatment should be available.

The principles of surgical treatment of endometriosis are:

1. To restore the normal anatomy of the pelvic organs so that optimum function of the tubes and ovaries is possible.
2. To free the pouch of Douglas and excise or coagulate endometriotic areas.
3. To restore normal anatomy within the ovaries by draining excising and endocoagulating the endometriotic cyst that may be present.
4. To bring about hemostasis and adopt measures that would prevent the chances of recurrence of adhesions.

Superficial Endometriosis

There are two or three methods of treating peritoneal and superficial endometriosis—Laser vaporization, thermal endocoagulation and electrocoagulation. The surface endometriosis is ablated with the above modalities but it is generally believed that the deeper lesions are not adequately treated. These methods of treatment lack long-term follow-up to be able to gauge their efficacy in the total extirpation of the lesion.

Redwine (1991)[16] first proposed that surgical excision of the peritoneal lesions should be carried out using scissors and monopolar current to actually denude the peritoneum and along with it the endometriosis. This superficial excision of endometriosis is not possible with laser vaporization or endocoagulation.

Resection of the uterosacral ligaments may be required in some cases where deep fibrotic endometriosis exists. Blunt dissection to determine the extent of endometriosis followed by sharp dissection to excise the lesions is carried out.

Endometriosis in the Pouch of Douglas

Adhesions between the Fallopian tube and Pouch of Douglas, ovarian fossa and posterior aspect of the uterus should be meticulously divided and cauterized to prevent recurrence.

An obliterated pouch of Douglas should also be dissected out so that free movement of the Fallopian tubes is possible and also the dyspareunia that many of these patients suffer from is reduced. Incase a rectovaginal endometriotic nodule exists in the posterior cervix cul de sac uterosacral ligaments and anterior bowel wall excision of the nodule should be carried out with proper dissection in the rectovaginal space.

Laparoscopic excision of endometriosis results in durable relief of pain in these patients if properly carried out. Recurrence of disease can occur but is less than expected.

Endometrioma

Endometriomas are a manifestation of an advanced stage of the disease. The role of surgery in cases of endometrioma associated with infertility is not well outlined. In patients with severe dysmenorrhea and dyspareunia who are not interested in fertility the treatment of choice is drainage of the endometrioma excision of the lining of the cyst and establishing hemostasis. This is by far more effective than simple drainage and cauterization of the cyst wall as far as relief of symptoms and rate of recurrence is concerned.

Beretta[18] reported better pregnancy rates after laparoscopic ovarian cystectomy than simple coagulation of the cyst wall.

Several conflicting findings are reported by workers who have treated women with endometriosis prior to subjecting them to ART procedures.

One of the reasons in not treating endometriomas adequately, i.e. by carrying out cystwall excision is that the ovarian stroma may be adversely affected and as a result the reproductive outcome of subsequent cycles of IUI IVF or ICSI may be impaired.

Garcia et al (2000)[17] investigated whether conservative surgery on endometriomas prior to an IVF cycle improves fertility outcome. They concluded that it does not improve the outcome Infact proceeding directly to hyperstimulation and IVF may confer better results reducing the cost and time to pregnancy. Canis et al (2001)[19] stressed that conservative treatment, i.e. drainage and coagulation per se does not reduce the IVF or ICSI success rates. The expertise of the endoscopic surgeon is essential to prevent damage to the ovarian stroma. A similar finding has been quoted by Donnez et al[20] (2001). Further studies are required to establish the exact place and extent of endometriosis surgery in an infertile patient.

The general opinion favors the treatment of endometriosis especially moderate to severe disease prior to subjecting the patient to fertility promoting technology.

LAPAROSCOPIC MYOMECTOMY

The presence of a fibroid or fibroids in the uterine cavity can impair the pregnancy rates due to various factors:

1. Intramural myomas in the cornual region may block the tubal ostia.
2. Abnormal endometrial maturation due to vascular changes.
3. Distortion of the uterine cavity may cause reduced implantation rate.
4. Inflammatory changes in the endometrium may cause reduced endometrial receptivity.
5. Sperm transport may be hampered due to abnormal contractility of the uterus.

The location of the myoma and its size will certainly have a bearing on the infertility potential of the myoma, e.g. implantation on the surface of the myoma will lead to miscarriage, or if the myoma is submucous it may cause a inflammatory reaction.

It must be remembered that there are several women with myomas that do conceive and that makes the correlation between the presence of leiomyomas and infertility rather debatable.

Buttram and Reiter[15] reviewed 1699 cases of myomectomy and found that 27 percent of these women were also infertile. After ruling out all other possible factors myomas were found to be responsible for the infertility in only 2.4 percent of cases.

Infact when it is not sure if the fibroid is the cause of infertility it may be detrimental to perform the myomectomy which can result in adhesions between the Fallopian tubes and the uterus.

There are workers who believe that if a patient with a myoma has to undergo an ART cycle it may be preferable for the patient to undergo a myomectomy prior to the ART cycle. The general opinion is that if there is a submucous myoma or intramural myoma larger than 3 cm the patient should undergo a myomectomy.

Elder Geva T (1998) et al found in their study that women with subserous myomas had pregnancy rates of 30.1 percent whereas those with intramural myomas had rates of 16.4 percent. The pregnancy rates were also lower when there was a submucous component to the myoma.

The procedure of myomectomy is not altogether and innocuous one as it may lead to the development of adhesions and distortion of the tubo-ovarian relationship leading to a drop in spontaneous conception rates hence the decision to perform the myomectomy should be undertaken only after due consideration.

Many authors have suggested the use of GnRH analogs in the preoperative phase to reduce the size and vascularity however this is a controversial topic and at present should be considered only if the patient is anemic and the hemoglobin is below 10 gm percent and the patient needs to be given time for the buildup of the Hb.

The exact location size and number of the myomas should be known so that as many myomas that can be removed should be taken out. In fact an MRI may be advisable if a USG does not show the myomas clearly. The procedure should also be undertaken only by a surgeon who is well versed with endoscopic suturing techniques as the scar that results should be able to withstand the distention during the pregnancy that would follow.

Procedure

The procedure follows proper preoperative care and is usually carried out in the immediate postmenstrual phase. The patient under general anesthesia is subjected to a laparoscopy with three or four punctures. Vasopressin is injected in the myometrium to bring about hemostasis.

The procedure involves incising the myometrium covering the myoma with monopolar cautery or with scissors to expose the surface of the myoma.

A myoma screw is inserted to give traction and the myoma is gradually enucleated with sharp and blunt dissection. The sheaf of blood vessels supplying the myoma are cauterized to reduce hemorrhage.

Two toothed forceps are used to hold the edges of the myometrium/fibroid capsule. The suction irrigator is used as a blunt probe to lever out the leiomyoma from its capsule; sharp scissors may be used as required.

If there are multiple myomas, efforts should be made as far as possible to remove them through one incision. If the myometrial defect is deep or large, it is repaired with 1-0 or 2-0 vicryl suture followed by serosal repair with 2-0 vicryl. The myometrium is sutured in two layers. The sutures are taken at 1 cm intervals using intracorporeal knot tying. The standard approach is a vertical incision in the uterus.

The suturing could also be done in two or three layers using the Brill suture which affords good apposition of the edges and hemostasis.

Removal of the myoma may be carried out using the Morcellators available or by delivering the tumors through a colpotomy.

Postoperatively healing of the scar takes place in 6 to 8 weeks and it will be prudent to plan the pregnancy thereafter.

The myomectomy should be carried out with minimal trauma to the myometrium and endometrium keeping in mind the importance of the tubal ostia and cornual region. The number of incisions on the surface of the uterus should be restricted so that the incidence of adhesions is minimized. Proper hemostasis and coaptation of the edges gives the patient the best chances of conception and safe pregnancy and delivery.

It is expected that a myoma up to 5 to 7 cm can be removed easily and the larger myomas may require a laparotomy to complete the removal satisfactorily.

To evaluate reproductive outcome after laparoscopic myomectomy for intramural myomas in infertile women Mineto Morita and Yasuyuki Asakawa[21] carried out a a retrospective study was carried out in 30 infertile women with intramural myomas measuring ≥ 50 mm in diameter. The overall rate of spontaneous intrauterine pregnancy was 50.0 percent (15 patients). Of 13 patients with infertility factors associated with the uterine myomas, three (23.1%) became pregnant, whereas 12 of 17 patients (70.6%) with no other associated infertility factor became pregnant. No uterine ruptures were observed. All pregnancies were spontaneous and 13 occurred within 1 year of the operation. In the 10 patients who gave birth by cesarean section, no adhesions were found on the myomectomy scar.

Miller et al reported that inspite of the high risk of adhesion formation, myomectomy seems to improve the reproductive outcome.[22] The reported conception rates for abdominal myomectomy in infertile patients have been up to 58 percent.[23] After laparoscopic myomectomy, conception rates have been quoted to be 71 percent and 75 percent respectively in two different series.[24,25]

If no associated factor for infertility is found, laparoscopic myomectomy enhances fertility rate.[26] In a series reported by Seinera et al,[23] 65 pregnancies were achieved in 54 patients with no case of uterine rupture. In another study by Dubuisson et al,[27] the estimated risk of uterine rupture has been reported to be 1.0 percent (95% CI 0.0-5.5%). However, particular care however must be given to the uterine closure.

PCOD CAUTERIZATION

In many an infertile patient the problem of polycystic ovaries prevents conception by altering the hormonal milieu within the ovary leading to anovulation. It has been estimated that genetic and environmental factors are responsible and the underlying hyperandrogenism due to ovarian dysfunction can lead to hyperinsulinemia and obesity.

The treatment for this problem is basically medical with ovulation promoting agents, e.g. Clomiphene citrate and Letrozole being most commonly prescribed alongwith efforts to reduce weight.

For those women who do not respond to these medications gonadotropin injections, e.g. pure FSH and recombinant FSH have been recommended.

However, the risk of OHSS with gonadotropins exists and that is why surgical intervention is preferable. It has also been shown that a single event of cauterization can lead to the patient having 10 to 12 ovulatory cycles and proves more economical than the administration of gonadotropins.

Procedure

Ovarian drilling or laparoscopic electro-cauterization of the ovarian surface (LEOS) as the procedure is sometimes referred to is a simple laparoscopic procedure carried out under general anesthesia by laparoscopy. About 5 to 7 punctures 1 or 2 mm deep are made on the ovarian surface with a PCOD monopolar needle with the intention of altering the hormonal milieu within the stroma The monopolar current is set at 50 to 75 watts.

Care is taken that the punctures are away from the hilum of the ovary and adequate irrigation of the ovaries is carried out.

Overzealous cauterization has been known to bring about premature menopause and this should be guarded against.

This procedure should be advised in women resistant to Clomiphene citrate and Letrozole and is especially effective in patients who are lean and have a high LH level in the menstrual cycle or in response to Clomiphene.

It may also be recommended when the patient has concomitant pathology, e.g. leiomyomas or endometriosis and polycystic ovaries are noted at the time of operative laparoscopy.

The results following this procedure show a high incidence of ovulation and conception.

In 50 percent of LEOS treated women adjuvant therapy may be required for ovulation induction.

A drawback is that in 20 percent of cases there are adhesions that develop between the tube and ovary hence this procedure should not be undertaken lightly and recommended only when Clomiphene or Letrozole fail to achieve results.

LAPAROSCOPIC CORRECTION OF UTERINE ANOMALIES

Patients with infertility may present with uterine anomalies such as Bicornuate uterus and Rudimentary Horn Many of these patients would have associated symptoms such as dysmenorrhea and a history of recurrent miscarriages or preterm labor due to cervical incompetence.

Repair of some of these problems can be carried out laparoscopically such as excision of a rudimentary horn but some procedures such as reconstruction of a Bicornuate uterus are best subjected to a laparotomy.

REFERENCES

1. Israel R, March CM. Hysteroscopic incision of the septate uterus. Am J Obstet Gynecol.
2. DeCherney AH, Russell JB, Giaeb RA. Resectoscopic management of Mullerian Fusion defects. Fertil. Steril 1986;45:726.
3. Birinyi L, Gyenes O, Major T. Orv Hetil Debrecent Egyetem Orvos es Egeszsegtudomanyi Centrum. Altalanos Orvostudomanyi Kar 2003;144(20):979-83.
4. Magos A. Reprod Biomed Online Hysteroscopic treatment of Asherman's syndrome 2002;9(Suppl 3) 46-51.
5. Liberis V, Dafopoulos K, Tsikouras P. Removal of endometrial polyps by use of grasping forceps and curettage after diagnostic hysteroscopy: Clin Exp Obstet Gynecol 2003;30(1): 29-31.
6. Neuwirth RS, Amin HK. Excision of submucous fibroids with hysteroscopic control. Am J Obstet Gynaecol 1976,126:95-99.
7. Coddington CC, Collins RL, Shawker TH. Long acting analogue used to treat uteri. Fertil Steril 1986;45:624.
8. Donnez J, Nisolle M. Casanas-Roux Endometriosis associated infertility: evaluation of preoperative use of Danazol Gestrinone and Buserelin Int J Fertil 1990;297-301.
9. Fernandez H, Sefrioui O, Virelizier C. Hysteroscopic resection of submucous myomas in patients with infertility;Hum Reprod 2001:16 (7) 1489-92.
10. Weidmann Sterzik K, Combisch V, Sturkensen J, Montag M. Beyond recanalising Proximal Tubal Obstruction. Hum Reprod 1996;11(5):986-91.
11. Donnez and Casanas-Roux. A prognostic factor in Proximal tubal Obstruction. Eur J Obstet Gynecol Reprod Biol 1988;29:53.
12. Novy MJ, Thurmond AJ, Patton P. Diagnosis of corneal obstruction by transcervical fallopian tube cannulation. Fertil Steril 1998;50:434.
13. Gomel V. Salpingo-ovariolysis by laparoscopy in infertility. Fertil Steril 1983;40:607.
14. Mettler L, Giesel H, Semm K. Treatment of female infertility due to tubal obstruction by operative laparoscopy. Fertil Steril 1979;32:384.
15. Buttram Jr VC, Reiter RX. Uterine leiomyomata etiology symptomatology and management. Fertil Steril 1981;36:433-45.
16. Redwine DB. Conservative laparoscopic excision of endometriosis by sharp dissection. Fertil Steril 1991;56:628-34.
17. Garcia Velasco JA, Mahutte NG, Corona J, Zuniga V, Giles J, Arici A. Removal of endometriomas before in vitro fertilization does not improve fertility outcomes a matched case control study; Fertil Steril 2001; 81(5): 1194-7.

18. Beretta P, Franchi M, Ghezzi F, Busacca M, Zupi E, Bolis P. Randomised clinical trial of two laparoscopic treatments of endometriomas. Cystectomy vs drainage and coagulation. Fertil Steril 1998;70:1176-80.
19. Canis M, Pouly JL, Tamburro S, Mage G, Wattiez A, Bruhat MA. Ovarian response during IVF—Embryo transfer cycles after laparoscopic ovarian cystectomy of endometriotic cysts >3 cm in diameter. Hum Reprod 2001;16(12):2583-6.
20. Donnez J, Wyns C, Nisolle M. Does ovarian surgery for endometriomas impair the ovarian response to gonadotropins? Fertil Steril 2001;76(4): 662-5.
21. Mineto Morita, Asakawa Y. Reproductive outcome after laparoscopic myomectomy for intramural myomas in infertile women with or without associated factors. Reprod Med and Biol 2006;5:31-35.
22. Miller CE, Johnston M, Rundell M. Laparoscopic myomectomy in infertile women. J Am Assoc Gynecol Laparoscop 1996;3:525-9.
23. Seinera P, Farina C, Todros T. Laparoscopic myomectomy and subsequent pregnancy:result in 54 patients. Human Reprod 2000;15(9):993-6.
24. Li TC, Mortimer R, Cook ID. Myomectomy: a retrospective study to examine reproductive performance before and after surgery. Human Reprod 1999;14(7):1735-40.
25. Verkauf BS. Myomectomy for fertility enhancement and preservation. Fertil Steril 1992;58:1-15.
26. Hasson HM, Rotman C, Rana N, Sistos F, Dmowski WP. Laparoscopic myomectomy. Obstet Gynecol 1992;80:884-8.
27. Dubuisson JB, Chapron C, Fauconnier A, Babaki-Fard K. Laparoscopic myomectomy fertility results: Ann N Y Acad Sci 2001;943:269-75.

Chapter

10

Endometriosis and Infertility

Sonal Karia, Ian S Fraser

INTRODUCTION

Endometriosis is a complex, chronic and often recurring condition with wide variability in age and mode of presentation, symptomatology, anatomical sites, response to treatment and rate of recurrence. In spite of the advances in diagnosis and management, it is a potentially challenging disease with devastating effects on lifestyle in a minority of patients. Endometriosis can have a range of effects from minimal or no symptoms to severe and excruciating pelvic pain, menstrual disturbances, infertility and systemic symptoms. In this chapter, we will focus mainly on the relationship between endometriosis and infertility, with specific emphasis on diagnosis and management of infertility related to endometriosis.

DEFINITION

Endometriosis is defined as the presence of tissue lesions and nodules which are histologically similar to the eutopic endometrium, but at sites outside the uterus. It is difficult to assess the prevalence of endometriosis due to difficulties related to diagnosis but the overall prevalence is thought to be ≈ 10 percent in the reproductive age group.[1] The disease is thought to be associated with pelvic pain and infertility in up to 90 million women in the world. It is thought to affect 50 to 60 percent of women and teenagers with pelvic pain and up to 50 percent of women with infertility.[1,2] It is probably common in all cultures, although there may be some differences in genetic influence and in the effects of repeated pregnancy and prolonged lactation.

Etiology and theories of origin of endometriosis:

Various theories of origin of endometriosis have been proposed, but the exact etiology still remains unclear and somewhat controversial. The current evidence supports a multifactorial origin of the disease including support for strong familial component with genomic, genetic and epigenetic mechanisms almost certainly playing a significant role.

1. Retrograde menstruation:
   - Still remains the most widely accepted theory of development of endometriosis
   - Retrograde menstruation of viable endometrial fragments via the fallopian tubes with attachment to the peritoneal surfaces, involving expression of extracellular membrane adhesion molecules and their co-receptors, and subsequent angiogenesis.[3,4]
   - Supported by the fact that the incidence is higher in women with outflow tract obstruction

- Reduced risk of recurrence in women with known endometriosis following endometrial ablation at the same time as excision of ectopic lesions.[5]

2. Coelomic metaplasia:
   - Cells from both the peritoneum and the endometrium derive from a common precursor, the coelomic epithelium.
   - Difficult to support the theory scientifically
   - Postulated as the most likely source of deep endometriotic nodules in the rectovaginal septum and some ovarian endometriomas.[6,7]
3. Genomics, Genetics and Epigenetics:
   - Possible polygenic mode of hereditary transmission with involvement of multiple loci including genes involved in oxidative stress and MAP (mitogen-activated protein kinase),[8] early growth response-1,[9] tumor suppressor gene TOB1[10] etc.
4. Shedding of endometrial stem cells:
   - Newer concept proposing the shedding of endometrial stem cells from basal endometrium which have the ability to form progenitor cells and potential to initiate a lesion from a single cell.

PATHOPHYSIOLOGY OF ENDOMETRIOSIS

There seems to be no single molecular abnormality responsible for the development of endometriosis. It is believed that endometriosis occurs as a result of multigene activation resulting in multiple and possibly simultaneous molecular abnormalities. The development of endometriosis involves complex and often multiple pathological mechanisms in the endometrium, peritoneum, and peritoneal fluid and in the ectopic lesions. There is increasing evidence that endometriosis is primarily an endometrial disease. In the endometrium, there is increased aromatase activity resulting in high local estrogen levels along with increased production of intracellular adhesion molecules and angiogenic molecules resulting in new blood and lymph vessel formation. In addition, there is a likely increase in the secretion of neurogenic factors resulting in development of new sensory nerve fibers. There is a probable reduction in apoptosis which allows greater viability of the shed endometrial fragments. Changes in the immune cell populations and generation of free oxygen radicals, structural proteins, growth and signalling molecules are also believed to play a role. As far as the peritoneum, peritoneal fluid and ectopic lesions are concerned; there may be increased number of macrophages but reduced macrophage scavenger activity and other immune cell disturbances (including dendritic cells, regulatory T cells and uterine natural killer cells) with increased expression of a wide range of molecules. Nerve growth factor and prostaglandins from different leukocytes potentially stimulate nociceptors on sensory nerve fibers responsible for pain generation.[11]

MECHANISM OF ENDOMETRIOSIS ASSOCIATED INFERTILITY

1. Distortion of pelvic anatomy due to inflammation and adhesion formation leading to alteration of tubo-ovarian relationship affecting release of the oocyte or the pickup and the transportation of the oocyte via the fallopian tube.
2. Factors in the peritoneal fluid
   - Increased concentration of activated peritoneal fluid macrophages with enhanced phagocytosis for sperm (but not necessarily for shed endometrial cells) and increase in local concentration of cytokines, proteolytic enzymes, etc.

- Sperm phagocytosis by peritoneal macrophages.[12]
- Increased concentration of interleukins, cytokines, growth factors and TNF-α affecting folliculogenesis, oocyte quality, ovulation,[13] sperm function and transport.[14]
- Conflicting data regarding the effect on fertilization as evidenced by a study of 980 patients undergoing ICSI which showed no difference in fertilization rates in patients with endometriosis compared to patients with other subfertility factors.[15] However, as all these patients underwent ICSI, it would be difficult to assess the true effect on fertilization and other studies have reported reduced fertilization rates.

3. Oocyte quality
   - Poor oocyte quality in patients with endometriosis as evidenced by the fact that pregnancy rates in patients with endometriosis did not differ significantly from other patients when donor oocytes were used.[16]
4. Implantation
   - There are histologic and biochemical alterations in the endometrium with altered cytokine and immune cell infiltration in patients with endometriosis.[17,18] There is some evidence of down regulation of certain gene products such as $\alpha v\beta 3$,[19] HOX genes[20] and others which play a role in implantation.

DIAGNOSIS

The diagnosis of endometriosis remains a challenge in spite of continuing attempts and efforts by various international research groups to formulate algorithms and diagnostic tools to simplify the diagnosis. Endometrial nerve fibers are present in almost all women with endometriosis, but are not present in women without endometriosis (Tokushige et al 2006). This could offer the basis of a research test for endometriosis when laparoscopy is not indicated (Al-Jefout et al 2009). Much research is being investigated in the serum and urinary biomarkers. Laparoscopy by an experienced gynecologist remains the gold standard for diagnosis. The diagnostic accuracy of laparoscopy is improved by concomitant histological examination of suspicious lesions.

Clinical

Endometriosis is a condition with highly variable symptomatology. Women experience a wide range of symptoms, from being asymptomatic (although rare) or having relatively mild symptoms through to experiencing a full variety of symptoms including severe dysmenorrhea, dyspareunia, chronic pelvic pain, menstrual disturbances, etc. The commonest symptom is progressive secondary dysmenorrhea. The pain usually begins premenstrually and usually continues through the duration of the menstrual bleeding. Depending on the anatomical site and extent of involvement, women may experience symptoms related to bowel viz dyschezia, hematochezia, painful abdominal bloating or to the bladder viz hematuria, dysuria, etc. The range and severity of symptoms often do not reflect the severity of the disease. A high index of suspicion is required because although the spectrum of symptoms is highly variable, most women with endometriosis present with some form of pelvic pain with or without other associated symptoms. Occasionally the primary presenting complaint may be infertility or an incidental diagnosis of endometriosis may be made on laparoscopy done for some other indication. D'Hoogee, et al reported that the prevalence of endometriosis among infertile patients was higher compared to fertile patients (33 v/s 4%).[21]

Clinical examination may be of limited value and precision in the diagnosis of endometriosis. Abdominal examination usually does not reveal diagnostic features except in cases of unusually large endometriomas which may be palpable abdominally or presence of nonspecific and vague tenderness. However, endometriomas which are large enough to be palpable abdominally would usually be associated with other symptoms. Bimanual examination may reveal induration and tenderness in the cul de sac. Tender nodules may be palpable in the cul de sac, rectovaginal septum or along the uterosacral ligaments.

Role of Imaging

There is a continuing attempt to develop reliable noninvasive tests for the diagnosis of endometriosis. Transvaginal ultrasound (TVUS) and magnetic resonance imaging (MRI) are the two imaging modalities that received attention and have shown some promise.

Transvaginal ultrasound may be useful in making a strong presumptive diagnosis of ovarian endometriomas but its usefulness in diagnosis of other forms of endometriosis remains a subject of ongoing debate. The classical picture of an ovarian endometrioma reveals diffuse low amplitude internal echoes with enhanced sound transmission and a visible uniform wall.[22] Additionally, some bright reflectors may be seen possibly representing products of red cell breakdown. The findings are not always classical and it may be difficult to distinguish endometriomas from ovarian neoplasms. Occasionally some solid components may be present as a result of bleeding with surrounding inflammation and accumulation of debris. Also, endometriomas are sometimes well vascularized lesions and hence may be confused with ovarian neoplasms on color Doppler imaging. Transvaginal and transrectal ultrasounds are increasingly being used in diagnosis of deep infiltrating lesions involving the rectosigmoid. In a recent meta-analysis a total of 10 studies fulfilled predefined inclusion criteria involving 1106 patients with suspected endometriosis. After obtaining the likelihood ratios and pooled estimates of sensitivities, specificities, positive and negative predictive values the authors concluded that TVS with or without the use of prior bowel preparation is an accurate test for noninvasive, presurgical detection of deep infiltrating endometriosis of the rectosigmoid.[23]

MRI has been proposed to be the best imaging modality at present for the identification of ovarian endometriomas, but does not have enough sensitivity and specificity for other endometriotic lesions. Compared to a reasonably high sensitivity of 90-92 percent and specificity of 91-98 percent for endometriomas, the sensitivity and specificity of MRI for other endometriotic lesions is 77 and 78 percent respectively.[24]

Studies comparing the utility of endorectal ultrasounds, transvaginal ultrasounds and MRI suggest that MRI performs similarly to TVS and rectal endoscopic sonography (RES) for the diagnosis of intestinal endometriosis but has higher sensitivity and likelihood ratios for utero-sacral ligament and vaginal endometriosis.[25]

Serum Markers in Endometriosis

Serum biomarkers have been a matter of continuing research to diagnose, measure disease severity and to monitor the effect of treatment. The best studied marker to date is the serum level of CA125.

However, CA125 lacks the sensitivity and specificity for diagnosis or even to be a screening test but high levels may reflect the severity of advanced disease.[26] The levels correlate better with large active endometriotic lesions compared to peritoneal adhesions and scarring.[27] Other serum markers (or combination of markers) like ICAM-1,

IL-6, monocyte chemoattractant protein-1, and IL-6 are gaining more attention in recent times. Othman et al reported significantly higher levels of these markers in patients with laparoscopic evidence of endometriosis compared to infertile women without endometriosis. Among these markers, IL-6 was found to have higher predictive value than others.[28]

Endometrial Nerve Fibers

Detection of nerve fibers in the functional layer of the endometrium is being investigated for use as a diagnostic test for endometriosis. M. Al-Jefout et al conducted a study on 99 consecutive women presenting with pelvic pain and/or infertility undergoing laparoscopy. The specificity and sensitivity of detection of nerve fibers in the endometrium were 83 and 98 percent respectively, with positive and negative predictive values of 91 and 96 percent respectively. The authors concluded that detection of nerve fibers on endometrial biopsy (under research conditions) provided a reliability of diagnosis of endometriosis which is close to the accuracy of laparoscopy.[29]

Laparoscopy

Endometriosis can exhibit a variety of appearances at laparoscopy in the form of peritoneal colorless papules, flare lesions showing active angiogenesis, black (with hemosiderin deposits) or scarred white implants, peritoneal windows, ovarian endometriomas, deep nodules, etc. The appearance is highly variable from person to person. Superficial lesions are usually located on the peritoneal surfaces of the pelvic organs with a conventional or blue or a blue-black "powder burn" appearance, as described by surgeons in the days gone past. Modern "classic" and highly active lesions have a red flame like or white scarred appearance. Ovarian endometriomas are formed by the invagination of endometriosis from the pelvic side wall into the ovarian cortex and contain thick brown chocolate like material. Deep infiltrating nodules are primarily found in the utero-sacral ligaments and the rectovaginal septum. Visual diagnosis in the absence of histological confirmation may be unreliable. A meta-analysis in 2004 which assumed a prevalence of 20 percent for endometriosis revealed that a finding of endometriosis on laparoscopy was incorrect in about half the cases.[30]

MANAGEMENT

The management of endometriosis entirely depends on the indication for treatment viz pain, menstrual disturbances, infertility or symptoms related to the other organ systems. In this chapter, we will focus on the management of endometriosis related infertility. Typically, successful management requires a combination of medical and surgical management. However, medical management plays no role in the management of infertility related to endometriosis except for down regulation prior to controlled ovarian hyperstimulation for assisted reproduction with superovulation +/- IUI or *in vitro* fertilization in patients with advanced disease.

Expectant Management

Patients with severe disease have a limited chance of spontaneous conception. However, the chance of spontaneous conception with mild to moderate disease without other subfertility factors is reasonable. Conception rates are similar in patients with mild to moderate disease to patients with unexplained infertility. Adamson D et al reported an average pregnancy rate of 45 percent with expectant management in patients with < stage 2 disease.[31] Expectant management remains a reasonable option in relatively young patients with mild to moderate disease with short duration of infertility and with no other subfertility factors.

When counseling patients for expectant management, it is important to clarify some of the risks with such an approach namely chance of progression of disease or complications related to endometriomas (like rupture or rarely torsion and even more rarely development of ovarian abscess from an endometrioma). Patients also need to be counselled about the possibility of failure of such an approach with possible need for surgical intervention or assisted reproduction in future.

Medical Management

Most of the medical therapies used for the treatment of endometriosis aim to inhibit ovulation and thereby suppress the hormonal stimulation of endometriotic lesions. As a result, these therapies can be effectively used for pain control or other symptoms of endometriosis but cannot be applied for the treatment of infertility related to the disease. A Cochrane review in which 24 trials were included revealed that the odds ratio for pregnancy following ovulation suppression versus placebo or no treatment for all women randomised was 0.79 (95% CI 0.54 to 1.14), P = 0.21 and 0.80 (95% CI 0.51 to 1.24), P = 0.32 respectively for subfertile couples only despite the use of a variety of suppression agents. There was no evidence of benefit from these infertility treatments.[32] Ovulation suppression was carried out using oral contraceptive pills, progestogen supplements, danazol or GnRH analogs. Hence, conventional hormonal treatment is not recommended except for short-term control of other symptoms in women who wish to conceive in the near future.

Surgical Management

The aim of surgical intervention in endometriosis related infertility is to excise endometriotic lesions and restore distorted pelvic anatomy along with restoration of the 'normal' hormonal and immune environment in the pelvis. The mode of surgical intervention can be via laparoscopy or laparotomy. Laparoscopic surgery is becoming more and more popular all over the world, as experience and expertise in the field continues to increase. The benefits of laparoscopy in the form of better clarity and magnification, quicker recovery resulting in shorter duration of hospital stay, reduced postoperative adhesion formation and relatively low incidence of complications in experienced hands outweigh the perceived disadvantages like the inability to palpate and feel structures, absence of 3 dimensional view and sometimes increased operative time. With advancing laparoscopic technique and increasing experience, more complicated endometriosis surgery is being performed laparoscopically in many places, including bowel resection, removal of moderately large and densely adherent endometriomas and excision requiring extensive ureterolysis.

Outcomes of Surgical Treatment

The pregnancy outcomes after surgical treatment depend not only on the stage of the disease but also on the presence of other subfertility factors, age of the female partner and possibly the duration of infertility. A Cochrane systematic review was conducted by Jacobson TZ et al[33] to evaluate the role of laparoscopic surgery for subfertility associated with endometriosis. Only 2 studies were eligible for inclusion and both the studies compared laparoscopic surgical treatment of minimal and mild endometriosis compared with diagnostic laparoscopy only. The main outcome measures were live birth, pregnancy, fetal losses, and complications of surgery. When combining live birth rate and ongoing pregnancy after 20 weeks, meta-analysis demonstrated an advantage of laparoscopic surgery when compared to diagnostic laparoscopy only, with an odds ratio (OR) of 1.64 (95% confidence interval 1.05 to 2.57) in favor of laparoscopic surgery. The odds ratio for clinical pregnancy was 1.66 (95% CI 1.09 to 2.51) favoring laparoscopic surgery. When considering fetal losses, there was no significant difference between laparoscopic surgery and diagnostic laparoscopy only. The OR was 1.33 (95% CI 0.60 to 2.94) favoring diagnostic laparoscopy only. The authors concluded that the use of laparoscopic surgery in the treatment of subfertility related to minimal and mild endometriosis may improve future fertility.[33] There is some evidence to support surgical management over medical or expectant management in cases of moderate to severe endometriosis. Apart from trying to restore anatomy, removal of adhesions containing foci of disease and making the ovaries accessible for future oocyte pick up for *in vitro* fertilization provide strong justification for surgical management. There is not enough evidence to justify repeated episodes of surgery and such patients may benefit more from assisted reproductive technologies.[34]

Surgery for Endometriomas

Surgical management of endometriomas has been a debatable issue due to concerns of reduced ovarian reserve as a result of surgery. A Cochrane systematic review comparing laparoscopic excision to ablation and drainage of endometriomas including two randomized studies for management of ovarian endometriomata of greater than 3 cm in size, for the primary symptom of pain revealed that laparoscopic excision of the cyst wall of the endometrioma was associated with reduced recurrence rate of the symptoms and reduced rate of recurrence of the endometrioma. For those women subsequently attempting to conceive it was also associated with a greatly increased spontaneous pregnancy rate in women who had documented prior sub-fertility (OR 5.21 CI 2.04-13.29).[35] There is also some evidence revealing improved response to gonadotropin treatment after excision but more RCT evidence is needed. There is growing evidence that ovarian reserve decreases as a result of excision of ovarian endometriomas with particular concern regarding the response to ovarian stimulation for ART following surgery. Laura Benaglia et al conducted a study on 93 women undergoing surgery for unilateral endometriomas and followed up the ones proceeding to IVF to monitor follicular growth. Absence of follicular growth in the operated ovary was seen in 12 patients with no effect on the contralateral ovary.[36]

Assisted Reproduction for Treatment of Endometriosis Related Infertility

Controlled Ovarian Hyperstimulation and IUI

Controlled ovarian hyperstimulation (COH) with or without IUI can be attempted using clomiphene citrate or gonadotropins in patients with patent fallopian tubes and normal semen parameters. Deaton JI et al conducted a RCT involving 67 couples comparing COH with clomiphene citrate and IUI with no intervention in patients with unexplained infertility or surgically corrected endometriosis. During the study, there were 14 pregnancies in 148 treated cycles (fecundity = 0.095) compared with 5 pregnancies in 150 untreated cycles (fecundity = 0.033). Using life-table analysis and the log-rank test, the difference in fecundities was statistically significant although there was no difference in pregnancy outcomes.[37] As per the ESHRE 2005 guidelines, treatment with IUI improves outcomes in minimal to mild endometriosis in stimulated cycles although the role of unstimulated IUI remains doubtful.[38] There is some evidence showing that endometriosis reduces the effectiveness of controlled ovarian stimulation and IUI.[39]

In vitro Fertilization

Endometriosis is a relatively common indication for IVF in modern infertility practice. Although IVF/ICSI can bypass most of the mechanisms of infertility related to endometriosis, studies have shown some important adverse effects of endometriosis on ART. The 2005 ESHRE guidelines recommended that IVF is an appropriate treatment especially if tubal function is compromised, if there is also male factor infertility and/or other treatments have failed.[38] Barnhart et al conducted a meta-analysis in 2002 including twenty-two published studies. The chance of achieving pregnancy was significantly lower for endometriosis patients (odds ratio, 0.56; 95% confidence interval, 0.44-0.70) when compared with tubal factor controls. They also reported a decrease in fertilization and implantation rates, and a significant decrease in the number of oocytes retrieved for endometriosis patients. Pregnancy rates for women with severe endometriosis were significantly lower than for women with mild disease (odds ratio, 0.60; 95% confidence interval, 0.42-0.87).[40]

Effect of Pre IVF Treatment on IVF Outcome

Presence of endometriomas or severe active peritoneal disease is thought to interfere with IVF outcomes. Until recently, the approach to endometriomas prior to ART was surgical treatment. A recent Cochrane systematic review of interventions for women with endometriomas prior to ART showed no effect of aspiration or cystectomy on clinical pregnancy rates compared to expectant management. The ovarian response was better in patients undergoing aspiration and poorer in patients undergoing cystectomy compared to expectant management. Surgical treatment of endometriomas has become a controversial issue due to the effects of surgery on ovarian reserve. This effect is further enhanced by surgery for bilateral endometriomas compared to unilateral ones. (Busacca et al 2006).

The review also included 1 trial comparing the effect of GnRH agonists v/s GnRH antagonists revealing no evidence of difference in the clinical pregnancy rates between the 2 groups. The number of mature oocytes retrieved and the ovarian response (E2 levels on the day of hcg trigger) was higher in the GnRH agonist group.[41]

Challenges Related to the Management of Endometriosis in Low-resource Settings

The main problem with management of endometriosis in low resource settings is related to the high cost of diagnostic measures and management. Laparoscopy is the gold standard for diagnosis but may not be easily available or affordable. It also has a reasonably long and difficult learning curve making it more challenging in low resource settings. This necessitates research to identify reliable, cheap and if possible non-invasive methods of diagnosis. The cost of ART remains another major issue in these settings. Undoubtedly, acceptance of minimal ovarian stimulation protocols for ART without affecting the outcome would reduce the total cost due to reduced need for gonadotropins. The concept of "soft IVF" is fast becoming popular in these settings.

CONCLUSION

Successful management of endometriosis remains one of the bigger challenges in current gynecology and infertility practice in spite of huge technical and medical advances. A greater awareness of the variability of the condition with respect to its clinical presentation will favorably affect the social, health and economic impacts of endometriosis. The highly complex and variable nature of the condition demands ongoing research for newer and simpler diagnostic and treatment modalities.

REFERENCES

1. Eskenazi B, Warner M. Epidemiology of endometriosis. Obstet Gynecol Clin North Am 1997; 24:235-58.
2. Goldstein DP, deCholnoky C, Emans SJ, Levantahl JM. Laparoscopy in the diagnosis and management of pelvic pain in adolescents. J Reprod Med 1980; 25:251-6
3. Halme J, Hammond M, Hulka J, et al. Retrograde menstruation in healthy women and in patients with endometriosis. Obstet Gynecol 1984; 64:151-4.
4. Witz C, Thomas M, Montoya-Rodriguez I, et al. Short-term culture of peritoneum explants confirms attachment of endometrium to intact peritoneal mesothelium. Fertil Steril 2001;75:385-90.
5. Bulletti C, DeZiegler D, Stefanetti M, et al. Endometriosis: Absence of recurrence in patients after endometrial ablation. Hum Reprod 2001; 16:2676-9.
6. Nisolle M, Donnez J. Peritoneal endometriosis, ovarian endometriosis, and adenomyotic nodules of the rectovaginal septum are three different entities. Fertil Steril 1997; 68:585-96.
7. Zheng W, Li N, Wang J, et al. Initial endometriosis showing direct morphologic evidence of metaplasia in the pathogenesis of ovarian endometriosis. Int J Gynecol Pathol 2005; 24:164-72.
8. Wu Y, Kajdacsy-Balla A, Strawn E, et al. Transcriptional characterizations of differences between eutopic and ectopic endometrium. Endocrinology 2006; 147:232-46.
9. Taylor R, Lundeen S, Giudice L. Emerging role of genomics in endometriosis research. Fertil Steril 2002;78:694-8.
10. Lebovic D, Baldocchi RA, Mueller MD, Taylor RN. Altered expression of a cell-cycle suppressor gene, Tob-1, in endometriotic cells by cDNA array analyses. Fertil Steril 2002;78:849-54.
11. Fraser I. Recognising, understanding and managing endometriosis. J Hum Reprod Sci; Issue 2, volume 1, 56-64.
12. Muscato JJ, Haney AF, Weinberg JB. Sperm phagocytosis by human peritoneal macrophages: A possible cause of infertility in endometriosis. Am J Obstet gynecol 1982; 144:503-10.
13. Yamashita Y, Ueda M, Takehara M, et al. Influence of severe endometriosis on gene expression of vascular endothelial growth factor and interleukin-6 in granulosa cells from patients undergoing controlled ovarian hyper stimulation for *in vitro* fertilization-embryo transfer. Fertil Steril 2002;78:865-71.
14. Oral E, Arici A, Olive DL, et al. Peritoneal fluid from women with moderate or severe endometriosis inhibits sperm motility: the role of seminal fluid components. Fertil Steril 1996;66:787-92.
15. Minguez Y, Rubio C, Bernal A, et al. The impact of endometriosis on couples undergoing intracytoplasmic sperm injection because of male infertility. Hum Reprod 1997;12:2282-5.
16. Diaz I, Navarro J, Blasco L, Simon C, Pellicer A, Remohi J. Impact of stage III – IV endometriosis on recipients of sibling oocytes: matched case control study. Fertil steril 2000;71:31-4.
17. Cirkel U, Ochs H, Mues B, et al. Inflammatory reaction in endometriotic tissue: an immunohistochemical study. Eur J Obstet Gynecol Reprod Biol 1993;48:43-50.
18. Klein N, Pergola G, Rao-Tekmal R, et al. Enhanced expression of resident leukocyte interferon gamma mRNA in endometriosis. Am J Reprod Immunol 1993; 30:74-81.
19. Lessey BA, Castelbaum AJ, Sawin SW, et al. Aberrant integrin expression in the endometrium of women with endometriosis. J Clin Endocrinol Metab 1994; 79:643-9.
20. Taylor HS, Bagot C, Kardana A, et al. HOX gene expression is altered in the endometrium of women with endometriosis. Hum Reprod 1999;14:1328-31.
21. D'Hooghe TM, Debrock S, Hill JA, Meuleman C. Endometriosis and subfertility: is the relationship resolved? Semin Reprod Med 2003;21:243-54.
22. Asch E, Levine D. Variations in appearance of endometriomas. J Ultrasound Med 2007;26:993-1002.
23. Hudelist G, English J, Thomas AE, Tinelli A, Singer CF, Keckstein J. Diagnostic accuracy of transvaginal ultrasound for non-invasive diagnosis of bowel endometriosis: Systematic review and meta-analysis. Ultrasound Obstet Gynecol. 2011 Mar; 37(3):257-63. doi: 10.1002/uog.8858.
24. Serra A, Hricak H. Gynaecologic imaging: Practical applications for magnetic resonance imaging. Curr Opin Obstet Gynecol Fertil 1997; 20:166-181.
25. Bazot M, Lafont C, Rouzier R, Roseau G, Thomassin-Naggara I, Daraï E. Diagnostic accuracy of physical examination, transvaginal sonography, rectal endoscopic sonography, and magnetic resonance imaging to diagnose deep infiltrating endometriosis. Fertil Steril. 2009 Dec; 92(6):1825-33. Epub 2008 Nov 18.
26. Cheng YM, Wang ST, Chou CY. Serum CA-125 in preoperative patients at high risk for endometriosis. Obstet Gynecol 2002;99:375-80.

27. Nagamani M, Kelver ME, Smith ER. CA 125 levels in monitoring therapy for endometriosis and in prediction of recurrence. Int J Fertil 1992; 37:227-31.
28. Othman EE, Hornung D, Salem HT, et al. Serum cytokines as biomarkers for nonsurgical prediction of endometriosis. Eur J Obstet Gynecol Reprod Biol 2008;137(2):240-46.
29. Al-Jefout M, Dezarnaulds G, Cooper M, Tokushige N, Luscombe GM, Markham R, Fraser I. diagnosis of endometriosis by detection of nerve fibres in an endometrial biopsy: A double blind study. Hum Reprod 2009, vol 24, No 12: 3019-24.
30. Wykes CB, Clark TJ, Khan KS. Accuracy of laparoscopy in the diagnosis of endometriosis: A systematic quantitative review: BJOG 2004; 11(11): 1204-12.
31. Adamson D. Surgical management of endometriosis. Semin Reprod Med 2003; 21:224-33.
32. Hughes E, Brown J, Collins JJ, Farquhar C, Fedorkow DM, Vandekerckhove P. Ovulation suppression for endometriosis. Cochrane Database Syst Rev. 2007 Jul 18 ;(3):CD000155.
33. Jacobson TZ, Duffy JM, Barlow D, Farquhar C, Koninckx PR, Olive D. Laparoscopic surgery for subfertility associated with endometriosis. Cochrane Database Syst Rev. 2010 Jan 20;(1):CD001398.
34. Adamson GD, Pasta DJ. Surgical treatment of endometriosis-associated infertility: Meta-analysis compared with survival analysis. Am J Obstet Gynecol 1994;171(6):1488-504; discussion 1504-5.
35. Hart RJ, Hickey M, Maouris P, Buckett W. Excisional surgery versus ablative surgery for ovarian endometriomata. Cochrane Database Syst Rev. 2008 Apr 16 ;(2):CD004992.
36. Benaglia L, Somigliana E, Vighi V, Ragni G, Vercellini P, Fedele L. Rate of severe ovarian damage following surgery for endometriomas. Hum Reprod. 2010 Mar; 25(3):678-82. Epub 2010 Jan 17.
37. Deaton JL, Gibson M, Blackmer KM, Nakajima ST, Badger GJ, Brumsted JR. A randomized, controlled trial of clomiphene citrate and intrauterine insemination in couples with unexplained infertility or surgically corrected endometriosis. Fertil Steril 1990; 54(6):1083-8.
38. Kennedy S, Bergqvist A, Chapron C, D'Googee T, Dunselman G, Greb R, Hummelshoj L, Prentice A, Saridogan E; on behalf of the special interest group for endometriosis and endometrium guideline development group. ESHRE guideline for the diagnosis and treatment of endometriosis. Hum Reprod 2005;20:2698-704.
39. Hughes EG. The effectiveness of ovulation induction and intrauterine insemination in the treatment of persistent infertility: A meta-analysis. Hum Reprod. 1997;12(9):1865-72.
40. Barnhart K, Dunsmoor-Su R, Coutifaris C. Effect of endometriosis on *in vitro* fertilization. Fertil Steril. 2002;77(6):1148-55.
41. Benschop L, Farquhar C, van der Poel N, Heineman MJ. Interventions for women with endometrioma prior to assisted reproductive technology. Cochrane Database Syst Rev. 2010 Nov 10;(11):CD008571.

Chapter

11

Polycystic Ovary Syndrome and Infertility

Hang Wun Raymond Li, Ernest Hung Yu Ng, PC Ho

INTRODUCTION

Polycystic ovary syndrome (PCOS) is the most common reproductive endocrine disorder in women of reproductive age, affecting about 4 to 8 percent of premenopausal women in Western countries.[1] Its true prevalence in Asian-Oceanic populations is not precisely known.

PCOS is a heterogeneous group of clinical features which may include oligo-anovulation and hence menstrual irregularity and subfertility, hyperandrogenism, and metabolic disorders such as obesity, insulin resistance and other features constituting the metabolic syndrome. Apart from ethnic differences, the heterogeneity could also be due to different criteria that have been used to define the condition. In recent years, the revised diagnostic criteria as agreed upon in the Rotterdam consensus meeting (the Rotterdam criteria) have been widely adopted. According to this, the diagnosis of PCOS is established in the presence of at least two of the following three criteria: (i) Oligo- and/or anovulation; (ii) Clinical and/or biochemical features of hyperandrogenism; and (iii) The presence of polycystic ovary (PCO) morphology, with the exclusion of other etiologies of hyperandrogenism.[2]

Although the main theme of this book is on managing infertility, as we understand that PCOS is not purely a fertility problem, we shall also briefly discuss the management of related health issues such as menstrual problems, clinical hyperandrogenism and metabolic dysfunction, which very often coexist with fertility problem and are not to be neglected.

INITIAL ASSESSMENT AND INVESTIGATIONS

History

Menstrual irregularity is the most common clinical feature that women with PCOS present with. A detailed menstrual history needs to be taken, including the cycle length, regularity and the last menstrual period. Usually women with PCOS have oligo-amenorrhea dating back to their adolescent years. Any history of abnormal intermenstrual bleeding should be noted since women with chronic anovulation are at a higher risk of endometrial pathology. As for all patients presenting with oligo-amenorrhea, symptoms associated with hyperprolactinemia (galactorrhea, headache, visual disturbance), thyroid dysfunction and climacteric symptoms should be enquired as well, in addition to any related drug or medical history which might have precipitated the menstrual cycle disturbance.

Hyperandrogenic symptoms, such as hirsutism, acne, greasy skin, and male pattern alopecia should be enquired about. Any self-remedies like shaving, waxing or cosmetic treatments for hirsutism should be documented. Also ask for any rapidly progressing symptoms of virilization for which we need to exclude adrenal or ovarian androgen-secreting tumors which in general are rare causes of androgen excess.

Other relevant history would include any recent weight changes, diet and exercise pattern, family history of PCOS and metabolic syndrome.

Physical Examination

The following would be the relevant physical findings to record:

i. Height, weight and body-mass index.
ii. *Waist-to-hip ratio (WHR):* In the WHO definition, WHR > 0.85 in women is part of diagnostic criteria of metabolic syndrome. In the American Heart Association definition, only the waist circumference is used and a value of > 80 cm in Asian women is part of metabolic syndrome.
iii. Blood pressure.
iv. Hirsutism assessed by Ferriman-Gallwey scoring, acne and male pattern baldness.
v. Acanthosis nigricans (marker of insulin resistance).
vi. Galactorrhea and goiter.
vii. Pelvic examination.
viii. Sign of virilization, e.g. clitormegaly.

Investigations

In the Rotterdam criteria, pelvic ultrasound scan provides one of the cardinal feature for diagnosing PCOS. The transvaginal scan is usually preferred as it can provide a better resolution of ovarian morphology. In women who have no sexual exposure or cannot tolerate a transvaginal scan, a transrectal or transabdominal scan may be the alternative. The ultrasound criteria for PCO morphology has been defined as either 12 or more follicles measuring 2 to 9 mm in diameter, and/or increased ovarian volume (>10 ml); only one ovary fitting this definition is sufficient for defining PCO.[3] If there is a dominant follicle (>10 mm) or a corpus luteum, the scan should be repeated in the next cycle.

A blood test for serum follicle-stimulating hormone (FSH), thyroid-stimulating hormone (TSH) and prolactin are the basic work-up for oligo-amenorrhea. Serum total testosterone can be checked, and in case of severe hyperandrogenemia (total testosterone > 5 nmol/l)[4] or signs of severe hirsutism or virilization, it needs to be followed by checking 17-hydroxyprogesterone to exclude late-onset congenital adrenal hyperplasia, an overnight dexamethasone suppression test to exclude Cushing's syndrome, as well as appropriate imaging (ultrasound scan of the pelvis and CT scan of the adrenals) to exclude an androgen-secreting tumor.

Tests like free testosterone or serum sex-hormone binding globulin (SHBG) to calculate the free androgen index are more of academic value but do not usually influence clinical management, and can hence be skipped in low-cost settings.

Before managing anovulatory subfertility due to PCOS, semen analysis of the male partner is recommended to exclude severe male factors which could influence on the choice of treatment. Simple oral medical treatment like antiestrogens with or without metformin can be commenced without tubal assessment unless tuboperitoneal factor is strongly suggested by history.

TREATMENT OF ANOVULATORY SUBFERTILITY IN PCOS

Weight Reduction

According to the WHO definition, overweight is defined as BMI $\geq$=25 kg/m^2, and obesity as BMI $\geq$=30 kg/m^2. Obesity is associated with poor response to fertility treatment, pregnancy loss and late-pregnancy complications. Weight loss should be advised prior to fertility treatment if the woman has a body mass index (BMI) above 25 kg/m^2. Weight loss helps to improve insulin resistance, lipid profile and hyperandrogenism. It also improves ovulation rates and possibly pregnancy rate.[5-7] There is limited data on its effect on pregnancy complications. Weight loss should be achieved with lifestyle modification by caloric restriction and increased physical exercise. Caloric restriction by a 500 to 1000 kcal/day reduction has been suggested to be effective, aiming at reducing the body weight by 7 to 10 percent over a period of 6 to 12 months. Moderate exercise lasting for 30 minutes or more per day is advisable.[6] The effects of caloric restriction, excessive physical exertion or pharmacological intervention during early pregnancy are not yet known, hence those interventions should precede ovulation induction.[8] It has been suggested that a modest weight loss of 5 percent may restore ovulation and fertility.

Clomiphene Citrate (CC)

Clomiphene citrate should be offered as a first-line therapy. It should be started at a dose of 50 mg daily on day 2 to 6 following a spontaneous or progestogen-induced bleeding. Ovarian response should be monitored by ultrasound on day 12 in the first cycle to assess the follicular development and endometrial thickness. If there are three or more mature follicles, the treatment cycle should be cancelled and the couple is advised to abstain from intercourse in order to reduce the risk of high-order multiple pregnancy. Ovulation can be confirmed in the mid-luteal phase with measurement of the serum progesterone concentration. If ovulation is confirmed, treatment at the same dosage can be maintained up to a maximum of 6 to 12 ovulatory cycles. The dose can be stepped up to 100 to 150 mg per day for 5 days per cycle if there is no ovulatory response. The reported ovulation rate is 75 to 80 percent, conception rate is 22 percent per ovulatory cycle, and cumulative live-birth rate is about 50 to 60 percent for up to 6 cycles.[8] Side effects may include hot flushes, headaches and visual disturbance although these are uncommon; multiple pregnancy rate can be up to 8 to 10 percent, and the risk of ovarian hyperstimulation syndrome (OHSS) is rare.

Metformin

A Cochrane review[9] assessed the effectiveness of insulin sensitizing drugs in fertility treatment for women with PCOS. The routine use of metformin either alone or in combination with CC appears to have limited efficacy in improving fertility. Although metformin alone improves the ovulation and clinical pregnancy rates than placebo or no treatment, its efficacy is inferior to CC alone. Co-treatment with metformin and CC improves the ovulation rate and clinical pregnancy rate, but not the livebirth rate in general, compared with CC alone.

In a subgroup of PCOS patients who are obese or CC-resistant, cotreatment with metformin and CC may improve clinical pregnancy rate[10,11] and can be a second-line option before gonadotropin induction or ovarian drilling is considered, especially in low resources settings. The recommended dose is 500 mg t.d.s. or 850 mg b.d. with meals. Side effects include dose-dependent gastrointestinal upset including nausea, vomiting, diarrhea. Lactic acidosis is a rare though serious complication, and hence metformin should not be prescribed to patients with renal, hepatic or major cardiovascular disease or hypoxia. When metformin is used in combination with CC, follicular response and ovulation should be monitored in the usual way as in CC treatment. There is some evidence from observational studies that the risk of miscarriage may be reduced if metformin is continued in pregnancy.[12,13] However, there is as yet no randomized trial reported in the literature on the use of metformin in pregnancy in women with PCOS. The use of metformin in pregnancy is classified by the United States FDA as Class B, but in view of inadequate evidence on its use in pregnancy, discontinuation is recommended when pregnancy is confirmed.

There is currently no evidence to support the use of other insulin sensitizers for fertility treatment in PCOS patients.

Laparoscopic Ovarian Drilling (LOD)

LOD can be offered as an alternative to gonadotropin treatment in anovulatory PCOS subjects who are resistant to CC. It may be of value in low-resource settings since it is less costly than gonadotropin treatment. It also provides laparoscopic pelvic/tubal assessment, and in case where tubo-peritoneal factor is identified, therapeutic surgery in the form of adhesiolysis or tubal reconstruction may be attempted, which can be more cost-saving compared to assisted reproduction. Another advantage with LOD is that it can achieve monofollicular ovulation with no risk of OHSS or multiple pregnancy,[14] and there is no need for intensive monitoring compared with gonadotropin induction, which are again valuable in low resource settings. Current evidence suggested that the efficacy of LOD is equivalent to that of gonadotropin in inducing ovulation.[14] A pregnancy rate of 67 percent has been reported after LOD in CC-resistant PCOS women.[15] About 50 percent will need post-operative adjuvants. CC can be added after 3 months and gonadotropin considered after 6 months if there is no ovulation.

A recommended method of LOD makes use of monopolar diathermy needle to make 4 punctures (7-8 mm in depth) into each ovary, using a 30W current for 5 seconds in each puncture.[15]

There is no evidence that LOD is useful for non-fertility indications, e.g. treating menstrual irregularity or hyperandrogenism.

Gonadotropin

Gonadotropin, like LOD, can be a second-line treatment for patients who do not respond to the maximum dose of CC (CC resistance) or who do not conceive despite being ovulatory on CC (CC failure), with or without metformin co-treatment where appropriate. Compared to LOD, the use of gonadotropins for ovulation induction usually involves higher cost, and hence may also be reserved as a third-line treatment option in low-resources settings before assisted reproduction is considered. Assessment of the tubal status is necessary before gonadotropin therapy if this has not already been done already.

The principle of using exogenous gonadotropins is to overcome the FSH threshold required for the follicular development.

There is no difference between urinary FSH (uFSH) and recombinant FSH (rFSH) in ovulation and pregnancy rates, as well as in the incidence of miscarriage, OHSS, multiple pregnancy and duration of stimulation.[16] Therefore, the use of uFSH preparations, e.g. human menopausal gonadotropin (hMG), may be preferred in low-resources settings due to its significantly lower cost compared to rFSH, except when the patient develops local allergic reactions which are sometimes related to the protein impurities in the uFSH products.

The chronic low dose step-up regimen is currently the recommended protocol by many authorities worldwide. By determining the FSH threshold gradually, such protocol tries to avoid excessive stimulation and multifollicular development. FSH is administered at a low starting dose (37.5-75 IU/day) for at least 10-14 days[8] and the daily dose is increased by 37.5 IU at weekly intervals up to a maximum of 225 IU if there is no ovarian response. The same dose is maintained once follicular growth is observed. Once 1 or 2 dominant follicles reach a mean diameter of 18 mm, human chorionic gonadotropin (hCG) is administered at a dose of 5000 to 10000 IU to trigger final maturation and ovulation, and timed intercourse will be advised. It may take several weeks to achieve an ovarian response in women with a high FSH threshold, particularly during the first treatment cycle. In subsequent cycles, the starting dose can be adjusted according to the ovarian response in previous cycles. If there are three or more dominant follicles, the treatment cycle should be cancelled and the couple should be advised to abstain from intercourse.

Ovarian response must be monitored during gonadotropin treatment to allow for dose adjustment, timing of hCG trigger and safeguard against excessive response where the cycle should be cancelled. Ultrasound scan offers a direct assessment of the number of dominant follicles and their sizes, and should be adopted as the preferred monitoring tool, whereas serum estradiol determination does not usually add in additional information and hence can be skipped to save cost.[17]

The use of GnRH analog (GnRHa) prior to gonadotropin administration may theoretically lower the basal LH tone and prevent premature LH surge. However, a meta-analysis[18] of three randomized trials showed no clear benefit in the routine use of GnRHa in conjunction with gonadotropin for ovulation induction. Moreover, the use of GnRHa will increase the cost both from its own cost as well the increased dose of gonadotropins usually required when GnRHa is used. Hence, the use of GnRHa should be considered only in patients with a previous history of premature luteinization.

Ovulation induction by gonadotropins in PCOS can result in a 6-month cumulative pregnancy rate of about 50-60 percent with a miscarriage rate of 30-40 percent. With the chronic low dose step-up protocol, the rates of severe OHSS and multiple pregnancy can be as low as <0.1 percent and 6 percent respectively. This is superior to the conventional regimens using higher dose of gonadotropins, and is particularly important in low-resources settings where managing complications like OHSS and multiple pregnancy would impose a tremendous burden to the medical resources.

Combined ovulation induction and intrauterine insemination (IUI) can be considered when there is concomitant mild male factor.

In Vitro Fertilization (IVF)

IVF should be reserved as the final treatment option for those failing ovulation induction treatment or those with other concurrent indications for IVF such as severe male factor or tuboperitoneal factor. Apart from the cost involved in assisted reproduction technology, the risks of OHSS and multiple pregnancies and their burden on the medical resources should be borne in mind. Reference can be made to the rest of this book regarding assisted reproduction treatment in the low-cost setting.

The main problem with IVF in patients with PCOS is the increased risk of excessive response and OHSS. As the incidence of OHSS in women undergoing IVF with the use of GnRH antagonists is significantly lower than that in women down-regulated with GnRH agonists, GnRH antagonists should be used in women with PCOS to prevent the premature rise of serum LH. There is also evidence that the use of metformin before ovarian stimulation with gonadotropins would reduce the risk of OHSS.[19] Therefore, metformin may also be used in women with PCOS undergoing IVF treatment if there is no contraindication.

If the ovarian response is excessive despite the above precautions, the final maturation of oocytes may be induced with a dose of GnRH agonist instead of hCG. When GnRH antagonist is used, the pituitary is still capable of responding to GnRH agonist with the release of endogenous LH which has a shorter half-life than hCG. This will reduce the risk of OHSS. Oocytes may be retrieved and fertilized *in vitro* but all the embryos are cryopreserved and not replaced in the stimulated cycle. This will eliminate the risk of late-onset OHSS associated with a pregnancy.

A meta-analysis showed that in women with PCOS undergoing IVF, when compared to non-PCOS women, there was a significant increase in cancellation rate (2.8% vs 4.1%), a significantly longer duration of stimulation (1.2 days), and significantly more oocytes being obtained (2.9). However, the fertilization rates and pregnancy rates were similar.[20]

Flow chart 11.1: Ovulation induction in PCOS patients with anovulatory subfertility

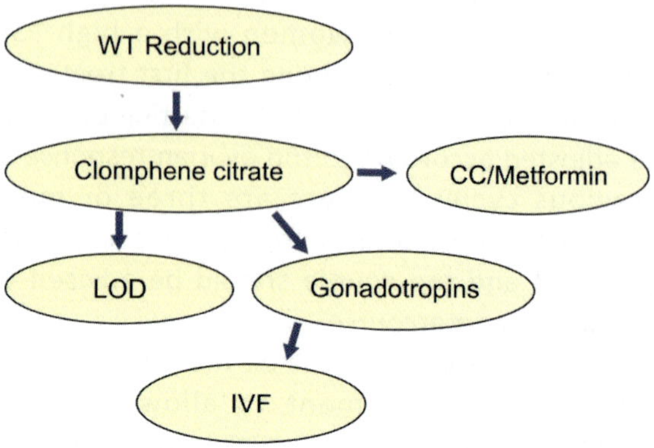

SUMMARY

Weight reduction should be the first step in treating anovulatory subfertility in women with PCOS who are obese. In those who are slim or those who remain anovulatory after optimal weight control, an oral anti-estrogen such as clomiphene citrate would be the first-line medical treatment for ovulation induction. In clomiphene-resistant patients, metformin co-treatment may be attempted. Both LOD and gonadotropin can be the second-line treatment with equal efficacy, but the former is less costly and can offer the opportunity for tubo-peritoneal assessment and therapeutic surgery. For those who fail these or those with concurrent severe male factor or tubo-peritoneal pathology, IVF would be the final resort (Flow chart 11.1).

OTHER HEALTH PROBLEMS IN PCOS

Apart from managing their fertility problem which is the main focus of this book, women with PCOS also commonly suffers from oligo-amenorrhea and would have increased risk of endometrial hyperplasia and cancer secondary to chronic unopposed estrogen stimulation. Hence it is important for them to have periodic induction of withdrawal bleeding with either combined oral contraceptive pills or progestogen when they are not undergoing fertility treatment. They may also have hyperandrogenic symptoms such as acne, seborrhea and hirsutism. They also have increased risk of metabolic syndrome in the long-term, and it would be sensible to advise adoption of a healthy lifestyle, regular monitoring of blood pressure, body weight, as well as blood sugar and lipid profile. The optimal interval to monitor blood sugar and lipids for the best cost-effectiveness is yet to be determined. An oral glucose tolerance test every 2 years can be suggested, especially in those who are obese, over 40 years of age, having history of gestational diabetes mellitus or family history of type 2 diabetes mellitus. This could be repeated earlier if additional risk factors emerge. Blood pressure monitoring during every visit, as well as biannual screening of lipid profile may be suggested. It should be noted that the use of fasting glucose alone has been shown to under-estimate diabetes prevalence and cardiovascular risk when compared to the use of oral glucose tolerance test, particularly among obese women.[21]

REFERENCES

1. Azziz R, Woods KS, Reyna R, Key TJ, Knochenhauer ES, Yildiz BO. The prevalence and features of the polycystic ovary syndrome in an unselected population. J Clin Endocrinol Metab 2004;89: 2745-9.
2. The Rotterdam ESHRE/ASRM-sponsored PCOS Consensus Workshop Group. Revised 2003 consensus on diagnostic criteria and long-term health risks related to polycystic ovary syndrome. Hum Reprod 2004;19:41-7.
3. Balen AH, Laven JSE, Tan SL, Dewailly D. Ultrasound assessment of the polycystic ovary: international consensus definitions. Hum Reprod Update 2003; 9:505-14.
4. Balan A. The Polycystic Ovary Syndrome: Guidance for Diagnosis and Management. Polycystic Ovary Syndrome UK, January 2006.
5. Norman RJ, Davies MJ, Lord J, Moran LJ. The role of lifestyle modification in polycystic ovary syndrome. Trends Endocrinol Metab 2002;13:251-7.
6. Moran LJ, Pasquali R, Teede HJ, Hoeger KM, Norman RJ. Treatment of obesity in polycystic ovary syndrome: a position statement of the Androgen Excess and Polycystic Ovary Syndrome Society. Fertil Steril 2009; 92(6):1966-82.
7. Moran LJ, Hutchison SK, Norman RJ, Teede HJ. Lifestyle changes in women with polycystic ovary syndrome. Cochrane Database Syst Rev 2011;(2): CD007506.
8. The Thessaloniki ESHRE/ASRM-Sponsored PCOS Consensus Workshop Group. Consensus on infertility treatment related to polycystic ovary syndrome. Hum Reprod 2008;23(3):462-77.
9. Tang T, Lord JM, Norman RJ, Yasmin E, Balen AH. Insulin-sensitising drugs (metformin, rosiglitazone, pioglitazone, D-chiro-inositol) for women with polycystic ovary syndrome, oligo-amenorrhoea and subfertility. Cochrane Database Syst Rev 2010; (1):CD003053.
10. Moll E, van der Veen F, van Wely M. The role of metformin in polycystic ovary syndrome: a systematic review. Hum Reprod Update 2007;13(6):527-37.
11. Creanga AA, Bradley HM, McCormick C, Witkop CT. Use of metformin in polycystic ovary syndrome: a meta-analysis. Obstet Gynecol 2008;111:959-68.
12. Glueck CJ, Philips H, Cameron D, Sieve-Smith L, Wang P. Continuing metformin throughout pregnancy in women with polycystic ovary syndrome appears to safely reduce first-trimester spontaneous abortion: a pilot study. Fertil Steril 2001;75(1):46-52.
13. Jakubowicz DJ, Iuorno MJ, Jakubowicz S, Roberts KA, Nestler JE. Effects of metformin on early pregnancy loss in the polycystic ovary syndrome. J Clin Endocrinol Metab 2002;87(2):524-9.
14. Farquhar C, Lilford R, Marjoribanks J, Vanderkerchove P. Laparoscopic 'drilling' by diathermy or laser for ovulation induction in anovulatory polycystic ovary syndrome. Cochrane Database Syst Rev 2007; (3):CD001122.
15. Amer SAK, Li TC, Cooke ID. A prospective dose-finding study of the amount of thermal energy required for laparoscopic ovarian diathermy. Hum Reprod 2003; 18(8):1693-8.
16. Bayram N, van Wely M, Van der Veen F. Recombinant FSH versus urinary gonadotropins or recombinant FSH for ovulation induction in subfertility associated with polycystic ovary syndrome. Cochrane Database Syst Rev 2001;(2):CD002121.
17. Shoham Z, Di Carlo C, Patel A, Conway GS, Jacobs HS. Is it possible to run a successful ovulation induction program based solely on ultrasound monitoring? The importance of endometrial measurements. Fertil Steril 1991;56:836-41.
18. Hughes E, Collins J, Vandekerckhove P. Gonadotropin-releasing hormone analogue as an adjunct to gonadotropin therapy for clomiphene-resistant polycystic ovary syndrome. Cochrane Database Syst Rev 2000;(2):CD000097.
19. Tso LO, Costello MF, Albuquerque LE, Andriolo RB, Freitas V. Metformin treatment before and during IVF or ICSI in women with polycystic ovary syndrome. Cochrane Database Syst Rev 2009;(2):CD006105.
20. Heijnen EM, Eijkemans MJ, Hughes EG, Laven JS, Macklon NS, Fauser BC. A meta-analysis of outcomes of conventional IVF in women with polycystic ovary syndrome. Hum Reprod Update 2006;12(1):13-21.
21. Wild RA, Carmina E, Diamanti-Kandarakis E, Dokras A, Escobar-Morreale HF, Futterweit W, Lobo R, Norman RJ, Talbott E, Dumesic DA. Assessment of cardiovascular risk and prevention of cardiovascular disease in women with the polycystic syndrome: a consensus statement by the Androgen Excess and Polycystic Ovary Syndrome (AE-PCOS) Society. J Clin Endocrinol Metab 2010;95(5):2038-49.

Chapter

12

Fibroids and Infertility

Jaideep Malhotra, Lakhwinder Singh, Narendra Malhotra

Uterine leiomyomas are present in 20 to 40 percent of reproductive-age women. Only 5 percent of fibroids are believed to be located in the submucosa where they can distort the endometrial cavity or cause abnormal bleeding patterns.[1] Submucosal and intramural fibroids that protrude into the endometrial cavity (Figs 12.1 and 12.2) have been associated with decreased pregnancy rate (PR) and implantation rate (IR) in patients undergoing *in vitro* fertilization (IVF).[2]

Fibroids that distort the endometrial cavity may impair fertility by several mechanisms including the creation of an abnormal site for placental implantation and growth resulting in infertility, an increased risk of spontaneous abortions, preterm labor and delivery. The accepted standard of care for patients with cavity-distorting submucosal fibroids is myomectomy before IVF.[2-4]

Small intramural fibroids are associated with a significant reduction in the cumulative pregnancy, ongoing pregnancy and livebirth rates in women undergoing three cycles of IVF/ICSI compared with controls. This can have important implications, particularly for women failing to conceive after

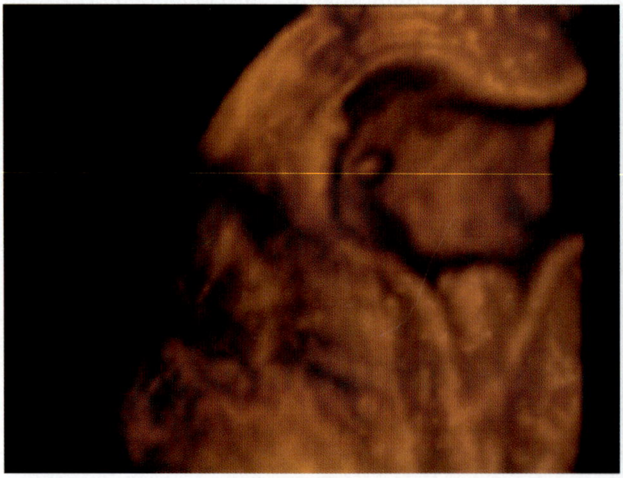

Fig. 12.1

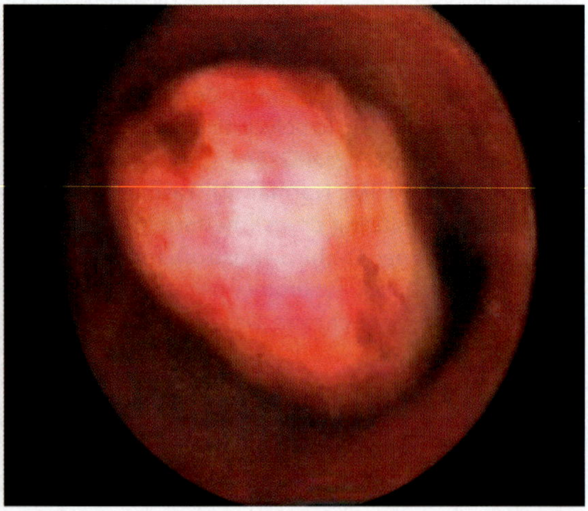

Fig. 12.2

Figs 12.1 and 12.2: Submucous fibroid seen by 3D-USG and hysteroscopy their first IVF cycle and considering further treatment attempts.[5-7]

The mechanisms by which small intramural fibroids exert their adverse effect on the success rate of IVF are unclear but may include altered myometrial contractility, uterine vascular distortion,[8,9] endometrial inflammation, thinning and atrophy[10,11] as well as exerting an adverse effect on gamete migration. Recently, alterations in gene expression (particularly those regulating retinoid synthesis and insulin-like growth factors metabolism) were found in myoma tissue compared with adjacent normal myometrium. Because the same genes are involved in implantation and post-implantation embryonic development, these findings may provide a link between the presence of fibroids and adverse reproductive outcome.[3,12,13]

The reproductive performance of women with small intramural fibroids following myomectomy should also consider the influence of other factors, such as female age and duration of infertility, on reproductive outcome after surgery.[14-16] Myoma size, location, number, age of patients, duration of infertility are key factors when discussing the outcomes after myomectomy (Fig. 12.3). Unfortunately, these factors are not separable for an individual patient, and the surgeon must weigh the cumulative impact of all three factors when deciding how and when to perform a myomectomy. It is important to clarify this issue, as myomectomy for intramural fibroids has a risk of morbidity and adhesion formation, and surgery should not be considered unless the benefits outweigh the risks.

MYOMAS AND OBSTETRICAL OUTCOMES

Obstetrical outcomes are compromised by uterine, according to a population-based retrospective study by Sheiner et al.[17,18] Compared to controls, women with uterine myomas during pregnancy had a 3.5-fold increase in the incidence of intrauterine growth restriction (6.8% vs 1.9%), a 4-fold increase in placental abruption (2.8% vs 0.7%), a 5-fold increase in the incidence of transverse lie or breech presentation (16.9% vs 2.4%), a 5-fold increase in the cesarean section rate (57.7% vs 10.8%), a 70 percent increase in premature rupture of membranes (9.6% vs 5.5%), and were three times more likely to receive transfusion (4.2% vs 1.4%). All of these outcomes were significant ($P < 0.001$). Adjusting for maternal age, parity, gestational age, and malpresentation, pregnancies in the myoma group still had a 6.7-fold risk of cesarean section (95% confidence interval [CI] 5.5–8.1, $P < 0.01$), 2.5-fold increase of placental abruption (95% CI 1.6–4.2, $P < 0.001$), and a 40 percent increase in preterm deliveries compared to pregnancies without uterine fibroids (95% CI 1.1–1.7, $P = 0.009$). The size and location of the myomas were not described in this study, but other studies have shown that fibroids adjacent to the placenta increase the risk of bleeding and premature rupture of membranes. It would appear that myomectomy could be justified in some circumstances to reduce the risk of adverse pregnancy outcomes in some patients.

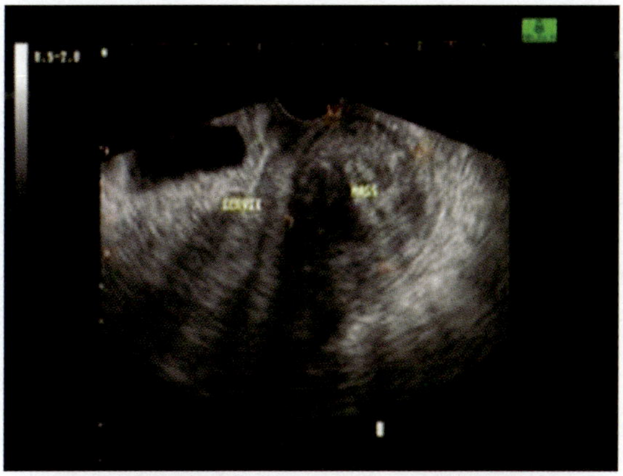

Fig. 12.3: Cervical fibroid seen on transvaginal sonography (TVS)

Laparoscopic versus Abdominal Myomectomy

Laparoscopic myomectomy is clearly associated with shorter hospitalization, faster recovery, less expense, less pain, less blood loss, less fever, and fewer surgical complications compared to abdominal myomectomy (Fig. 12.4). Pregnancy rates and recurrence rates appear to be comparable between laparoscopic and abdominal myomectomy. Surgical times may be longer than with open procedures, but the recovery time is shorter. In these studies, the conversion rate to laparotomy was typically less than 2 percent of cases, even large deep myomas were resected.

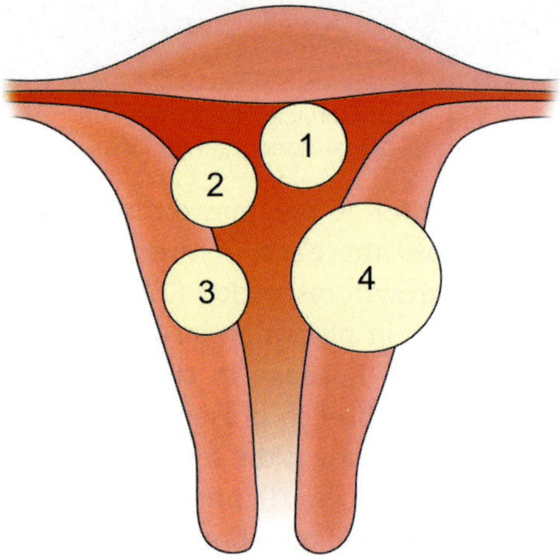

Fig. 12.4: 4 sites of myoma decides route of removal

"It is apparent that little remains in the reproductive surgeon's armamentarium that can't be accomplished through the use of a laparoscope"—Dr Alan DeCherney (Figs 12.5 and 12.6). A role for laparoscopy is well supported in the treatment of myoma associated subfertility.

ADHESIONS

Laparoscopic versus Abdominal Myomectomy

Dubuisson et al[15] performed second-look laparoscopy in 45 women after laparoscopic myomectomy and assessed 72 myomectomy sites. Adhesions were found in 36 percent of patients and at 17 percent of each myomectomy site. The adhesion rate was highest with posterior incisions, but the rate of adhesion formation was only 33 percent at this site. The sigmoid colon was the

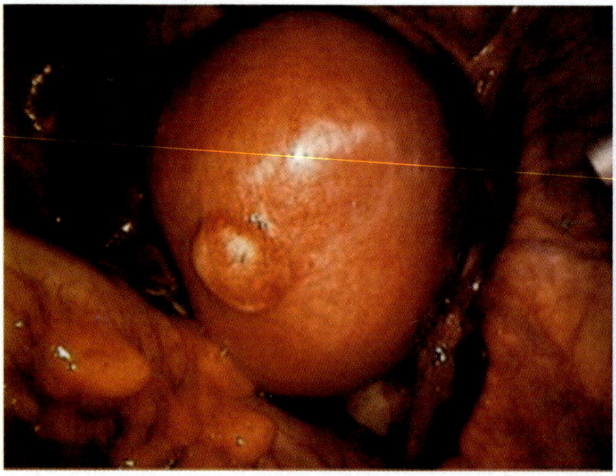

Fig. 12.5

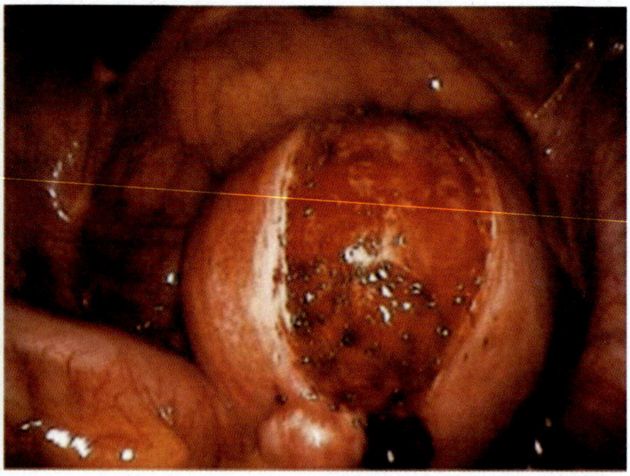

Fig. 12.6

Figs 12.5 and 12.6: Large fibroid laparoscopic removal

leading site for uterine adhesions, followed by the bladder, adnexa, small bowel, and peritoneum. Of those who had adnexal adhesions, most had preexisting adnexal adhesions, another surgical procedure carried out at the same time as myomectomy, or a posterior myomectomy site. The investigators concluded that the rate of adhesions after laparoscopic myomectomy was low and rarely involved the adnexa.

Adhesion rate with laparoscopic myomectomy is consistently lower than the rate expected with abdominal myomectomy. Oxygenized regenerated cellulose and autocrosslinked hyaluronic acid gel both appear to reduce adhesions, and GnRH—a therapy may also be effective for this purpose.

PREGNANCY AFTER LAPAROSCOPIC MYOMECTOMY

Overall pregnancy rates and spontaneous abortion (SAB) rates with laparoscopic myomectomy are comparable to abdominal myomectomy (Table 12.1). This appears to be true for patients who require laparoscopic repair of the endometrial cavity, have large myomas, and for those who require IVF.[19]

The only prospective randomized study to evaluate pregnancy rates after laparoscopic and abdominal myomectomy was published in 2000 by Seracchioli et al[18] and there was no difference in pregnancy rates or outcomes. The study included 56 women who attempted to conceive after laparoscopic myomectomy, and 59 after abdominal myomectomy. All women were instructed to delay pregnancy for 6 months postoperatively. The pregnancy rate was 54 percent with laparoscopic myomectomy, not different compared to 56 percent with abdominal myomectomy. The cumulative pregnancy rates by Kaplan-Meier analysis was approximately 26 percent by 12 months in both groups, approximately 45 percent by 2 years, and approximately 50 percent by 3 years. The abortion rate was 20 percent in the laparoscopic myomectomy group and 12 percent with open myomectomy, but this difference was not significant. There was no difference in the incidence of preterm deliveries. The cesarean section rate was 78 percent in the abdominal myomectomy group, and 65 percent with laparoscopic myomectomy corresponding to a vaginal delivery rate of 22 percent and 35 percent, respectively.

Three case control studies have evaluated pregnancy outcomes after laparoscopic myomectomy. Bulletti et at[21] retrospectively compared pregnancy outcomes in three groups of infertile women: (1) Women with uterine fibroids and no surgery, (2) Laparoscopic myomectomy, and (3) Unexplained infertility. Delivery rates were significantly higher with laparoscopic myomectomy (42%) compared to untreated women with fibroids (11%) and women with unexplained infertility (25%). The spontaneous abortion rate was higher in the untreated myoma group compared to either the laparoscopic myomectomy group or those with unexplained infertility, although the difference did not meet statistical significance.

Stringer and colleagues' retrospective case-control study compared 49 women with abdominal myomectomy and 49 women with laparoscopic myomectomy.[22] Seven pregnancies were reported in the laparoscopic group, including three who had delivered by the time of publication. All three were delivered by elective cesarean section at term, and no evidence of uterine dehiscence was found.

Campo and co-investigators[23] retrospectively studied 41 women with infertility attributed to uterine fibroids, including 22 treated with laparoscopic myomectomy, and 19 abdominal myomectomy patients. Postoperative outcomes were similar in both groups. Overall the pregnancy rate was 61 percent, and included a livebirth rate of 86 percent and a spontaneous abortion rate of

Table 12.1: Pregnancy outcomes after laparoscopic myomectomy (patients attempting pregnancy)

Study	Number pregnant	Pregnancy rate	SAB	Livebirth rate	C/S rate	Uterine rupture
RCTs	30 L/S	54%	20%	77%	65%	0
Seracchioli, 2000	33 abd	56%	12%	88%	78%	0
Case control	44 L/S	42%	7%	93%		0
Bulletti, 1999	12 No Tx	11%	45%	55%		0
	27 Unexpl	25%	7%	93%		0
Case series						
Ribeiro, 1999	18	64%	12%	78%	57%	0
Landi, 2003	72		17%	79%	46%	0
Campo, 1999	13	54%	15%	85%	45%	0
Malzoni, 2003	21	55%	15%	81%	57%	0
Seracchioli, 2003	9	39%	22%	78%		0
DiGregorio, 2002	65	44%	11%	86%	92%	0
Dubuisson, 2000	100	53%	31%	69%	42%	1 surgical site
Seinera, 1997, 2000	64		12%	86%	80%	0
Stringer, 1997, 2001	7		28%	72%	57%	0
Rossetti, 2001	21	66%	22%	78%	71%	0
Dessolle, 2001	44	41%	14%	82%	32%	0
Darai, 1997	17	39%	23%	58%	33%	0
Nezhat, 1999	42		20%	75%	78%	0
Dubuisson, 1996	7	33%	0%	100%	57%	0
Miller, 1996	30	75%	13%	87%		0
Campo, 2003	22	61%	14%	86%	40%	0
Total L/S (n)	626					1

Hurst. Laparoscopic myomectomy. Fertil Steril 2005.[19,20]

14 percent. Patients who conceived were younger, had larger myomas resected, and the myomas tended to be intramural. There were no cases of uterine rupture.

Goldberg et al[24] valuated published series and found more pregnancy complications in 53 pregnancies after uterine artery embolization compared to 139 pregnancies after laparoscopic myomectomy. Pregnancies after uterine artery embolization had significantly higher preterm delivery (odds ratio 6.2, 95% CI 1.4–27.7) and malpresentation rates (odds ratio 4.3, 95% CI 1.0–20.5). Postpartum hemorrhage and spontaneous abortion rates tended to be higher after embolization, but the sample size was too small to be conclusive.

These combined studies indicate that laparoscopic myomectomy is a feasible option for infertile women. The best prognosis for future fertility is found in young women with otherwise unexplained infertility when a myoma distorts the endometrial cavity.

Comparison of pregnancy outcome between women undergoing laparoscopy and those undergoing laparo-conversion. Delivery rate insignificantly higher after laparoscopic myomectomy than after laparoconversion. This difference may be explained by the smaller number and size of myomata removed by laparoscopy.[25]

Uterine Rupture After Laparoscopic Myomectomy

Uterine rupture appears to be a rare occurrence in large clinical series. Based on the clinical trials and case series, it would appear that the risk of uterine rupture during pregnancy is no higher than one percent when the myometrial incision is appropriately repaired.[16] Laparoscopically-assisted myomectomy (LAM) maybe performed if correct closure of the myometrium cannot be obtained by laparoscopy.[26,27]

Cesarean section should be routinely advised for delivery after resecting large, deep or multiple leiomyomata.

ENTRY INTO THE CAVITY

Entry into the endometrial cavity presents another technical challenge during laparoscopic myomectomy. Small series show that the cavity can be adequately repaired and the prognosis for future pregnancy is good in these circumstances. Delivery by cesarean section is generally recommended in these cases.

Seracchioli et al[24] reported on laparoscopic myomectomy in 34 women with uterine fibroids penetrating the uterine cavity. Of the 23 women who attempted pregnancy, nine conceived within one year, and seven delivered at term without complications. They concluded that laparoscopic myomectomy for fibroids penetrating into the uterine cavity was safe and provided the advantages of minimal access surgery.

Laparoscopy provides a mechanism to diagnose and treat underlying pelvic pathology that maybe causative for infertility as well as other symptoms, thereby optimizing both spontaneous and assisted PRs. Assisted reproductive technology (ART) and laparoscopy are not mutually exclusive, but coexisting and potentially complimentary treatments.

HYSTEROSCOPIC REMOVAL

All fibroids which are more than 50 percent in the cavity can be safely removed by hysteroscopy (resection or laser ablation or vaporization).

Management of Fibroids in Infertility

Epidemiological evidence on the relationship between infertility and fibroids is not conclusive due to methodological limitations. Conversely, two main pieces of clinical evidence support the vision that fibroids may interfere with fertility. First, insights from the IVF model suggest a detrimental effect on implantation: the delivery rate is reduced in patients with fibroids, while it is not affected in patients who had undergone myomectomy. Second, even if randomized studies are lacking, surgical treatment appears to increase the pregnancy rate: about one of two women undergoing myomectomy for infertility subsequently conceives.

The effect of myomas on reproductive outcome has been the subject of many studies; however, a definitive answer is still missing. Hart and colleagues[28] investigated the outcome of assisted reproduction in women who had intramural myomas that were up to 5 cm in diameter. In this study, 112 women who had myomas were compared with 322 women who did not have any uterine pathology. Pregnancy, implantation, and ongoing pregnancy rates were reduced significantly and were 23.3 percent, 11.9 percent, and 15.1 percent, respectively, compared with 34.1 percent, 20.2 percent, and 28.3 percent in the control group. When the results of logistic regression were adjusted for the number of embryos transferred and the women's age, the odds ratio (OR) of an ongoing pregnancy in the presence of an intramural fibroid that was up to 5 cm in diameter was halved (OR, 0.46; CI, 0.24–0.88), especially among women who were at least 40 years of age.

Hysteroscopic myomectomy is the gold standard for the treatment of submucous myomas. For other myomas, abdominal myomectomy, or laparoscopic myomectomy— when the experience of the surgeon and the facilities are sufficient—are the best alternatives. In most of the literature, the pregnancy rates were increased and the miscarriage rates were decreased after surgery with these two techniques. Other alternative treatment modalities, such as CUV, laparoscopic myolysis, or MRI-guided focused ultrasound, are to be monitored and evaluated thoroughly before they are applied as routine procedures.

A major point to be considered in this area is related to the severity of the disease. Uterine leiomyomata is a heterogeneous condition varying from a small single subserosal fibroid to multiple large lesions that radically distort pelvic anatomy. Whereas the effect on fertility of the former is irrelevant, the latter strongly impairs the probability of conception. Available evidence suggests that submucosal, intramural and subserosal fibroids interfere with fertility in decreasing order of importance. Although more limited, some evidence also supports an impact of the number and the dimension of the lesions.

The notion that fibroids affect fertility has to be translated into clinical practice. Drawing clear guidelines for the management of fibroids in infertile women is however difficult due to the lack of large randomized trials aimed to elucidate which patients may benefit from surgery. The Practice Committee of the American Society for Reproductive Medicine (2006) recommends surgical treatment after complete evaluation of other potential factors of infertility.[29] We believe that this view is somehow simplistic and we suggest to adopt a comprehensive and personalized approach in the decision-making process to identify the best option for the woman. At least four points have to be considered:

i. The age of the woman.
ii. The location, dimension and number of the fibroids.
iii. The concomitant presence of fibroids-related symptoms such as menorrhagia or hyper-menorrhea.
iv. The presence of other causes of infertility and whether or not there is an indication to IVF.

As previously underlined, in some cases the decision maybe an easy task. In contrast, many women may fall in a 'gray' zone. In these cases, it is suggested to adopt a personalized attitude clearly exposing the pros and cons of myomectomy to the patient, including risks associated to fibroids during pregnancy on one hand and those associated with surgery on the other hand. The ultimate aim is to assume a shared decision with the patient.

So some crude guidelines for the management of women who have uterine myomas are as follows. The location and size of the myomas are the two parameters that influence the success of a future pregnancy. Subserosal myomas seem to have little, if any, effect on reproductive outcome, especially if they are up to 5 to 7 cm in diameter. Intramural myomas that do not encroach upon the endometrium also can be considered to be relatively harmless to reproduction, if they are smaller than 4 to 5 cm in diameter. This is the ambiguous gray zone of the subject, and where research should be focused before a consensus can be established. Myomas that compress the uterine cavity with an intramural portion (submucous myoma type II) and submucous myomas significantly reduce pregnancy rates, and should be removed before assisted reproductive techniques are used.

REFERENCES

1. Lethaby A, Vollenhoven B. Fibroids (uterine myomatosis, leiomyomas). Clinical Evidence 2011;2011. Epub 2011/04/12.
2. Kroon B, Johnson N, Chapman M, Yazdani A, Hart R. Fibroids in infertility—consensus statement from ACCEPT (Australasian CREI Consensus Expert Panel on Trial evidence). The Australian and New Zealand Journal of Obstetrics and Gynaecology 2011;51(4): 289-95. Epub 2011/08/03.
3. Cakmak H, Taylor HS. Implantation failure: molecular mechanisms and clinical treatment. Human Reproduction Update 2011;17(2):242-53. Epub 2010/08/24.
4. Yazbeck C, Fauconnier A, Pouly JL. [Reproductive surgery]. Journal de gynecologie, obstetrique et biologie de la reproduction. 2010;39(8 Suppl 2):S75-87. Epub 2010/12/28. La chirurgie de la reproduction.
5. Olive DL. The surgical treatment of fibroids for infertility. Seminars in Reproductive Medicine 2011;29(2):113-23. Epub 2011/03/26.
6. Bettocchi S, Achilarre MT, Ceci O, Luigi S. Fertility-enhancing hysteroscopic surgery. Seminars in Reproductive Medicine 2011;29(2):75-82. Epub 2011/03/26.
7. Shokeir T, El-Shafei M, Yousef H, Allam AF, Sadek E. Submucous myomas and their implications in the pregnancy rates of patients with otherwise unexplained primary infertility undergoing hysteroscopic myomectomy: a randomized matched control study. Fertility and Sterility 2010;94(2):724-9. Epub 2009/05/02.
8. Olive DL, Pritts EA. Fibroids and reproduction. Seminars in Reproductive Medicine 2010;28(3):218-27. Epub 2010/04/24.
9. Malzoni M, Sizzi O, Rossetti A, Imperato F. Laparoscopic myomectomy: a report of 982 procedures. Surgical Technology International 2006;15:123-9. Epub 2006/10/10.
10. Rackow BW, Arici A. Fibroids and *in-vitro* fertilization: which comes first? Current Opinion in Obstetrics and Gynecology 2005;17(3):225-31. Epub 2005/05/05.
11. Porozhanova V, Porozhanova K. [Uterine fibromas and infertility]. Akusherstvo i ginekologiia. 2004;43(6):33-8. Epub 2005/01/27. Matochna leiomioma i infertilitet.
12. Yoshino O, Hayashi T, Osuga Y, Orisaka M, Asada H, Okuda S, et al. Decreased pregnancy rate is linked to abnormal uterine peristalsis caused by intramural fibroids. Hum Reprod 2010;25(10):2475-9. Epub 2010/08/20.
13. Ben-Nagi J, Miell J, Mavrelos D, Naftalin J, Lee C, Jurkovic D. Endometrial implantation factors in women with submucous uterine fibroids. Reproductive Biomedicine Online 2010;21(5):610-5. Epub 2010/10/01.
14. Roux I, Faivre E, Trichot C, Donnadieu AC, Fernandez H, Deffieux X. [Fertility following myomectomy by laparotomy in women aged over 38]. Journal de gynecologie, obstetrique et biologie de la reproduction. 2011;40(2):123-9. Epub 2010/11/06. Fertilite apres myomectomie par laparotomie pour les femmes de plus de 38 ans.
15. Horne AW, Critchley HO. The effect of uterine fibroids on embryo implantation. Seminars in Reproductive Medicine 2007;25(6):483-9. Epub 2007/10/26.
16. Benecke C, Kruger TF, Siebert TI, Van der Merwe JP, Steyn DW. Effect of fibroids on fertility in patients undergoing assisted reproduction. A structured literature review. Gynecologic and Obstetric Investigation 2005;59(4):225-30. Epub 2005/03/19.
17. Biderman-Madar T, Sheiner E, Levy A, Potashnik G, Mazor M. Uterine leiomyoma among women who conceived following fertility treatment. Archives of Gynecology and Obstetrics 2005;272(3):218-22. Epub 2005/06/23.
18. Sheiner E, Bashiri A, Levy A, Hershkovitz R, Katz M, Mazor M. Obstetric characteristics and perinatal outcome of pregnancies with uterine leiomyomas. The Journal of Reproductive Medicine 2004;49(3): 182-6. Epub 2004/04/22.
19. Peacock K, Hurst BS. Laparoscopic Myomectomy. Surgical Technology International 2006;15:141-5. Epub 2006/10/10.
20. Hurst BS, Matthews ML, Marshburn PB. Laparoscopic myomectomy for symptomatic uterine myomas. Fertility and Sterility 2005;83(1):1-23. Epub 2005/01/18.

21. Bulletti C, De Ziegler D, Polli V, Flamigni C. The role of leiomyomas in infertility. The Journal of the American Association of Gynecologic Laparoscopists 1999;6(4): 441-5. Epub 1999/11/05.
22. Stringer NH, Walker JC, Meyer PM. Comparison of 49 laparoscopic myomectomies with 49 open myomectomies. The Journal of the American Association of Gynecologic Laparoscopists 1997;4(4): 457-64. Epub 1997/08/01.
23. Campo S, Campo V, Gambadauro P. Reproductive outcome before and after laparoscopic or abdominal myomectomy for subserous or intramural myomas. European Journal of Obstetrics, Gynecology, and Reproductive Biology 2003;110(2):215-9. Epub 2003/09/13.
24. Goldberg J, Pereira L, Berghella V, Diamond J, Darai E, Seinera P, et al. Pregnancy outcomes after treatment for fibromyomata: uterine artery embolization versus laparoscopic myomectomy. American Journal of Obstetrics and Gynecology 2004;191(1):18-21. Epub 2004/08/06.
25. Nezhat FR, Roemisch M, Nezhat CH. Long-term follow-up of laparoscopic myomectomy. The Journal of the American Association of Gynecologic Laparoscopists 1996;3(4 Suppl.):S35. Epub 1996/08/01.
26. Dubuisson JB, Chapron C, Fauconnier A, Babaki-Fard K. Laparoscopic myomectomy fertility results. Annals of the New York Academy of Sciences 2001;943:269-75. Epub 2001/10/12.
27. Dubuisson JB, Chavet X, Chapron C, Gregorakis SS, Morice P. Uterine rupture during pregnancy after laparoscopic myomectomy. Hum Reprod 1995;10(6): 1475-7. Epub 1995/06/01.
28. Hart R, Khalaf Y, Yeong CT, Seed P, Taylor A, Braude P. A prospective controlled study of the effect of intramural uterine fibroids on the outcome of assisted conception. Hum Reprod 2001;16(11):2411-7. Epub 2001/10/27.
29. Myomas and reproductive function. Fertility and Sterility. 2006;86(5 Suppl 1):S194-9. Epub 2006/10/24.

Chapter 13

Managing Male Infertility Clinically in Low-resource Setting

Vijay Kulkarni

A clinician keeping himself abreast with latest knowledge and concepts from international conferences and journals, faces the reality of implementing those in his set up. More often than not, it is difficult if not impossible to convert those ideas in his surroundings mainly due to financial restrains. Hence clinically oriented and therapy guided strategies are required in low resource settings. These strategies may not exactly follow the algorithms[1] dealing with Male Infertility as given in textbooks or journals.

Following are some of the situations in male infertility clinic where such strategies can be implemented:

1. Hormonal assay
2. FSH
3. Testicular biopsy in CABVD, VEA, OAS, TESE
4. TRUS in CABVD
5. Vasography
6. Cryopreservation of sperms in situational anejaculation
7. Dedicated vibration device Vs locally available vibrators
8. Electroejaculation for diagnosis and cryopreservation
9. CDD for varicocele against simple Doppler probe
10. Prolonged medical trials

Hormonal Assay: Not every case of oligoasthenospermia (OAS) or oligoasthenoteratospermia (OATS) requires complete hormonal studies. If patient is clinically well androgenized with normal testicular volume, he does not need to get entire compliment of hormones. Such assay should be reserved for cases where clinical impression is that of hypogonadism where FSH alone could suffice.

FSH: Every case of OAS does not merit FSH levels. Only when the sperm count is between azoospermia to <5 mill/cc, then the FSH levels make sense. Clinical correlation with soft, small testes also decides the need to do the FSH levels.

Testicular Biopsy (TBx): It is the most over used investigation in andrology. It is an invasive investigation (Fig. 13.1). It has specific indications:

- If SA shows azoospermia (pseudoejaculation ruled out) but clinically it is equivocal for the diagnosis of primary testicular failure (Non-obstructive azoospermia) or obstructive azoospermia, then testicular biopsy is indicated.
- If IVF-ICSI is indicated and if the couple wishes to ascertain/confirm the presence of sperms prior to the procedure, only then Trial TESE or multi quadrant Needle Aspiration Biopsies may be performed.

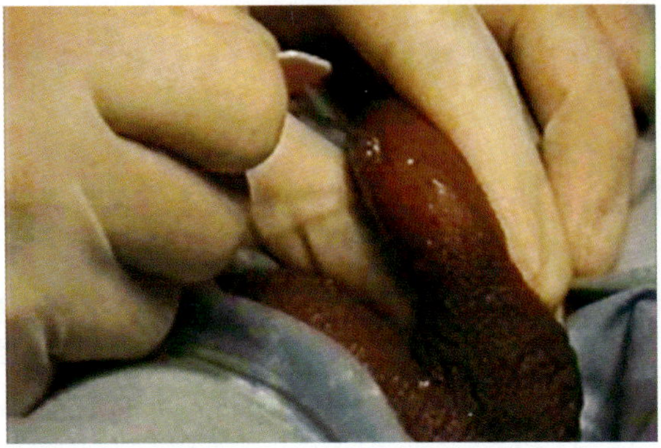

Fig. 13.1: Needle aspiration biopsy (NAB)—Testicular sperm retrieval technique

Type of TBx: Conventional open TBx under LA/GA can be replaced with Needle Aspiration Biopsy under LA. It requires less OT material and is histologically equally well interpretable. Besides, biopsies can be mapped for future reference when doing TESE at the time of IVF-ICSI.

Situations where clinical impressions can avoid unnecessary TBx in low resource settings:

- *TBx and CABVD (Congenital absence of bilateral vas deferens):* The diagnosis of CABVD is a clinical diagnosis. In addition, if the caput of epididymis are full/turgid, testicular biopsy is superfluous. One will almost certainly find sperms in percutaneous epididymal aspiration (PESA) at the time of IVF-ICSI.
- *TBx and Planned VEA (Vasoepididymal Anastomosis):* If the azoospermic patient displays clinically turgid epididymis, then TBx is not necessary. The sperms can be found in the serial incisions over epididymis during the surgery of VEA. If sperms are not found, then one can always perform the TBx in the same procedure.
- *TBx in OATS:* Testicular biopsy does not make the clinician wiser in cases of OAS as the biopsy would show various grades of hypospermatogenesis. He already knows that there is low production of sperms and the biopsy does not change the therapy.
- *Trial TESE:* If the couple does not insist on prior confirmation of presence of sperms, this additional procedure may be avoided and can be performed on the day of ovum pick-up for sperm retrieval. Normal or near normal FSH and fair sized testes are clinical prerequisites.

TRANSRECTAL ULTRASOUND (TRUS) TO CONFIRM CABVD

As mentioned earlier, CABVD is entirely clinical diagnosis. One does not require TRUS to confirm it. Low volume semen (<1 cc), -ve fructose and absence of palpable vasa are adequate clinical parameters for the diagnosis.

Vasography

This procedure is performed to check the patency of the distal vas. Vasography as a separate procedure is best avoided. It can be combined with the definitive procedure. For example, during the surgery of VEA or of ejaculatory duct block, the patency can be checked by saline irrigation or threading the dilated vas with a nylon thread. It is much easier to close the vas under microscope during open procedure; thus avoiding the risk of creating an iatrogenic block[2] at the site of vasal puncture/incision.

CRYOPRESERVATION OF SPERMS IN SITUATIONAL ANEJACULATION

Cryopreservation of sperm requires a set-up which may not be available at every center in low resource setting. The male can be trained to use vibrator to produce ejaculate and he can then give a fresh sample of semen using the vibrator on the day of IUI.

DEDICATED VIBRATION DEVICE VS LOCALLY AVAILABLE VIBRATORS

Dedicated vibration device is an expensive device and not easily available (Fig. 13.2).

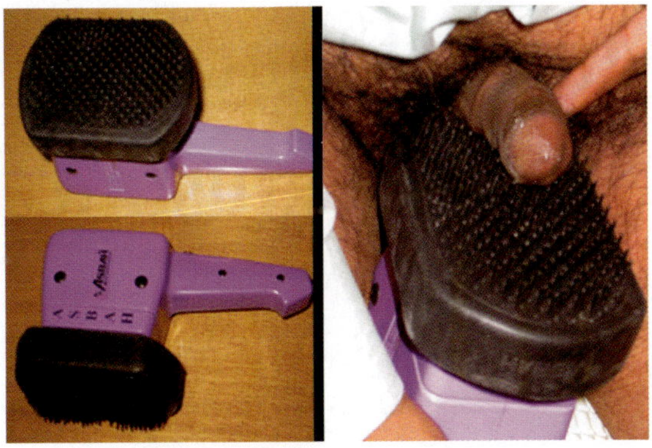

Fig. 13.2: Expensive vibrators

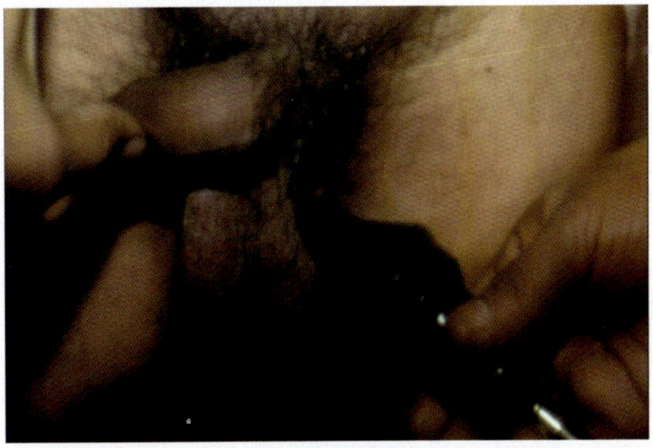

Fig. 13.3: Varicocele diagnosis (Use of inexpensive simple pocket/portable Doppler probe)

Similar results can be produced using locally available inexpensive body vibrators. Moreover, being inexpensive, the vibrator can be bought by the patient and used in his own home to facilitate the treatment of situational anejaculation.

ELECTROEJACULATION FOR DIAGNOSIS AND CRYOPRESERVATION

Some cases of anejaculation may be not respond to vibration therapy; hence electroejaculation (EE) may need to be resorted to. EE is expensive and needs GA. Also, elctroejaculated sperms when thawed out, have been observed to show poor motility. Hence it is much logical to plan the EE on the ovulation day of the female partner and utilize the fresh semen sample for IUI, rather than do the EE only for the diagnostic purpose and cryopreserve the sperms for later use.

Color Duplex Doppler (CDD) for Varicocele Against Simple Doppler Probe (Fig. 13.3)

The hallmark criterion for varicocele surgery is that the varicocele has to be clinically palpable.[3] Any palpable varicocele will emit enough auditory signals from simple pocket/portable Doppler probe to confirm the refluxing veins. Bidirectional Color Duplex Doppler (CDD) with imaging which is expensive, is not necessary.

Prolonged Medical Trials

Many drugs like antioxidants and micronutrients are aggressively marketed by the pharmaceutical companies. Utility of these drugs still cannot be precisely prognosticated. The indications for the use of such drugs are still unclear.[4] These drugs are expensive when given in prescribed dosages and the trial period is long. Hence in a low resource settings, the clinician needs to curb such trial and to choose the further step early, i.e. appropriate ART or varicocele surgery. This step spares the patient money as well as time.

Thus a good clinical examination and history can help take decisions which may not exactly conform to the algorithms given in the books, without compromising its correctness.

REFERENCES

1. Wein: Campbell-Walsh Urology, 9th edn. Saunders, Male Infertility: Mark Sigman, Jonathan P Jarrow (Eds). Chapter 19, Fig. 19.4, 2007;621.
2. Wein: Campbell-Walsh Urology, 9th edn. Saunders, Chapter 20—Surgical Management of Male Infertility: Larry I Lipshultz, Anthony J Thomas Jr, Mohit Khera (Eds). 2007;709.
3. Evolving Approach to the Varicocele: Mohit Khera, Larry I Lipshultz (Eds). Urol Clin N Am 2008;35:183-9.
4. An evidence-based perspective to the medical treatment of male infertility: A Short Review Hussein Ghanema, Rany Shamloul. Urol Int 2009;82:125-9.

Chapter

14

Milder Stimulation Only Justified

Shee-Uan Chen, Yu-Shih Yang

PHYSIOLOGICAL RECRUITMENT, SELECTION AND DOMINANCE OF OVARIAN FOLLICLES

A normal reproductive cycle includes recruitment of a cohort of antral follicles followed by the selection of a dominant follicle. During the late luteal phase of the previous cycle, estradiol, inhibin A, and progesterone levels fall because of the apoptosis of corpus luteum. These result in an increasing frequency of pulsatile gonadotropin-releasing hormone (GnRH) secretion that then induces follicle-stimulating hormone (FSH) secretion. When FSH levels rise over a threshold during the luteal-follicular transition of the cycle, a cohort of small antral follicles is recruited to develop.[1] After the initial rise from the late luteal phase, FSH levels are maintained during the early and mid-follicular phase (till around cycle day 7) for the selection of a pre-dominant follicle. The time where FSH levels remain above the threshold in the early and mid-follicular phase is referred as the FSH window.[2]

The FSH levels then decrease as a consequence of the negative feedback on the hypothalamic-pituitary axis acted by increasing inhibin B and estradiol from developing antral follicles. Decremented FSH level is essential for dominance of a single follicle from the recruited cohort. The follicle with the highest number of FSH receptors on granulosa cells achieves dominance over the others. The remaining recruited follicles undergo atresia. The dominant follicle continues to grow with expression of luteinizing hormone (LH) receptors and acquires responsiveness to LH. The increasing estradiol levels secreted from the dominant follicle reaches a threshold and then induces a LH surge from pituitary that triggers oocyte maturation and ovulation.[2]

PRINCIPLE OF STANDARD MAXIMAL STIMULATION AND MILDER STIMULATION

The ovarian stimulation is to create higher gonadotropin levels than the threshold in the early or mid-follicular phase (in the FSH window) to overcome the regular selection of a single pre-dominant follicle and to extend the FSH window throughout the follicular phase.[2] The purpose is to increase the number of dominant follicles containing oocytes and to increase the chance of pregnancy in the infertility treatment. Ovarian stimulation is a key step of assisted reproductive technology (ART) that needs an accurate determination of a regime for the patient. The medicines used for controlled ovarian stimulation include oral clomiphene citrate, aromatase inhibitor, subcutaneous human menopausal gonadotropin (hMG), recombinant FSH and LH, human chorionic gonadotropin (hCG), GnRH agonist and antagonist. The single use or combination use and their dosages are critical to achieve an optimal ovarian response.

The principle of standard maximal ovarian stimulation is to create high FSH levels since cycle day 2 or 3 of early follicular phase to recruit and select the cohort of follicles and to extend the FSH window to the late follicular phase, leading to growth of multiple dominant follicles. Three standard protocols are commonly used for IVF, including the long GnRH agonist plus gonadotropin protocol, the short GnRH agonist plus gonadotropin protocol, and the gonadotropin plus GnRH antagonist protocol. The long GnRH agonist protocol in combination with relatively high daily doses of gonadotropins, starting doses usually vary between 150 and 300 IU/day, remains the most commonly used stimulation protocol.[3] In the long protocol, patients are administered with GnRH agonist from the previous mid-luteal phase and with gonadotropins after attaining down-regulation. Patients in the short protocol are administered with GnRH agonist from day 2 of the menstrual cycle and with gonadotropin from day 5. The short protocol has advantage of the initial stimulatory effect of GnRH agonist on pituitary to induce gonadotropin release (the flare-up effect) that promotes follicular development. The total cost of gonadotropins was significantly lower in the short protocol, but there was no significant difference in live birth rates between the short and long protocols.[3] The gonadotropin plus GnRH antagonist protocol is gradually increasingly used.[4-6] The gonadotropin is administered since day 2 or 3 of the menstrual cycle. The GnRH antagonist, in a daily dose of 0.25 mg subcutaneously, is added when the lead follicle reaches 14 mm or since the cycle day 6, and it is continued until the day of induction of oocyte maturation. The recent meta-analysis demonstrated that the use of the antagonist protocols was associated with a reduction in ovarian hyperstimulation syndrome (OHSS), compared with the long GnRH agonist protocols and there was no significant difference in live-birth rates.[6] Yet, currently standard stimulations need high medicine cost. For the patients with low economics, the affordability should be concerned.

The principle of the milder stimulation is to create a moderate FSH elevation since the early or mid follicular-phase overcoming the selection of single predominant follicle and to extend the FSH window to the late follicular phase, leading to the growth of several follicles.[7] Milder stimulation is aimed to develop safer and more patient-friendly protocols in which the risks and discomforts of treatment are minimized. There is no standard protocol of milder stimulation in which oral medicine is used either alone or in combination with gonadotropins and GnRH antagonists. The gonadotropins are administered at a lower dose and for a shorter duration in the follicular phase.[8] The cost of medicines in the milder stimulation protocols is less than the standard maximal stimulation protocols.

The protocols of standard maximal ovarian stimulation and milder stimulation are summarized in Table 14.1.

Factors are Helpful to Determine the Regime of Ovarian Stimulation for Individuals

The age, body weight, body mass index, cycle length, antral follicle counts, baseline serum FSH, LH, estradiol, inhibin B or anti-Mullerian hormone (AMH) levels can assist in the determination of protocol and dosage for individual patient.[9-12] Excessive dosage is not necessary and may result in OHSS for high responders. Insufficient dosage may lead to cancellation of treatment cycle. For

Table 14.1: Protocols of standard maximal ovarian stimulation and milder stimulation

Standard maximal ovarian stimulation	*Milder ovarian stimulation*
Long GnRHa plus gonadotropin protocol	Clomiphene
Short GnRHa plus gonadotropin protocol	Aromatase inhibitor
Gonadotropin plus antagonist protocol	Gonadotropin in the alternate days
	Clomiphene plus gonadotropin
	Clomiphene plus gonadotropin and GnRH antagonist
	Delayed low-dose gonadotropin plus GnRH antagonist protocol
	hCG administration in the late follicular phase

low economic patients, the cost of medicine is an important determining factor.

In consideration of patients' safety and fitness, milder stimulation has its potential role in IVF and would be method of choice for the low economic patients. Methods of milder stimulation are described as followings:

CLOMIPHENE CITRATE

Clomiphene citrate, an estrogen antagonist, binds estrogen receptors of hypothalamus and pituitary and blocks the negative feedback of estrogen. Thus, it enhances endogenous pituitary FSH and LH secretion and gives moderate gonadotropin stimulation to the ovaries. Clomiphene has been used induce ovulation for a long period and is still appreciated for its oral administration and low price, compared with gonadotropins. Branigan et al reported a protocol using oral contraceptives followed by clomiphene 100 mg since cycle day 3 for 8 days, hCG triggering oocyte maturation, IVF, and embryo transfer.[13] No LH surges occurred in this series. A mean number of mature oocytes of 3.2 were retrieved. They achieved 32.8 percent of pregnancy rate. That was not significantly different from the matched stimulated IVF group. Clomiphene only protocol for IVF/ICSI can be effectively used in selected patients with development of several follicles, tubal factor or severe oligoasthenospermia. For patients of normal ovarian reserve who are mono-follicular response to clomiphene, the gonadotropin co-treatment can be used.

AROMATASE INHIBITOR

Aromatase converts androstenedione to estrone and testosterone to estradiol. When aromatase inhibitor is administered in the early follicular phase, it can decrease the conversion of androgens to estrogens in granulosa cells of developing ovarian follicles, resulting in increase of intra-ovarian androgens and reduction of a rise in estrogens.[14] Due to a reduced negative feedback of estrogen, it leads to increasing endogenous FSH and LH secretion from pituitary and offers moderate gonadotropin stimulation to the ovaries. Like clomiphene for ovulation induction, aromatase inhibitors are orally taken and are cheap. Letrozole has been found to be as effective as clomiphene for ovulation induction.[14] Compared with clomiphene, they may offer the potential advantage of endometrial thickness due to not blocking estrogen receptors of endometrium and are more rapidly cleared from the body because of their shorter half-life (45 hours instead of a few weeks).[15] Recent data have raised concerns regarding possible teratogenicity of aromatase inhibitors.[16] But these findings were not confirmed in a larger group of patients.[17] Due to the short half-life, the teratogenic effects from aromatase inhibitors used in the early follicular phase are not likely. Aromatase inhibitor for ovarian stimulation is now an off-label use.

Gonadotropin in the Alternative Days or Clomiphene Plus Gonadotropin

Gonadotropin (150-225 IU) in the alternative days may reduce the incidence of OHSS for high responders and save the cost of medicine. The combination of clomiphene and gonadotropins may counterbalance undesired anti-estrogenic effect of clomiphene on the endometrium and may reduce the amount of gonadotropins required due to the synergistic effect on the ovaries. Regarding the optimal gonadotropin regimen in the milder stimulation, most studies vary in the starting dose, day of initiation, daily injections or on alternate days. A study showed that a stimulation regimen combining clomiphene of 100 mg/day for 5 days during the early follicular phase with 225 IU FSH and 75 IU of LH on alternate days resulted in comparable cancellation and ongoing pregnancy rates per cycle to those following a standard long GnRH agonist plus gonadotropin protocol.[18] The average dosage of FSH used was significantly reduced in the former group. Al-Inany et al observed that the number of patients who had a premature LH surge was significantly lower in the hMG plus clomiphene group than the hMG only group (5% vs. 16%).[19] The rationale is that the anti-estrogenic effect of clomiphene may inhibit premature LH rise while maintaining a positive effect on ovarian follicle development.

CLOMIPHENE PLUS GONADOTROPIN AND ANTAGONIST PROTOCOL

The availability of GnRH antagonists has allowed for the prevention of premature LH rises in combination with clomiphene or letrozole and gonadotropins.[20,21] It facilitates the development of simpler, milder and safer stimulation protocols.[22] Equally high pregnancy rates have been obtained with the clomiphene plus gonadotropin and GnRH antagonist protocol, compared with standard ovarian stimulation with a significant reduction in the total dose of gonadotropins needed.[23-25] A randomized controlled study observed similar ongoing pregnancy rates of clomiphene plus gonadotropin with and without the use of GnRH antagonist.[26] Therefore, considering the cost and patient friendliness, the clomiphene plus gonadotropin protocol would be feasible for IVF treatment.

DELAYED LOW-DOSE GONADOTROPIN PLUS GnRH ANTAGONIST PROTOCOL

A milder stimulation regimen, modified from the standard FSH plus antagonist protocol, using a daily dose of 150 IU FSH starting from cycle day 5 with GnRH antagonist co-treatment from a follicle size of 14 mm, has been developed for IVF.[27-29] The low-dose gonadotropin administration delayed until the mid-follicular phase is based on the FSH window concept for allowing fewer follicles to continue their development.[2] Verberg et al performed a meta-analysis and reported a 35 percent reduction in the number of oocytes retrieved with a median of 6 compared with 9 following standard stimulation.[22] With a reduction of FSH needed, this protocol resulted in pregnancy rates comparable to those of standard GnRH agonist protocol. When ovarian stimulation was initiated on cycle day 5, a daily dose of 150 IU FSH, compared with 100 IU/day, was found to induce multiple follicular developments more consistently.[30] Even though using 150 IU FSH from cycle day 5, the mono- or bi-follicular response was 15 to 20 percent.[22] However, this protocol is still not cheap from economic consideration.

hCG ADMINISTRATION IN THE LATE FOLLICULAR PHASE

The use of micro-dose hCG (200 IU/day) after clomiphene in the late follicular phase (follicle size> 12 mm) results in continuing follicular growth, increasing estradiol levels, ovulation and pregnancy.[31] This treatment offers a cost-effective alternative before gonadotropin therapy for patients with previous failure of ovulation by clomiphene. The use of hCG (or LH) in the late follicular phase is based on the expression of LH receptors of granulosa cells in dominant follicles that acquiring LH responsiveness.[2] The efficacy of the strategy with initial standard stimulation protocols and complete replacement of FSH with hCG in the late follicular phase has been investigated by Filicori et al.[32] They reported that this approach resulted in a significant reduction in FSH needed and less small follicles at final oocyte maturation without compromising the pregnancy rate, compared with the standard long protocol. The increments of progesterone secretion or premature LH surges of follicular phase in this micro-dose hCG late administration protocol were not found. This strategy might theoretically reduce the incidence of OHSS but data to support this point has not been established.[33]

NATURAL CYCLE IVF

The first successful IVF treatment was performed in a natural cycle.[34] Natural cycle IVF consists of simple monitor of follicular growth and retrieval of a single oocyte. This strategy avoids multiple pregnancies and OHSS. Natural cycle IVF does not require frequent injections and saves the medicine cost. Ongoing pregnancy rates per started natural cycle IVF have been estimated to be 7.2 percent.[35] This may be different based on the population selected. The use of hCG for trigger of oocyte maturation permits timing of retrieval. Flushing of the follicle may enhance the efficiency of the oocyte retrieval. Natural cycle is a safe and patient friendly option. However, despite some advantages of this method, low efficacy has limited its widespread use. Natural cycle IVF in a selected population, such as young patients with tubal factor, male factor, or female with very poor ovarian reserve, has its essential place.[36]

ORAL CONTRACEPTIVE PRETREATMENT FOR SYNCHRONIZATION

During recruitment at the luteal-follicular shift, some early antral follicles with various sizes may be more responsive to FSH and may start growing faster. This may lead to some follicles reaching maturity or postmaturity ahead of the rest of the cohort during ovarian stimulation. Induction of a hypogonadotropic state with synthetic estrogen and progestin may be helpful to synchronize follicle development. Synchronization of follicular growth before ovarian stimulation allows simultaneous follicular growth during stimulation and ovulation to be triggered when the majority of follicles have reached concomitant maturation.[2,37] The other advantage using oral contraceptive is programing the timing for start of IVF cycle and conduct of oocyte retrieval. In addition, in patients who were previously resistant to clomiphene, suppression of the ovary with oral contraceptives before administration of clomiphene results in excellent rates of ovulation and pregnancy.[38] The decreases in LH and ovarian androgens may be responsible for the improved response.

Milder Stimulation Benefits for Endometrial Receptivity

The window of implantation in the reproductive cycle is defined between 6 and 10 day after the LH surge based on the existing evidences.[39] The endometrium, by the effect of progesterone and estrogen secreted from corpus luteum of the implantation window acquires a functional capability to support blastocyst adhesion and development. Ovarian stimulation may have negative effect on the endometrium for embryo implantation compared with natural cycles using frozen-thawed embryos or oocyte donation.[40] The supraphysiological estradiol level and earlier elevation of progesterone during ovarian stimulation could result in reduced implantation rates independent of embryo quality.[41,42] The mechanism underlying this deleterious effect is thought to be an abnormally accelerated endometrial maturation leading to change of implantation window and impaired endometrial receptivity. Some studies showed that the gene expression profiling of the endometrium in high responder is different from that of a natural cycle.[43-45] Increased pregnancy rates have been observed following a FSH step-down regimen for high responder when estradiol levels were not too high.[46] Milder stimulation, aiming at a more physiological response, may improve embryo implantation rates through benefits of better endometrial receptivity.[47]

Milder Stimulation may Benefit for Oocyte Quality

Standard ovarian stimulation induces a larger number of oocytes that may not be equal to a larger number of euploid embryos. The chromosomal constituents of human embryos assessed by fluorescent *in situ* hybridization revealed a significantly higher proportion of euploid embryos following mild ovarian stimulation compared with conventional stimulation.[29] This phenomenon could be the outcome of interference with the natural selection of oocytes or the exposure of growing follicles to the potentially negative effects of stimulation. Ovarian stimulation might disrupt mechanisms involved in maintaining accurate chromosome segregation.[48,49] These observations suggest that through maximal stimulation, the supernumerary oocytes and embryos may have lower quality. Comparable pregnancy rates were achieved between standard ovarian stimulation and milder stimulation using FSH 150 IU daily since cycle day 5.[27-29] The improved embryo quality may compensate for fewer embryos obtained.

Milder Stimulation Benefits for Luteal Function

In a normal ovulatory cycle, the function of corpus luteum is maintained by the pituitary gonadotropins, mainly LH, throughout the luteal phase. Slowing down of the GnRH pulse generator accompanied with diminished LH secretion is responsible for the apoptosis of the corpus luteum at the late luteal phase.[50] The luteal phase defect is common in standard ovarian stimulation protocol, and luteal support is routinely used in the IVF cycle. The main cause of luteal phase defect in standard IVF cycles is related to the supraphysiological levels of steroids secreted by a large number of corpora lutea during the early and mid-luteal phase, which inhibit the LH release via negative feedback actions on the hypothalamic-pituitary axis.[51] The other cause of earlier luteolysis is the prolonged pituitary suppression from GnRH agonist co-treatment for the prevention of spontaneous LH surge in standard long protocol.[3] The function of corpus luteum of a milder stimulation regime would be better.[52]

Milder Stimulation Reduces Cost, Complexity, Discomfort and Drop-out Rates

Standard stimulation with a long protocol is complex and expensive. It requires weeks of daily injections and demanding monitoring is needed that may influence a woman's daily life. Frequent injections may induce pain and emotional stress, and hyper-response of ovaries will result in abdominal discomfort. Considerable drop-out rates (28%) has been attributed to the physical or psychological burden of treatment.[53] Milder stimulation, using oral medicine or lower doses and fewer days of gonadotropins, is less complex and improves compliance. This will reduce patient distress and requires fewer visits for monitoring with less interruption to the working life.[54] Milder stimulation protocols have been shown to decrease drop-out rates and to allow a higher acceptance of repetitive IVF cycles.[53] These observations support that patients are willing to accept milder stimulation cycles.

Milder Stimulation Reduces OHSS and Improves Safety

The standard ovarian stimulation protocol is associated with risk of severe OHSS with an incidence of 1 to 5 percent.[55] A critical condition develops with massive ascites or pleural effusion, dyspnea, hemoconcentration and oliguria that can be life-threatening. Patients are hospitalized because of severe OHSS with a high cost. Females with young age, lean, longer interval of mense, polycystic ovaries and higher AMH are risk for OHSS. Milder stimulation significantly reduces the risk of OHSS, compared to standard maximal stimulation.[28,56] Nevertheless, even mild ovarian stimulation may sometimes elicit excessive follicular response in a proportion of women and may not totally eradicate OHSS. hCG is the standard medicine for trigger of oocyte maturation. However, hCG has sustained luteotropic action because of its prolonged circulating half-life that may predispose to OHSS. Reducing the trigger dose of hCG may lower the incidence of OHSS.[57] The risk of severe OHSS may be reduced to near zero if ovulation trigger is induced with a GnRH agonist instead of hCG.[5,58] An endogenous LH surge can be induced from the pituitary by a GnRH agonist. Compared to hCG, LH has a faster plasma metabolic clearance (half-life of hCG: 2.3 days vs. LH: 3-5 hours).[55] This strategy is applicable in the non-GnRH agonist cycle or in the GnRH antagonist cycle. These approaches reduce health risks for women and costs involved in hospitalization of OHSS.

Milder Stimulation Achieves Reasonable Pregnancy Potential

Increased quality of IVF laboratory and limited number of embryos transferred may reduce the need for large quantities of oocytes. In studies investigating the relationship between oocyte numbers and pregnancy rates, a modest number of oocytes are associated with a higher pregnancy rate.[59, 60] A recent meta-analysis suggests that the retrieval of a modest number of oocytes following mild stimulation is associated with a higher implantation rate (31% vs. 29%) compared with patients that more oocytes is retrieved following conventional stimulation.[22] The milder stimulation strategy may benefits for oocyte quality, endometrial receptivity, and luteal function. The fear of reducing the number of oocytes retrieved following mild ovarian stimulation resulting in reducing pregnancy potential would be unnecessary.[61]

Milder Stimulation with Single Embryo Transfer (SET) Prevents Complication from Multiple Pregnancy

SET is an important approach to avoid multiple pregnancy in IVF treatment. Zhang et al. (2007) reported a milder stimulation strategy that clomiphene (50 mg) was initiated orally each day, beginning on day 3, with subcutaneous administration of 75 to 150 IU of hMG every 48 hours, beginning on day 5 or 8. They observed that clinical pregnancy rate for SET in the fresh cycle was 18 percent and for SET frozen transfers was

35 percent. A large randomized efficacy study found a mild strategy using 150 FSH since day 5 and flexible GnRH antagonist co-treatment with SET achieving a similar live birth after 1 year (43.4% vs. 44.7%) compared with standard long protocol stimulation and the transfer of two embryos, while reducing patients' discomfort and multiple pregnancy.[28] When mild stimulation is combined with a SET strategy, medicine costs and potential expense associated with multiple pregnancy would be significantly reduced.[62]

Embryo Cryopreservation Using Vitrification is Helpful for the Milder Stimulation Strategy

Cryopreserved embryos can increase the cumulative pregnancy rate per oocyte retrieval. A lower numbers of oocytes in milder stimulation might decrease supernumerary embryos for cryopreservation, compared with standard stimulation. An efficient and costless method for embryo cryopreservation such as vitrification is required.[63-65] In the clomiphene treatment, the endometrial thinning has been observed in 15 to 50 percent patients because of the antiestrogenic effect of clomiphene on the endometrium.[66] Cryopreserved embryo transfers in this situation may yield higher pregnancy rates than fresh transfers.[67] A milder stimulation in combination with vitrification would be an important alternative of the standard stimulation protocols.

Milder Stimulation can be Used for High Responder, Normal Responder and Poor Ovarian Reserve

For high responder of young patient, high antral follicle count or AMH or history of OHSS, milder stimulation protocols is important to reduce abdominal discomfort and OHSS that improves safety.[55] The number of injection and the total amount of gonadotropins are reduced. Although the mean number of oocytes retrieved is less than standard stimulation, the proportion of high quality and euploid embryos would be sufficient and endometrial receptivity would be better. Clomiphene or gonadotropin (150 IU) in the alternative days can be used for high responder.

For normal responder, the milder stimulation using clomiphene or clomiphene plus gonadotropin could induce a few follicles to achieve the purpose of pregnancy. The pregnancy rates of a milder strategy of clomiphene plus gonadotropin with or without GnRH antagonist has been found to be comparable to the standard stimulation regimens, with a significant reduction in the total dose of gonadotropin needed and of the economical costs.[23-26]

For poor responders, milder stimulation or natural cycle IVF has been used as an alternative to conventional stimulation protocols. Acceptable results have been reported.[7] The strategy of using a high dose adjustment of the standard long protocol for women with poor ovarian reserve has not shown benefits.[68,69] High doses of FSH may recruit resistant follicles rescuing them from atresia. But the oocytes may be poor quality and may not generate good quality embryos.[7] Since the economical cost of gonadotropins is one of the major expenses in IVF treatment, the large increase in drug fee for high-dose gonadotropin regimens may not be justified in this situation. A standard short GnRHa plus gonadotropin protocol can be applied for poor ovarian reserve.[3] For patients with very poor ovarian reserve, the choice of a milder stimulation protocol or natural cycle, instead of a high dose regimen, is indicated.[36] Milder regimens with clomiphene or clomiphene plus gonadotropin can be used.

The potential advantages and disadvantages of standard maximal ovarian stimulation and milder stimulation are summarized in Table 14.2.

Table 14.2: Comparisons of standard maximal ovarian stimulation and milder stimulation

Parameters	*Standard stimulation*	*Mild stimulation*
Cost	higher	lower
Complexity	higher	lower
Discomfort	more	less
Drop-out rate	higher	lower
OHSS	higher	lower
Oocyte number	more	fewer
High quality oocyte	comparable	comparable
Endometrial receptivity	may be decreased	may be better
Luteal function	may be decreased	may be better
Cryopreservation	more	fewer
Cancellation due to single follicle development	lower	higher
Pregnancy rate perstimulatory cycle	comparable	comparable or lower

CONCLUSION

A milder ovarian stimulation achieves a moderate gonadotropin elevation during the early or mid-follicular phase (the FSH window) to overcome the single predominant follicle selection and extends the FSH window to enhance the growth of several follicles. It is administered with clomiphene either alone or in combination with gonadotropins, or hCG in the late follicular phase, with or without GnRH antagonist co-treatments. Milder stimulation can be used for intrauterine insemination and IVF. It can be used for high responder, normal responder or poor responder. The age, body weight, and antral follicle counts may assist to determine regime and dosage for individual patient. Pretreatment with oral contraceptives could be helpful for synchronization of cohort of follicles in the selected patients. Milder stimulation is more patient friendly and reduces cost, complexity, discomfort, and drop-out rate. It prevents OHSS and improves safety. The oocyte quality, endometrial receptivity and luteal function could be better in mild stimulation. A mild stimulation strategy with SET leads to a reasonable outcome as well as reduces multiple pregnancy and costs. Vitrification of embryos enhances the usefulness of milder stimulation protocols. Milder stimulation would be method of choice in the economic consideration facilitating its regular use in low-resource settings.

REFERENCES

1. McGee EA, Hsueh AJ. Initial and cyclic recruitment of ovarian follicles. Endocr Rev 2000;21:200-214.
2. Macklon NS, Stouffer RL, Giudice LC, Fauser BCJM. The science behind 25 years of ovarian stimulation for *in vitro* fertilization. Endocr Rev 2006;27:170-207.
3. Ho CH, Chen SU, Peng FS, Chang CY, Lien YL, Yang YS. Prospective comparison of the short and long GnRH agonist protocols using recombinant gonadotropins for IVF/ICSI treatments. Reprod BioMed Online 2008;16:632-39.
4. Lee TH, Wu MY, Chen HF, Chen MJ, Ho HN, Yang YS. Ovarian response and follicular development for single-dose and multiple-dose protocols for gonadotropin-releasing hormone antagonist administration. Fertil Steril 2005;83:1700-1707.
5. Engmann L, DiLuigi A, Schmidt D, Nulsen J, Maier D, Benadiva C. The use of gonadotropin-releasing hormone (GnRH) agonist to induce oocyte maturation after cotreatment with GnRH antagonist in high-risk patients undergoing *in vitro* fertilization prevents the risk of ovarian hyperstimulation syndrome: a prospective randomized controlled study. Fertil Steril 2008;89:84-91.
6. Al-Inany HG, Youssef MA, Aboulghar M, Broekmans F, Sterrenburg M, Smit J, Abou-Setta AM. Gonadotrophin-releasing hormone antagonists for

assisted reproductive technology. Cochrane Database Syst Rev 2011 May 11;5:CD001750.

7. Revelli A, Casano S, Salvagno F, Delle Piane L. Milder is better? Advantages and disadvantages of "mild" ovarian stimulation for human *in vitro* fertilization. Reprod Biol Endocrinol 2011;9:25.
8. Fauser BC, Nargund G, Andersen AN, Norman R, Tarlatzis B, Boivin J, Ledger W. Mild ovarian stimulation for IVF: 10 years later. Hum Reprod 2010;25:2678-84.
9. Hohmann FP, Laven JS, de Jong FH, Eijkemans MJ, Fauser BC. Low-dose exogenous FSH initiated during the early, mid or late follicular phase can induce multiple dominant follicle development. Hum Reprod 2001;16:846-54.
10. Chuang CC, Chen CD, Chao KH, Chen SU, Ho HN, Yang YS. Age is a better predictor of pregnancy potential than basal follicle-stimulating hormone levels in women undergoing *in vitro* fertilization Fertil Steril 2003;79:63-8.
11. Lee TH, Liu CH, Huang CC, Wu YL, Shih YT, Ho HN, Yang YS, Lee MS. Serum anti-Müllerian hormone and estradiol levels as predictors of ovarian hyperstimulation syndrome in assisted reproduction technology cycles. Hum Reprod 2008;23:160-67.
12. Yates AP, Rustamov O, Roberts SA, Lim HY, Pemberton PW, Smith A, Nardo LG. Anti-Mullerian hormone-tailored stimulation protocols improve outcomes whilst reducing adverse effects and costs of IVF. Hum Reprod 2011 Jun 13 [Epub ahead of print].
13. Branigan EF, Estes MA. Minimal stimulation IVF using clomiphene citrate and oral contraceptive pill treatment for LH suppression. Fertil Steril 2000;73:587-90.
14. He D and Jiang F. Meta-analysis of letrozole versus clomiphene citrate in polycystic ovary syndrome. Reprod Biomed Online 2011 April 3 [Epub ahead of print].
15. Requena A, Herrero J, Landeras J, Navarro E, Neyro JL, Salvador C, Tur R, Callejo J, Checa MA, Farre´ M, Espino´s JJ, Fa´bregues F, Gran˜a-Barcia M. Use of letrozole in assisted reproduction: a systematic review and meta-analysis. Hum Reprod Update 2008;6:571-82.
16. Biljan MM, Hemmings R, Brassard N. The outcome of 150 babies following the treatment with letrozole or letrozole and gonadotropins. Fertil Steril 2005;84 (Suppl. 1):S95.
17. Tulandi T, Martin J, Al-Fadhli R, Kabli N, Forman R, Hitkari J, Librach C, Greenblatt E, Casper RF. Congenital malformations among 911 newborns conceived after infertility treatment with letrozole or clomiphene citrate. Fertil Steril 2006;85:1761-65.
18. Weigert M, Krischker U, Pohl M, Poschalko G, Kindermann C, FeichtingerW. Comparison of stimulation with clomiphene citrate in combination with recombinant follicle-stimulating hormone and recombinant luteinizing hormone to stimulation with a gonadotropin-releasing hormone agonist protocol: a prospective, randomized study. Fertil Steril 2002;78:34-39.
19. Al-Inany H, Azab H, El-Khayat W, Nada A, El-Khattan E, Abou-Setta AM. The effectiveness of clomiphene citrate in LH surge suppression in women undergoing IUI: a randomized controlled trial. Fertil Steril 2010;94:2167-71.
20. Hwang JL, Huang LW, Hsieh BC, Tsai YL, Huang SC, Chen CY, et al. Ovarian stimulation by clomiphene citrate and hMG in combination with cetrorelix acetate for ICSI cycles. Hum Reprod 2003;18:45-49.
21. Lee TH, Lin YH, Seow KM, Hwang JL, Tzeng CR, Yang YS. Effectiveness of cetrorelix for the prevention of premature luteinizing hormone surge during controlled ovarian stimulation using letrozole and gonadotropins: a randomized trial. Fertil Steril 2008;90:113-20.
22. Verberg MF, Eijkemans MJ, Macklon NS, Heijnen EM, Baart EB, Hohmann FP, Fauser BC, Broekmans FJ. The clinical significance of the retrieval of a low number of oocytes following mild ovarian stimulation for IVF: A meta-analysis. Hum Reprod Update. 2009;15:5-12.
23. Williams SC, Gibbons WE, Muasher SJ, Oehninger S. Minimal ovarian hyperstimulation for *in vitro* fertilization using sequential clomiphene citrate and gonadotropin with or without the addition of a gonadotropin-releasing hormone antagonist. Fertil Steril 2002;78:1068-72.
24. Fiedler K, Ludwig M. Use of clomiphene citrate in *in vitro* fertilization (IVF) and IVF/intracytoplasmic sperm injection cycles. Fertil Steril 2003; 80:1521-23.
25. Lin YH, Hwang JL, Seow KM, Huang LW, Hsieh BC, Tzeng CR. Comparison of outcome of clomiphene citrate/human menopausal gonadotropin/cetrorelix protocol and buserelin long protocol: a randomized study. Gynecol Endocrinol 2006;22:297-302.
26. Fiedler K, Krusmann G, von Hertwig I, Schleyer M, Wurfel W. Comparison of Clomid/FSH/HMG for IVF with and without GnRH antagonist. Hum Reprod 2001;16:72.
27. Hohmann FP, Macklon NS, Fauser BC. A randomized comparison of two ovarian stimulation protocols with gonadotropin releasing hormone (GnRH) antagonist

cotreatment for *in vitro* fertilization commencing recombinant follicle-stimulating hormone on cycle day 2 or 5 with the standard long GnRH agonist protocol. J Clin Endocrinol Metab 2003;88:166-73.
28. Heijnen EM, Eijkemans MJ, De Klerk C, Polinder S, Beckers NG, Klinkert ER, et al. A mild treatment strategy for *in vitro* fertilization: a randomized non-inferiority trial. Lancet 2007;369:743-49.
29. Baart EB, Martini E, Eijkemans MJ, Van Opstal D, Beckers NG, Verhoeff A, Macklon NS, Fauser BC. Milder ovarian stimulation for *in vitro* fertilization reduces aneuploidy in the human preimplantation embryo: a randomized controlled trial. Hum Reprod 2007;22:980-88.
30. de Jong D, Macklon NS, Fauser BC. A pilot study involving minimal ovarian stimulation for *in vitro* fertilization: extending the follicle-stimulating hormone window' combined with the gonadotropin-releasing hormone antagonist cetrorelix. Fertil Steril 2000;73:1051-54.
31. Branigan EF, Estes A. Use of micro-dose human chorionic gonadotropin (hCG) after clomiphene citrate (CC) to complete folliculogenesis in previous CC-resistant anovulation. Am J Obstet Gynecol 2005;192:1890-94.
32. Filicori M, Cognigni GE, Gamberini E, Parmegiani L, Troilo E, Roset B. Efficacy of low-dose human chorionic gonadotropin alone to complete controlled ovarian stimulation. Fertil Steril 2005;84:394-401.
33. Verberg MF, Macklon NS, Nargund G, Frydman R, Devroey P, Broekmans FJ, Fauser BC. Mild ovarian stimulation for IVF. Hum Reprod Update 2009; 15:13-29.
34. Steptoe PC, Edwards RG. Birth after the preimplantation of a human embryo. Lancet 1978;2:366.
35. Pelinck MJ, Hoek A, Simons AH, Heineman MJ. Efficacy of natural cycle IVF: a review of the literature. Hum Reprod Update 2002;8:129-39.
36. Tarlatzis BC, Zepiridis L, Grimbizis G, Bontis J. Clinical management of low ovarian response to stimulation for IVF: a systematic review. Hum Reprod Update 2003;9:61-76.
37. Frydman R, Forman R, Rainhorn JD, Belaisch-Allart J, Hazout A, Testart J. A new approach to follicular stimulation for *in vitro* fertilization: programmed oocyte retrieval. Fertil Steril 1986;46:657-62.
38. Branigan EF, Estes MA. A randomized clinical trial of treatment of clomiphene citrate-resistant anovulation with the use of oral contraceptive pill suppression and repeat clomiphene citrate treatment. Am J Obstet Gynecol. 2003;188:1424-28.
39. Horcajadas JA, Sharkey AM, Catalano RD, Sherwin JRA, Domýnguez F, Burgos LA, Castro A, Peraza MR, Pellicer A, Simon C. Effect of an intrauterine device on the gene expression profile of the endometrium. J Clin Endocrinol Metab 2006;91:3199-207.
40. Paulson RJ, Sauer MV, Lobo RA. Embryo implantation after human *in vitro* fertilization: Importance of endometrial receptivity. Fertil Steril 1990; 53:870-74.
41. Simon C, Cano F, Valbuena D, Remohi J, Pellicer A. Clinical evidence for a detrimental effect on uterine receptivity of high serum oestradiol concentrations in high and normal responder patients. Hum Reprod 1995;10:2432-37.
42. Bosch E, Labarta E, Crespo J, Simon C, Remohi J, Jenkins J, Pellicer A. Circulating progesterone levels and ongoing pregnancy rates in controlled ovarian stimulation cycles for *in vitro* fertilization: analysis of over 4000 cycles. Hum Reprod 2010;25: 2092-2100.
43. Liu Y, Lee KF, Ng EH, Yeung WS, Ho PC. Gene expression profiling of human peri-implantation endometria between natural and stimulated cycles. Fertil Steril 2008;90:2152-64.
44. Van Vaerenbergh I, Van Lommel L, Ghislain V, In't Veld P, Schuit F, Fatemi HM, Devroey P, Bourgain C. In GnRH antagonist/rec-FSH stimulated cycles, advanced endometrial maturation on the day of oocyte retrieval correlates with altered gene expression. Hum Reprod 2009;24:1085-91.
45. Labarta E, Martínez-Conejero JA, Alamá P, Horcajadas JA, Pellicer A, Simon C, Bosch E. Endometrial receptivity is affected in women with high circulating progesterone levels at the end of the follicular phase: a functional genomics analysis. Hum Reprod 2011 May 2. Epub ahead of print.
46. Simon C, Garcia Velasco JJ, Valbuena D, Peinado JA, Moreno C, Remohi J, Pellicer A. Increasing uterine receptivity by decreasing estradiol levels during the preimplantation period in high responders with the use of a follicle-stimulating hormone step-down regimen. Fertil Steril 1998;70:234-39.
47. Devroey P, Bourgain C, Macklon NS, Fauser BC. Reproductive biology and IVF: Ovarian stimulation and endometrial receptivity. Trends Endocrinol Metab 2004;15:84-90.
48. Munne S, Magli C, Adler A, Wright G, de Boer K, Mortimer D, Tucker M, Cohen J, Gianaroli L. Treatment-related chromosome abnormalities in human embryos. Hum Reprod 1997;12:780-84.

49. Hodges CA, Ilagan A, Jennings D, Keri R, Nilson J, Hunt PA. Experimental evidence that changes in oocyte growth influence meiotic chromosome segregation. Hum Reprod 2002;17:1171-80.
50. Chen SU, Chen RJ, Shieh JY, Chou CH, Lin CW, Lu HF, Yang YS. Human chorionic gonadotropin up-regulates expression of myeloid cell leukemia-1 protein in human granulosa-lutein cells: implication of corpus luteum rescue and ovarian hyperstimulation syndrome. J Clin Endocrinol Metab 2010;95:3982-92.
51. Fatemi HM, Popovic-Todorovic B, Papanikolaou E, Donoso P, Devroey P. An update of luteal phase support in stimulated IVF cycles. Hum Reprod Update 2007;13:581-90.
52. Fauser BC, Devroey P. Reproductive biology and IVF: ovarian stimulation and luteal phase consequences. Trends Endocrinol Metab 2003;14:236-42.
53. Verberg MF, Eijkemans MJ, Heijnen EM, Broekmans FJ, De Klerk C, Fauser BC, Macklon NS. Why do couples drop-out from IVF treatment? A prospective cohort study. Hum Reprod 2008;23:2050-55.
54. de Klerk C, Macklon NS, Heijnen EM, Eijkemans MJ, Fauser BC, Paschier J, Hunfeld JA. The psychological impact of IVF failure after two or more cycles of IVF with a mild versus standard treatment strategy. Hum Reprod 2007;22:2554-58.
55. Chen SU, Chen CD, Yang YS. Ovarian hyperstimulation syndrome (OHSS): new strategies of prevention and treatment. J Formosan Med Assoc 2008;107:509-13.
56. Karimzadeh MA, Ahmadi S, Oskouian H, Rahmani E. Comparison of mild stimulation and conventional stimulation in ART outcome. Arch Gynecol Obstet 2010;281:741-46.
57. Nargund G, Hutchinson L, Scaramuzzi R, Campbell S. Low-dose HCG is useful in preventing OHSS in high-risk women without adversely affecting the outcome of IVF cycles. Reprod Biomed Online 2007;14:682-85.
58. Kol S, Dor J. Update on prediction and management and prevention of OHSS: GnRH agonist versus hCG to trigger ovulation. Reprod Biomed Online 2009;19:59-60.
59. Melie NA, Adeniyi OA, Igbineweka OM, Ajayi RA. Predictive value of the number of oocytes retrieved at ultrasound-directed follicular aspiration with regard to fertilization rates and pregnancy outcome in intracytoplasmic sperm injection treatment cycles. Fertil Steril 2003;80:1376-79.
60. van der Gaast MH, Eijkemans MJ, van der Net JB, de Boer EJ, Burger CW, van Leeuwen FE, Fauser BC, Macklon NS. Optimum number of oocytes for a successful first IVF treatment cycle. Reprod Biomed Online 2006;13:476-80.
61. Zhang J, Silber S, Kuwayama M, Kato K. Clinical update on clomiphene-citrate stimulated ivf with single embryo transfer. Hum Reprod 2007;22:I139-I139 Suppl. 1 P351
62. Polinder S, Heijnen EM, Macklon Habbema JD, Fauser BC, Eijkemans MJ. Cost-effectiveness of a mild compared with a standard strategy for IVF: a randomized comparison using cumulative term live birth as the primary endpoint. Hum Reprod 2008;23:316-23.
63. Huang CC, Lee TH, Chen SU, Chen HH, Cheng TC, Liu CH, Yang YS, Lee MS. Successful pregnancy following blastocyst cryopreservation using super-cooling ultra-rapid vitrification. Hum Reprod 2005;20:122-28.
64. Chen SU, Lee TH, Lien YL, Tsai YY, Chang LJ, Yang YS. Microsuction of blastocoelic fluid before vitrification increased survival and pregnancy of mouse expanded blastocysts, but pretreatment with the cytoskeletal stabilizer did not increase blastocyst survival. Fertil Steril 2005;84 Suppl. 2: 1156-62.
65. Chen SU, Yang YS. Vitrification of oocytes: Various procedures. In Tucker MJ and Liebermann Editions. Vitrification in Human Assisted Reproduction. 2007, pp 129-44.
66. Fisher SA, Reid RL, Van Vugt DA, Casper RF.A randomized double-blind comparison of the effects of clomiphene citrate and the aromatase inhibitor letrozole on ovulatory function in normal women. Fertil Steril 2002;78:280-85.
67. Zhang J, Chang L, Sone Y, Silber S. Minimal ovarian stimulation (mini-IVF) for IVF utilizing vitrification and cryopreserved embryo transfer. Reprod Biomed Online 2010;21:485-95.
68. Land JA, Yarmolinskaya MI, Dumoulin JC, Evers JL. High-dose human menopausal gonadotropin stimulation in poor responders does not improve *in vitro* fertilization outcome. Fertil Steril 1996;65: 961-65.
69. Lekamge DN, Lane M, Gilchrist RB, Tremellen KP. Increased gonadotrophin stimulation does not improve IVF outcomes in patients with predicted poor ovarian reserve. J Assist Reprod Genet 2008;25: 515-21.

Chapter 15

The Role of Intrauterine Insemination in Low-resource Setups

Sheila Loh, Yin Yin Yong

INTRODUCTION

The rationale behind intrauterine insemination (IUI) is increasing the gamete density at the time and site of potential fertilization, i.e. increasing the chances of spermatozoa meeting the oocyte in the fallopian tube after ovulation has occurred (Fig. 15.1). Initially, artificial insemination was developed for male factor infertility with the sites of insemination ranging from intravaginal, intracervical to intrauterine.

Nowadays, artificial insemination is practised for a wide range of indications, from male sexual dysfunction to male infertility to unexplained infertility, and the most commonly technique used is intrauterine insemination. In the era of highly successful assisted reproduction technique (ART) programs, this chapter examines the critical factors affecting success of an IUI program and the role of IUI in low resource setups.

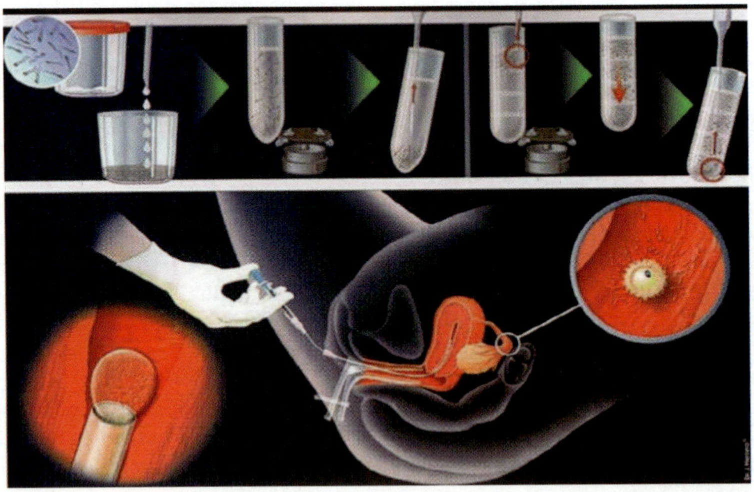

Fig. 15.1: The process of intrauterine insemination (IUI). (Illustration reproduced with permission from Dr J Herrero and reprinted from the Atlas of Assisted Reproduction, published by Merck-Serono, 2006)

INDICATIONS OF IUI[6]

The most common indications of IUI with husband's sperms are mild male factor infertility, cervical factor infertility and unexplained infertility. Other suitable indications include mild endometriosis (without significant anatomic distortion of the pelvic organs), immunological factor infertility and ovulatory dysfunction that has failed with ovulation induction alone.[1] IUI may also be performed for coital problems like ejaculatory disorders (Table 15.1).

Table 15.1: Indications for IUI

Main indications:	1. Unexplained infertility
	2. Cervical factor infertility
	3. Mild male factor
	4. Coital problems
Acceptable indications:	1. Immunological infertility
	2. Mild/minimal endometriosis
	3. Ovulatory disorders

Loh SKE et al, SMJ 1999[6]

Steures et al[2] performed a systemic review and meta-analyses of effectiveness of IUI in 3 situations: unexplained infertility, cervical factor infertility and male factor infertility. In couples with unexplained infertility, IUI was more effective than expectant management (relative risk (RR) 1.3 [95% CI 0.84 to 1.91]). In addition IUI with ovarian stimulation (in some studies, this was referred to as superovulation with IUI, SO-IUI) was more effective than IUI alone (RR 1.8, [95% CI 1.2 to 2.7]).

For cervical factor infertility, IUI alone had a higher success rate compared with expectant management (RR 1.6 [95% CI 0.87 to 3.1]) but ovarian stimulation did not increase the success rates further.[2] In male factor infertility, IUI seemed to be associated with a better pregnancy rate than expectant management, however, this difference did not reach statistical significance due to the limited power of the studies (RR 4.50 [95% CI 0.52 to 39.01].[2] For IUI with or without ovarian stimulation, a pregnancy rate of 3 to 18 percent per cycle has been reported, provided a yield of at least 1 million total motile sperm count (TMC) can be obtained.[3] For optimum results, the best results are obtained when the TMC is at least 5 million with normal sperm morphology.[4]

FACTORS AFFECTING IUI SUCCESS RATES

There are many variables which can affect the success rates of an IUI program. Table 15.2 summaries the most important factors.

Table 15.2: Factors affecting IUI success rates

- Etiology
- Woman's age
- Duration of infertility
- Ovarian stimulation
- Timing of insemination
- Sperm parameters
- Limited cycle attempts

Patient Characteristics and Pregnancy Rate with IUI

Age of the women significantly impacts on IUI success as does duration of infertility. Women aged above 40 years had a lower IUI success rate as did couples who had been infertile for longer than 5 years. Tables 15.3 and 15.4 summarize patient characteristics and pregnancy rate with IUI.

Table 15.3: Pregnancy rate by women's age at IUI

Age (years)	*PR / Patient (%)*
<26	18.9
26 – 30	13.9
31 – 35	12.4
36 – 40	11.1
41 – 45	4.7
46 – 51	0.5

Stone BA et al, *AJOG, 1999*[5]

Table 15.4: Pregnancy rate and duration of infertility

Duration of infertility (year)	*PR / Cycle (%)*
≤ 5 years	13
> 5 to 10 years	3
> 10 years	0

Loh SKE et al, *SMJ, 1999*[6]

Ovarian Stimulation

In general, ovarian stimulation with gonadotrophins result in significantly higher pregnancy rate per IUI cycle as compared with natural cycle-IUI and clomiphene-IUI.[7] The rational for ovarian stimulation being the possibility of overcoming subtle defects in ovulatory dysfunction and by increasing the number of oocytes available for fertilization, the chances of pregnancy may be enhanced albeit at the expense of higher multiple pregnancies and the need for more frequent monitoring scans. Similar pregnancy rates were achieved when comparing clomiphene-IUI (CC-IUI) with Letrozole-IUI.[8] Since Letrozole is more expensive than CC, the use of CC-IUI should be the first option in low-resource settings when ultrasound monitoring is not available or when cost of gonadotropins is an issue.

Follicle Monitoring Techniques and Timing of IUI

Serial ultrasound monitoring of follicle development is essential for timing of IUI and detection of over response, when cancellation of cycle should be discussed. Ultrasound follicle measurements may be started from day 8 in a gonadotrophin IUI cycle or day 10 in a CC-IUI cycle. The addition of a triggering injection of 5000 hCG or serial urinary LH surge detection when the lead follicle has reached ≥18 mm diameter will further optimize the success rate. In a low resource setting, measurement of serum estradiol or salivary estradiol is not recommended as it is relatively expensive, time-consuming and does not increase success rates. Timing IUI with basal body temperature charts was inaccurate and resulted in half the pregnancy rate of ultrasound monitoring alone.[9]

The exact timing of IUI is crucial to the success of the treatment. Cochrane[10] review showed that pregnancy rates were optimal between 32 and 40 hours after hCG trigger. When timing IUI by urinary LH test kits, highest pregnancy rates were achieved 24 to 42 hours after LH was detected.[11] hCG "boost" may be added 8 to 20 hours after the spontaneous LH surge to further optimize the pregnancy rates.[12]

A meta-analysis of 14 studies showed that absolute pregnancy rates were 8.4 percent for monofollicular growth and 15 percent for multifollicular growth.[13] When there were 3 or 4 follicles, there was no significant increase in pregnancy rates whereas the multiple pregnancy rates increased. International guidelines for cancellation show different cut-off points. We found the RCOG (Royal College of Obstetricians and Gynecologists) recommendation, of withholding hCG trigger injection and cycle cancellation when there are more than 3 follicles greater than 16 mm, to work very well in minimizing the risks of high-order multiple pregnancies (HOMP).[14] In situations where serial ultrasound follicle monitoring services are very basic, consideration should be given to offer only CC-IUI, Letrozole-IUI and natural cycle-IUI in order to avoid HOMP.

Type of IUI Catheter

In most of the studies, the catheter type did not influence the outcome of the IUI treatment, as long as the catheter was nontoxic and sterile. The rigid Tomcat catheter performed as well as the soft Cook catheter in a study by Miller et al (2005).[15] However, as in ART programs, we prefer a soft flexible catheter, e.g. Gynetic, for performing the insemination as we found it easy to use and suitable for most patients.

Number of Inseminations

Cochrane review[16] showed that there was no significant benefit in performing two or three inseminations over a single correctly-timed insemination. Hence, for cost-effectiveness, we advise performing only one insemination per cycle. The exception being if the total motile count (TMC) after sperm processing is less than 1 million on the insemination day, a second insemination may be offered within the next 24 hours.

Number of IUI Cycles

A significant decline in cycle fecundity after the third or fourth IUI cycle has been reported by several studies.[17-19]

Our own local data[6] supports this (Table 15.5) and we advice our patients to consider ART as the next step if they have failed to conceive with 3 optimally performed stimulated IUI cycles. Table 15.5 shows the results of cycle number and pregnancy rates for some studies.

Laboratory Factors

Initial evaluation of the sperm sample is important as only normal sperm samples or mild male factor infertility benefitted from the IUI program and patients who do not fulfill the minimum criteria should be offered ART. Many studies correlated total motile count (TMC) after sperm processing to pregnancy rate.

	TMC (Sperm Prep)
• Minimum to achieve pregnancy[20]	1 million
• Significant lower pregnancy rate[21]	< 2 million
• Likelihood of pregnancy[22]	≥ 4 to 5 million

There are various sperm preparation techniques for IUI, the most common being sperm washing, swim-up method and gradient processing method. All three methods require centrifugation to concentrate the final sperm preparation. There was no difference between pregnancy rates among these 3 basic techniques in a recent meta-analysis.[23] Hence, in a low-resource setting, the simplest technique, the swim-up technique, is recommended. In clinics which have no access to andrology laboratories, commercial kits, e.g. sperm select® kit (CooperSurgical) and Basic Sperm Wash System® (in vitro care) may be used for sperm processing in the office setup.

Luteal Phase Support

Generally, luteal phase support is not necessary in natural cycle-IUI or CC-IUI cycles. In normally ovulating women in gonadotrophin-IUI cycles, it is also not practised by most authors. However, Balasch et al (1996)[24] showed that the spontaneous abortion rate was reduced in gonadotropin-IUI

Table 15.5: Clinical pregnancy rate by cycle attempt

		Clinical Pregnancy Per cycle (%)					
		1st	2nd	3rd	4th	5th	6th
Loh SKE et al[6]	1999	13	13	3	0	0	NA
Dmowski PW et al[17]	2004	15	12	8	7	7	0
Custers IM et al[18]	2008	7.4	7.0	5.1	5.4	4.4	4.7
Aboulghar M et al[19]	2001	← 16.4 percent per cycle →			← 5.6 percent per cycle →		

cycles for WHO Type II anovulatory patients when luteal support was used. Hence, we routinely use vaginal progesterone to support the luteal phase in this group of patients.

Adjunctive Therapy with GnRH Agonists and Antagonists

Adjunctive therapy with GnRH agonists to prevent premature LH surges is[25] not necessary and will increase both costs and pain to patients. Two recent small studies have shown an increase in success rates with the addition of GnRH antagonist to gonadotrophin-stimulated IUI cycles but at an increased risk of multiple pregnancies. In low-resource settings, GnRH agonists and antagonists should not be used as it will increase costs significantly and increase the risk of multiple pregnancies as well as the need for more monitoring scans.

IUI VERSUS ART: COST-EFFECTIVENESS

A. Many studies have reported on the cost-effectiveness of IUI versus ART. A cohort study[26] found that the cost per delivery with ART was three to four fold higher than that with IUI. (Table 15.6).

However, ART was more cost effective than IUI in couples where the women were over the age of 40 years, where the male partner had extremely low sperm counts, couples with a long duration of infertility (>60 months) and severe endometriosis. When 3 previous cycles of IUI had failed, couples should be advised to consider ART rather than persist with IUI as the cost effectiveness favored ART. (Fast Track and Standard Treatment Trial (FASTT, 2009)[27]

B. A basic algorithm to triage patients into IUI or ART program is suggested in Flow chart 15.1.

CONCLUSION

IUI is a simple, cheap and noninvasive fertility treatment. In low resource settings, IUI still has a major role as first line treatment of infertility, provided there are sufficient sperms and there is no tubal disease. Success rates range from 3 percent to 20 percent, with most centres averaging between 8 to 14 percent per cycle. Success rates can be optimized by patient selection, using some form of ovarian stimulation and timing the insemination appropriately. Careful and judicious monitoring of follicle response with a strict cancellation criteria is important in minimizing multiple pregnancies. For cost-effectiveness, it is important to limit the number of IUI cycles and to offer ART where available, if the couple have not been successful after 3 cycles of IUI.

Table 15.6: Relative cost-effectives of various infertility treatment at one academic medical center (Van Voorhis *et al*, 1997)[26]

Procedure	*No. of couples*	*No. of procedures*	*No. (%) of deliveries*	*Multiple birth rate (%)*	*Cost per delivery ($)*
IUI	54	103	6 (5.8)	0	8,674
CC-IUI	91	188	12 (6.3)	8.3	7,808
HMG-IUI	52	80	14 (17.5)	21.0	10,282
ART	136	155	43 (27.7)	30.0	37,028

Flow chart 15.1: Algorithm for patient selection in IUI program

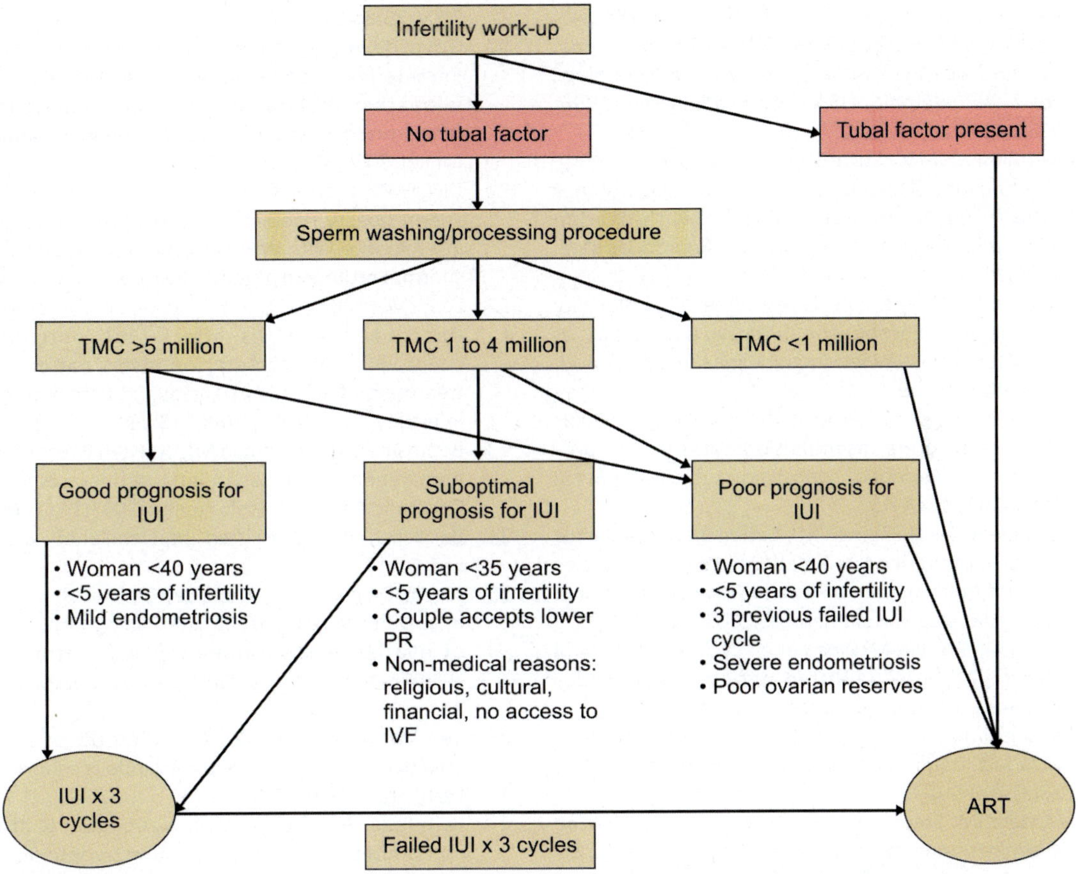

REFERENCES

1. Balasch J, Homburg R. Practical Guide to PCOS and IUI, CMP Medica Pacific, 2007; 33.
2. Steures P, Van der Steeg JW, Hompes PGA et al. Intrauterine Insemination, what do we really know? A critical appraisal of the literature, F, V and V in OBGYN, 2010;13-28.
3. Ombelet W, andeput H, Van de Putte G et al. Intrauterine insemination after ovarian stimulation with clomiphene citrate: predictive potential of inseminating motile count and sperm morphology? Hum. Reprod. 1997;12:1458-63.
4. Balasch J, Homburg R. Practical Guide to PCOS and IUI. CMP Medica Pacific, 2007;33-4.
5. Stone BA, Vargyas JM, Ringler GE *et al*. Determination of the outcome of intrauterine insemination: analysis of outcomes of 9963 consecutive cycles. Am J Obstet Gynecol 1999;180:1522-34.
6. Loh SKE, Leong NKY. Superovulation-intrauterine insemination: an additional tool in the treatment of infertility Signapore Med J 1996;37:66-8.
7. Balasch J. Reprod. Biomed Online 2004; 9: 664-72.
8. Al-Fozan H, Al-Khadouri M. Tan SL et al. A randomized trial of letrozole versus clomiphene citrate in women undergoing superovulation. Fertile Steril. 2004;1561-63.
9. Marinho AO, Sallam HN, Goessens LK et al. Real time pelvic ultrasonography during the periovulatory period of patients attending an artificial insemination clinic. Fertil. Steril. 1982;37:633-38
10. R. Cantineau AE et al. Cochrane Database Syst. Rev 2003;(i):CD 003854.

11. Khattas AF, Mustafa FA, Taylor PJ. The use of Urine LH detection kits to time intrauterine insemination with donor sperm. Hum Reprod. 2005;20(9):2542-45.
12. Dodson WC, Harey AF. In: Adashi EY et al. eds. Reproductive Endocrinology, Surgery and Technology vol 2. Philadelphia, USA: Lippincott-Raven. 1996; 2234-43.
13. van Rumste MM, Custers IM, van der Veen F et al. The influence of the number of follicles on pregnancy rates in intrauterine insemination with ovarian stimulation: a meta-analysis. Hum Reprod Update. 2008;14:563-70.
14. Haagen EC, Hermens RP, Nelen WL et al. Subfertility guidelines in Europe: the quantity and quality of intrauterine insemination guidelines. Hum Reprod. 2006;21:2103-09.
15. Miller PB, Acres ML, Proctor JG et al. Flexible versus rigid intrauterine insemination catheters: a prospective, randomized, controlled study. Fertil Steril 2005;83(5):1544-46.
16. Cantineau AE, Heineman MJ, Cohen BJ. Single versus double intrauterine insemination in stimulated cycles for subfertile couples: a systemic review based on a Cochrane review. Hum Reprod. 2003;18:941-46.
17. Dmowski WP, Pry M, Ding J et al. Cycle – specific and cummulative fecundity in patients with endometriosis who are undergoing controlled ovarian hyperstimulation – intrauterine insemination or *in vitro* fertilization embryo transfer. Fertil Steril 2002; 78(4):750-56.
18. Custers IM, Steures P, Hompes P et al. Intrauterine insemination: how many cycles should we perform? Hum Reprod. 2008;23(4):885-8.
19. Aboulghar M, Mansour R, Serour G et al. Controlled ovarian hyper-stimulation and intrauterine insemination for treatment of unexplained infertility should be limited to a maximum of three trials. Fertil Steril 2001;75:88-91.
20. Goverde AJ, McDonnell J, Vermeiden JP et al. Intrauterine insemination or *in vitro* fertilization in idiopathic subfertility and male subfertility: a randomized trial and cost effectiveness analysis. Lancet 2000;355(9197):13-18.
21. Dickey RP, Pyrzok R, Lu PY et al. Comparison of the sperm quality necessary for successful intrauterine insemination with WHO threshold values for normal sperm. Fertil Steril 1999;71:864-69.
22. Lee VMS, Wong JSY, Loh SK et al. sperm motility in the semen analysis affects the outcome of superovulation intrauterine insemination in the treatment of infertile Asian couples with male factor infertility. BJOG 2002; 109: 115-20.
23. Boomsma CM, Heineman MJ, Cohleen BJ et al. Semen preparation techniques for intrauterine insemination. Cochrane Database Syst. Review 2007;17:CD 04507.
24. Balasch J, et al. J Assisted Reprod Genet 1996;13: 551-6.
25. Barros-Delgadillo JC, Trejo-Castandeda H, E-Ormsby et al. Differing response to GnRH antagonists in cycles of ovarian hyperstimulation plus intrauterine insemination. Gynecol Obstet. Max. 2010;78(1):15-28.
26. Van Voorhis BJ, Sparks AE, Allen BD et al. Cost effectiveness of infertility treatments: a cohort study. Fertil Steril 1997;67:830-36.
27. Reindollar RH, Regan MM, Neumann PG et al. A randomized clinical trial to evaluate optimal treatment for unexplained infertility: the fast track and standard treatment (FASTT) trial. Fertil Steril 2009; 16:1395-1445.

Chapter 16

In Vitro Maturation

Seung-Yup Ku, Shin Yong Moon

INTRODUCTION

In vitro maturation (IVM) has been focused as an alternative source of competent oocytes without use of gonadotropin. Especially, women with hyper-response to ovulation induction would be appropriate candidates for IVM.

Human oocytes obtained for *in vitro* maturation (IVM) are usually obtained from 6 to 14 mm sized follicles which are of immature status. Therefore, adequate maturation is key procedure of this technology and the ultimate goal of IVM would be to artificially provide the original intrafollicular maturation conditions.

WHY IVM?

Nowadays, it has become a trend to use gonadotropin for superovulation carefully to minimize the side effects. However, one of the most serious complications, ovarian hyperstimulation syndrome (OHSS) is not yet preventable. Oocyte IVM technology involves retrieving immature oocytes from antral follicles and culturing in a 'cumulus-enclosed fashion.' Further studies are needed for IVM to be considered an effective and safe method compared to conventional ART treatment.

There are some factors that are known to influence the success rate of IVM, and they are as follow: selection of the patients, priming of the follicles, preparing endometrium, and condition of the culture (Gardner, 2009).

Until now, about 1000 IVM-babies have been born and 400 of them have been registered. There have not been any reports regarding the complications related to pregnancy or malformation as yet (Mikkelsen et al, 2005). Although the hypothesis that IVM can result in imprinting disturbances has not been proved wrong, cytogenetic evaluation of embryos is probably a reasonable predictor of the risks caused by IVM method (Gardner, 2009).

OOCYTES FROM ANTRAL FOLLICLES

Small antral follicles of 2 to 8 mm are recruited by FSH concentration that rises after regression of the corpus luteal cyst of the previous menstrual cycle. Each follicle has different capacity for its growth. The recruited antral follicle each grows differently due to paracrine interactions and FSH levels, which decrease with the growth of a dominant follicle. When immature oocytes are aspirated, some of the follicles might be about to go through atretic changes. Some of the small follicles' oocyte-granulosa complexes may lack inhibitory signals which lead to reactivation.

The induction of the atretic process can be prevented by maintaining increased FSH concentrations and higher MII maturation was yielded after gonadotropin priming. In young volunteers who were treated with oral pills after which maximum of 4 to 5 days of rFSH was given, when three or more follicles of size >6 mm was monitored, oocytes were retrieved the following day. As part of the outcomes, an average of 6.5 oocytes had been retrieved per cycle, and the follicles >7 mm in diameter had a better maturation capacity than that of the smaller follicles. In addition to that, maturation rate to MII stage as in the range of 70 to 80 percent.

Follicular diameter at the time of oocyte pick-up seems to be important in further development. Oocytes were well developed when they were aspirated before the dominant follicle reached 10 mm (Gardner, 2009).

HOW TO DO IVM?

The technique of immature oocyte retrieval involves the following. First, aspiration of immature oocytes should be performed with a transvaginal ultrasound that has good resolution so that small antral follicles are detected without difficulty. Second, a double-lumen needle would be of good use for flushing when cumulus-oocyte complexes (COCs) are not readily detached from its follicular wall. Third, pre-warmed buffer solution containing 2 to 10 U/ml heparin is generally used to flush the punctured follicles. Last but not least, aspiration pressure should be reduced to 60 mm Hg from 100 mm Hg during aspiration of the immature oocytes, in order to prevent the detachment of cumulus from the oocyte and for a more delicate oocyte aspiration.

Identification and typing of cumulus-corona-oocyte complexes requires careful process. The morphology of the aspirated COCs from smaller follicles less than 12 mm does not exactly resemble the mature oocytes, but is rather enclosed within compacted layers of cumulus mass. One has to be able to differentiate more compact masses of mural granulosa cells from the clumps of COCs, for identification of the COCs. Moreover, since it is much more time consuming searching and evaluating COCs compared to that of the conventional IVF method, it is important to keep control of temperature, and pH. Since, the mucification process does not happen in most of the cases in the follicle of small size, detachment of COCs from the follicle wall is not as easy and multiple flushings are required to obtain immature oocyte.

The manipulation of the COCs is generally performed as in the following manner. Entire petri dish is overviewed at a magnification of 5X, then, the isolation of immature COCs from the red blood cells can be attempted through filtering via cell-strainer device with 70 um pores. The clumps which seem to be containing an oocyte is then sucked up using the pipette and replace them to a new plate to rinse debris off. The oocytes are washed in three steps in buffered media before being placed in IVM media for incubation.

To perform a more thorough evaluation, inverted microscope with Hoffman modulation contrast system can be adapted. A magnification of 200X is done, and germinal vesicle is sought for to grade nuclear maturation. Maintenance of physiologic temperature of 37°C is another condition which should be considered, and it is possible with heating stages on the stereo-microscope as well as inverted microscope. Laminar flow is necessary for a gassed table mini-incubator to maintain optimal temperature and pH of the culture medium outside the incubator.

Depending on the type of clinical protocol applied, the COCs are cultured for 24-36 or even 48 hours. The oocyte, when matured enough, is scored according to three criteria: cumulus expansion, nuclear maturation, and oocyte morphology.

Optimal culture medium as well as effective strategy for culturing oocytes is what we strive to distinguish among many known available methods. As with other ART treatment, culturing method should be individualized according to the condition of the oocyte to improve the quality.

IVM of oocytes drawn from small antral follicles carry possibility of having increased risk of aneuploidy, but there exists few information regarding cytogenetic constitution of IVM. There have been several studies which concluded that oocytes retrieved from small antral follicles have less capacity to undergo correct chromosome segregation (Gardner, 2009).

CYTOPLASMIC MATURITY IN OOCYTES

After sperm penetrates oocyte, cortical granule (CG) exocytosis happens as a result of intracellular calcium mobilization. Then, CG releases hydrolytic enzymes, which modifies zona pellucida to harden, and thus polyspermy prohibited. In a mature oocyte, CGs are lined up below oolemma. Incomplete dispersion of CGs, thus, relates to incomplete cytoplasmic maturation.

CGs may be localized by electron microscope analysis. Another way to identify the location of CGs would be to stain CGs with a fluorescent marker and analyze them on a confocal laser microscope.

Although what microfilaments do in primate oocyte maturation is unclear, the formation and localization of microfilaments may provide information about maturity of oocyte. Microfilaments are needed in chromosome movements during first and second meiosis, in the movement of the sperm after fertilization, and for syngamy as well. Microtubules are tubulin protein which forms meiotic spindle during maturation. Microtubules are known to be sensitive to changes in surrounding environment including temperature. Segregation and alignment of the chromosomes during meiosis involve interaction between chromosomes and cytoskeleton, and thus disturbance of the spindle microtubules can be irreversible and eventually affect the genetic balance. Evaluation of the abnormal spindle structures after oocyte maturation is important in many aspects. During culture of the oocytes, such evaluation may provide information regarding control of manipulation, and checkpoint for assessing the environment surrounding the oocyte (Table 16.1).

Table 16.1: List of recent culture conditions used by IVF laboratories

	Basal Media	*Protein*	*Gonadotropin*	*Others*	*Reference*
Manufactured medium	Maturation medium (Maria fertility hospital)	–	0.075 IU/mL FSH, 0.075 IU/mL LH	–	Lim et al, 2009
	TCM-199	20 percent FBS	0.075 IU/mL FSH, 0.5 IU/mL hCG, 1 g/mL E2	–	Cha et al, 2005
Commercial medium	IVM medium Medicult® IVM System	10 percent patient serum	0.075 IU/mL FSH, 0.1 IU/mL hCG	–	Origio medicult media
	IVM media kit SAGE®	–	0.075 IU/mL FSH, 0.075 IU/mL hCG	–	SAGE Media

Mitochondrial redistribution was shown to induce structural changes in hamster oocytes after fertilization. Changes in the pattern of mitochondrial distribution are known to be associated with abnormal development of the embryo. Thus, by analyzing mitochondrial distribution of an oocyte, one could roughly predict the quality of embryo.

Proteins are needed for regulation of nuclear and cytoplasmic maturation to happen, which eventually leads to maturation of mammalian oocyte. 2D gel electrophoresis may enable us to explore about factors involved in cytoplasmic maturation. Since some aspects of cytoplasmic maturation are controlled by cytoplasm, reviewing the pattern of proteins synthesized after oocyte maturation with specific culture may help us as well.

INSEMINATION AFTER IVM

The time of maturation is important in many aspects. It affects the fertilization and developmental capacity of the oocyte. Also, it depends on the type of hormonal treatment given to the patient and the conditions in which the oocyte has been cultured.

PolScope was used to examine the spindles in *in vitro* matured denuded oocytes, and after 24 hours, 77 percent of the oocytes reached the metaphase II. A study in which *in vitro* matured cumulus-enclosed MII oocytes retrieved from small follicles are used, is necessitated to check these data accordingly.

Several studies conclude that immature oocytes from ICSI cycles have a low developmental potential.

Insemination via conventional IVF of *in vitro* matured oocytes has shown lower success rate compared with that of *in vivo* mature oocytes. Prolonged culture period resulting in hardening of the zona pellucid of the oocyte might be associated with the decreased fertilization.

In one study, higher fertilization rates by ICSI and similar embryonic quality compared to that of IVF were observed. Lately, a higher fertilization rate with ICSI, and higher pregnancy and implantation rates with IVF had been noted. With the outcomes of these studies, we may conclude that the functional mechanisms required for the fertilization have been accomplished in *in vitro* matured oocytes, comparable with those of oocytes in *in vivo*.

After polar body (PB) extrusion, the oocyte requires a short period of time to form its second meiotic spindle. This process is necessary for preparing the oocyte for the entrance of sperm. When should we perform microinjection of IVM? Between 2 and 6 hours after PB extrusion is thought be the most optimal time for microinjection of IVM oocytes. Highest fertilization rates may be accomplished when oocytes are injected between 1 and 2 hours after PB extrusion. However, embryonic quality was shown to be similar if oocytes were injected earlier or later (Gardner, 2009).

OOCYTE AGING

What happens when the oocytes are aged *in vitro*? When the oocytes become post-mature, changes in localization of cytoplasmic organelles may take place. Moreover, after fertilization, post-mature oocytes may even inhibit the release of cortical granule or show poor zona reaction. In aged oocytes, clumping of mitochondria, an increase in the electron density along with changes in shape, and the association with large vacuoles become more distinct (Gardner, 2009) (Figures 16.1A to C).

Metaphase I oocytes failed to complete maturation or MII oocytes aged in culture tend to show deep-seated spindles with less number of microtubules or spindles with attenuated poles. Chromosomes often form clusters or disperse in the cytoplasm (Van Blerkom et al, 1994). Fragmentation of PB may be a sign of aging in human oocytes (Gardner, 2009). A study about

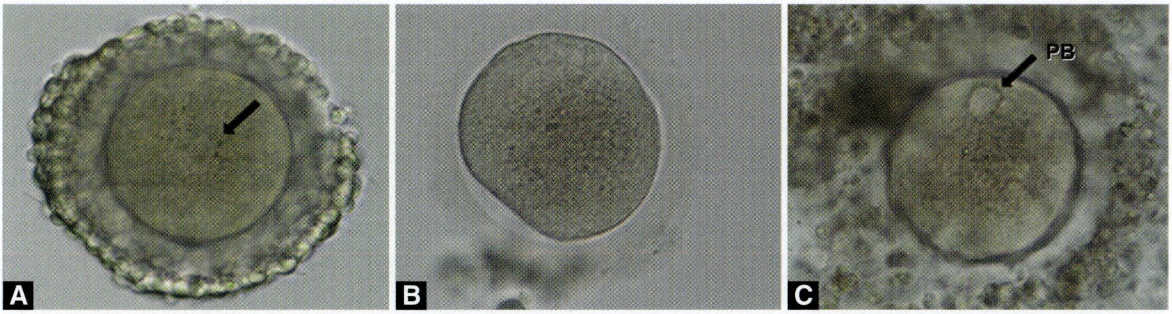

Figs 16.1A to C: Photomicrographs of IVM oocytes. (A) Cumulus-corona-oocyte complex (COC) has the GV (arrow). (B) Metaphase I oocyte after *in vitro* maturation (24–30 hours of culture). (C) Metaphase II oocyte after *in vitro* maturation (24–30 hours of culture) (PB: polar body). X200

spontaneous zona hardening by Fukuda et al concluded that hardening of zona is an indicator of oocyte aging (Fukuda et al, 1992).

Calcium signaling is associated with important consequences in oocytes, including acquiring meiotic competence and oocyte activation (Carroll et al, 1994; Homa et al, 1993). Modification in the regulation of intracellular Ca is one of the major changes taking place during oocyte maturation (Carroll et al, 1996). Recently, *in vitro* aging-related changes in Ca release after fertilization have been observed (Gardner, 2009).

EMBRYONIC DEVELOPMENT

The quality of oocyte, which has undergone IVM, may be evaluated by reviewing its fertilizability and its capacity in embryo development.

Many studies have shown a high incidence of cleavage arrest after IVM and increased multinucleation due to cell division arrest (Nogueira et al, 2000). Possible reasons causing cleavage arrest are inadequate conditions of culture, abnormalities, and failure of embryonic gene expression. PCO patients were observed to have a low cleavage rate from IVM of oocytes (Gardner, 2009).

Cell division arrest may also cause the increased incidence of polyploidy and mosaicism. Chromosomal abnormalities have been blamed for its partial associated with multinuclear blastomeres. This kind of poor embryo quality is seen mainly in people with the immature oocytes such as GVs, from superovulation and ICSI. These less than optimal oocytes from ICSI cycles should not be compared with immature oocytes retrieved from small follicles of 6 to 12 mm, without stimulation but rather with an aid of small amount of gonadotropin. IVM oocytes yield good quality embryos, and satisfactory pregnancy rates were made possible with a maximum of 2 to 3 embryos transferred (Mikkelsen et al, 2000).

Another method that may be applied in evaluating embryo quality is the spreading technique for the FISH method. Chromosome analysis via FISH reveals nuclear status of the embryo. At last, evaluation of blastocyst formation rate can be another substitute.

IVM MEDIA

It is needless to say that media and laboratory conditions affect nuclear and cytoplasmic maturation of oocytes during IVM. Among many factors of culture medium, pH affects internal pH of the oocyte. How is pH an important factor during IVM of oocytes? According to Cicirelli et al, increasing pH leads to resumption of meiosis (Cicirelli et al, 1983). Changes in pH during isolation resulted in alteration of the developmental capacity (Imoedemhe et al, 1993). In one study where different culture media, or culture conditions with minor changes were used for IVM of mouse oocytes, spontaneous oocyte maturation, meiotic inhibitors suppressing germinal vesicle breakdown (GVBD) or ligands inducing meiosis were shown to be affected and led to significant changes (Downs et al, 1997). Maintenance of essential metabolism, growth and molecular expression patterns, preimplantation embryo development can be achieved. In the near future, culture conditions that enable generation of factors which are critical for further embryo development shall be available.

IVM FOR FERTILITY PRESERVATION

In vitro fertilization and embryo cryopreservation are considered as the only available method for fertility preservation in female patients who have been diagnosed with cancer and planning to undergo treatment. However, delay in the treatment of cancer and exposure to above normal level of estrogen caused by ovarian hyperstimulation may have negative effect on patients. *In vitro* maturation, which does not necessary delay cancer treatment, nor exposes patients to increased estradiol level has been a new option which has been available recently.

Brief overview of an IVM cycle for fertility preservation is as follows. Monitoring begins between days 2 and 5 of a menstrual cycle, with a baseline scan of uterus and ovaries for any abnormalities, and for IVM, endometrium and antral follicles. About a week later, when it is time for largest follicle to reach 10 to 12 mm in diameter, patients should visit the clinic for the second scan. 10,000 IU of hCG should be administered intramuscularly 38 hours before the collection of the oocytes. Cycles for fertility preservation, do not require paying attention to endometrial thickness, since embryo transfer will not take place. Multiple punctures usually take place and flushing the needle between punctures is often necessary (Ata et al, 2010).

PERSPECTIVES

The reserves necessary for early development of embryo are gained late in oogenesis, right before the incidence of ovulation. Also, the oocyte is known to produce RNA species with prolonged stability that is only functional in different levels at different times. IVM may be yielding less number of clinical pregnancies owing to lack of these different mechanisms required at different times. Heterogeneous pool of oocytes and the oocytes retrieved from the smallest follicles which may not have necessary reserves for proper preimplantation development are some of the possible reasons contributing to above-mentioned difficulty.

There have been studies asserting that nuclear and cytoplasmic maturation have to happen in relation to one another for normal development. Disturbances in nuclear meiotic maturation rate, inadequate redistribution of organelles, and disability to decondense sperm chromatin after sperm aster formation are some of the consequences when their course maturations are in discordance (328-330).

Also, we cannot make such abrupt statement that today's culture techniques provide the most adequate environment to enhance the outcome of IVM. Thus, further studies to elucidate the critical mechanisms of oocyte maturation should be planned.

When meiotically competent oocyte is retrieved, meiosis is reinitiated resulting in immediate arrest of transcription leading to discontinuation of cytoplasmic maturation. If cytoplasmic maturation is to be continued, then the reinitiation of meiosis should be inhibited, along with optimal culture environment provided. In order to attempt this, we should first be able to grade cytoplasmic maturation. Moreover, research needs to be done to enable routine practice that allows grading of oocyte maturity. This way, we could have an idea of exactly how far certain oocyte has gone in the course of its maturation, and provide culture environment accordingly.

Some of the possible causes that seem to be resulting in deficient quality of the oocytes such as aneuploidy as well as the failure of embryonic development are as follows. Even before the retrieval of the oocyte, intrafollicular environment may be suboptimal leading to defects originating in GV oocyte. *In vitro* environment of oocyte, where oocyte is cultured, might cause defects. GV oocyte retrieved from the follicle with cytoplasmic immaturity might be another reason (Gardner, 2009).

An ideal culture system in which a prolonged period of *in vitro* development before the beginning of meiosis, namely prematuration culture, and an optimal *in vitro* environment before and during maturation should be provided. This culture system might be a requisite to enable a synchronized nuclear and cytoplasmic maturation of oocytes. The regulation of the nuclear maturation of human oocyte might provide the first step towards favorable medium conditions that enhance cytoplasmic maturity during a prematuration phase.

CONCLUSIONS

Immature oocyte should be retrieved before the intraovarian selection processes happen or after FSH is given. Prolonged so-called prematuration system may be advantageous for IVM since follicles of 6 to 12 mm still proceed with a growth phase of 4 to 5 days before ovulation, *in vivo*.

For immature oocytes to be well-developed, oocyte nuclear and cytoplasmic maturation should be coordinated. Hence, the transzonal connection between granulosa cells and oocyte should be held patent, so that regulatory substances may be transferred between them. In order for the cytoplasmic maturation of the oocyte to be achieved, oocytes should be in meiotically arrested state, and growth factors and hormonal supplements provided. Once cytoplasmic maturation is completed, the development after fertilization may be improved.

Safety restricts the use of protein sources obtained from other species. Serum substitutes may be necessary to cover the serum functions, as mentioned above.

Steroids in culture medium may play important role in maintenance of intercellular contacts, namely estrogens and progesterone, as well as for the oocyte's cytoplasmic maturation. In addition to that, meiosis-activating sterol, growth hormone, activin/inhibin ratios, or enhancers of glutathione synthesis in the cytoplasm are some of the methods to improve cytoplasmic maturation (Gardner, 2009).

Safety should be tested on the reinitiation of meiosis by performing karyotyping of MII oocytes. If proven safe, matured oocytes should be injected with sperm and the incidence of aneuploidy checked in day 3 embryos. Blastocyst quality obtained after IVM should be emphasized, and transferred embryos should be monitored closely during implantation for a successful outcome.

BIBLIOGRAPHY

1. Ata B, Shalom-Paz E, Chian RC, Tan SL. *In vitro* maturation of oocytes as a strategy for fertility preservation. Clin Obstet Gynecol 2010;53(4):775-86.

2. Carroll J, Swann K, Whittingham D, Whitaker M. Spatiotemporal dynamics of intracellular [Ca2+]i oscillations during the growth and meiotic maturation of mouse oocytes. Development 1994;120(12): 3507-17.
3. Carroll J, Jones KT, Whittingham DG. Ca2+ release and the development of Ca2+ release mechanisms during oocyte maturation: a prelude to fertilization. Rev Reprod 1996;1(3):137-43.
4. Cha KY, Chung HM, Lee DR, Kwon H, Chung MK, Park LS, Choi DH, Yoon TK. Obstetric outcome of patients with polycystic ovary syndrome treated by *in vitro* maturation and *in vitro* fertilization-embryo transfer. Fertil Steril 2005;83(5):1461-5
5. Cicirelli MF, Robinson KR, Smith LD. Internal pH of Xenopus oocytes: a study of the mechanism and role of pH changes during meiotic maturation. Dev Biol 1983;100(1):133-46.
6. Fukuda A, Roudebush WE, Thatcher SS. Influences of *in vitro* oocyte aging on microfertilization in the mouse with reference to zona hardening. J Assist Reprod Genet 1992;9(4):378-83.
7. Gardner DK. Textbook of assisted reproductive technologies. 3rd ed. London: Informa Healthcare; 2009;111-53.
8. Homa ST, Carroll J, Swann K. The role of calcium in mammalian oocyte maturation and egg activation. Hum Reprod 1993;8(8):1274-81.
9. Imoedemhe DA, Chan RC, Ramadan IA, Sigue AB. Changes in follicular fluid gas and pH during carbon dioxide pneumoperitoneum for laparoscopic aspiration and their effect on human oocyte fertilizability. Fertil Steril 1993;59(1):177-82.
10. Lim JH, Yang SH, Xu Y, Yoon SH, Chian RC. Selection of patients for natural cycle *in vitro* fertilization combined with *in vitro* maturation of immature oocytes. Fertil Steril 2009;91:1050-5.
11. Mikkelsen AL, Smith S, Lindenberg S. Impact of oestradiol and inhibin A concentrations on pregnancy rate in *in-vitro* oocyte maturation. Hum Reprod 2000;15(8):1685-90.
12. Mikkelsen AL. Strategies in human *in-vitro* maturation and their clinical outcome. Reprod Biomed Online 2005;10(5):593-9.
13. Nogueira D, Staessen C, Van de Velde H, Van Steirteghem A. Nuclear status and cytogenetics of embryos derived from *in vitro*-matured oocytes. Fertil Steril 2000;74(2):295-8.
14. Van Blerkom J, Davis PW. Cytogenetic, cellular, and developmental consequences of cryopreservation of immature and mature mouse and human oocytes. Microsc Res Tech 1994;27(2):165-93.

Chapter 17

Advances in Assisted Reproductive Technologies in Low-resource Settings

Hrishikesh Pai, Rishma Pai, Nandita Palshetkar, Nandan Roongta, Rutvij Dalal

INTRODUCTION

Assisted reproductive technologies (ARTs) primarily aim at assisting in achievement of conception. It is our ethical responsibility to make these technologies available to all who seek ART, irrespective of their socioeconomic status or location. This should be done irrespective of the available resources, with no compromise on the methodology or technology used.

There has been a belief that assisted reproductive technology (ART) is technically too demanding for the capacity and expertise available in developing countries. It has always been considered too costly for the low-resources of the developing nations. To add to these factors, there are the sociocultural factors that cannot be ignored. In most such settings, children are so highly valued that a woman's status is often majorly defined through motherhood, with infertility being a terrible stigma. Such circumstances exacerbate suffering, and cause desperation.[17]

The World Health Organization (WHO) in a 2001 meeting challenged some of the popular assertions about infertility and the developing world. It recommended that infertility be considered a global health problem and called for more innovative approaches in treatment, such as development of low-cost ART for low-resource settings.[1] An attitude shift in the past decade has resulted in innovative attempts exploring low-cost ART. Also medical technology transfer has been accelerated through globalization. Future steps should offer infertility services within comprehensive reproductive health programs, and equitable access.[2]

As per the European Society for Human Reproduction and Embryology (ESHRE), the cornerstones in the treatment of infertility in low-resource settings, are the simplification of techniques, minimizing of complications, training for health care workers, and the incorporation of fertility treatments into existing health care programs.

In this article we will throw light upon the innovations in the various aspects of the ART cycle, which ultimately culminate into a very high pregnancy rate in couples undergoing treatment.

PRETREATMENT

Pretreatment[3] is the foundation on which the results of ART are based. It is essential to first eliminate or improve the causative and contributory factors of infertility, so as to offer optimum ART results to patients. Considering that patients would not be desirous of repetitive attempts, more so in a low-resource setting for accessory reasons, it is amongst the most important steps with appropriate prior counseling.

Uterine Myomas

Myomas located in close proximity (less than 5 mm) to the endometrial cavity, and those that distort the uterine cavity, and larger intramural myomas may have adverse effects on IVF outcomes. Intramural myomas larger than 4 cm in diameter should be removed by laparotomy or laparoscopy irrespective of whether or not they distort the uterine cavity. In patients with submucous myomas, a hysteroscopy for ruling out distortion of the endometrium and a myomectomy where indicated is associated with improved outcomes in ART results.[4]

Endometriosis

Various studies have shown that cases of minimal and mild endometriosis undergoing ART treatment have a shorter time to pregnancy and higher live-birth rate if all visible endometriosis is completely eliminated before the start of treatment.[5] However moderate to severe endometriosis, need to be considered differently. Especially ovarian endometriomas and the associated injury to the ovarian reserve is still elusive. Current evidence indicates that laparoscopic removal of endometriomas does not improve IVF results. On the contrary, it may cause a decrease of ovarian responsiveness to gonadotropins.[6] Hence, it is more prudent to proceed to IVF directly to reduce time to pregnancy, and avoid potential surgical compromise to the ovary and its reserve.

Hydrosalpinges

The deleterious effects of large hydrosalpinges on IVF outcome and the advantages of disconnecting the tube from them have been well documented. As per the Cochrane review 2010,[7] surgical treatment should be considered for all women with hydrosalpinges prior to IVF treatment. Previous evidence supported only unilateral salpingectomy for a unilateral hydrosalpinx (bilateral salpingectomy for bilateral hydrosalpinges). This review now provides evidence that laparoscopic tubal occlusion is an alternative to laparoscopic salpingectomy in improving IVF pregnancy rates in women with hydrosalpinges. Further research is required to assess the value of placement of an occlusive microinsert into the proximal portion of the tube, tubal aspiration of hydrosalpinges prior to or during IVF procedures and also the value of tubal restorative surgery as an alternative (or as a preliminary) to IVF.

PCOD

Metformin as an adjunct to IVF treatment for women with PCOS has to be considered keeping the following aspects in mind, i.e. the BMI, proven insulin resistance, and previous evidence of resistance to clomiphene citrate. Patients, who had previously demonstrated clomiphene resistance, did benefit from adjunctive metformin. Also, hyperinsulinemic lean women with PCOD display a higher ovulation rate with metformin.[8] The Cochrane review 2009[9] found no evidence that metformin treatment before or during ART cycles improves live birth or pregnancy rates. However, the risk of OHSS in women with PCOS and undergoing IVF or ICSI cycles was reduced with metformin. Weight loss / Bariatric surgery also play a contributory role.

OVULATION INDUCTION

With the challenging aim to achieve a low-cost protocol close to the ideal, multiple permutations and combinations have been attempted. This being one of the most important aspects of the ART cycle, special emphasis has been placed on it.

Special considerations in the low-resource setting:
- Optimum stimulation (considering that the patient might not opt for a repeat attempt)
- Natural cycle IVF
- Minimal stimulation protocols in cases where applicable
- Prevention of ovarian hyperstimulation syndrome (OHSS)
- Prevention of multiple embryo pregnancies[16]

An ideal low-cost protocol would be:
- Low-cost
- Simple
- Without compromise in quality
- Success rates at par with the standard protocols.

The International Society for Mild Approaches in Assisted Reproduction (ISMAAR) has proposed the following classification for ovulation stimulation during ART procedures (Table 17.1).

1. *Natural cycle/Modified natural cycle protocols:* The natural cycle protocol involves no drugs whatsoever, and the LH surge is used to decide the timing of the oocyte retrieval. The modified natural cycle protocol is also with no stimulation medications, but only the hCG trigger is used, prior to the oocyte retrieval.

Table 17.1: International Society for Mild Approaches in Assisted Reproduction (ISMAAR) definitions[14]

Terminology	*Aim*	*Methodology*
Natural cycle IVF	Single oocyte	No medication
Modified natural cycle IVF	Single oocyte	hCG only Antagonist and FSH/HMG add-back
Mild IVF	2 to 7 oocytes	Low-dose FSH/HMG/oral compounds and antagonist
Conventional IVF	≥ 8 oocytes	Agonist or Antagonist Conventional FSH/HMG dose

Several studies published recently have shown that natural/modified natural cycles are beneficial in poor responders, those with repeated failure of implantation, and in those where stimulation is contraindicated.[12,13] It should preferably be offered as a series of cycles, as it is safer, cost-effective and less stressful to the patient.

2. *Antagonist vs agonist protocol:* Comparing both protocols the differences found included longer duration of treatment and higher consumption of gonadotropins, higher E2 levels on the day of hCG administration in the GnRH agonist compared to GnRH antagonist group. GnRH antagonists suppress gonadotropin secretion resulting in dramatic reduction in treatment cycle duration. A Cochrane review 2007, concluded that GnRH antagonist protocols are short, simple, with good clinical outcomes and significant reduction in severe OHSS incidence and gonadotropin amount; however, the lower pregnancy rate compared with the GnRH agonist long protocol necessitates counseling subfertile couples before recommending change from GnRH agonist to antagonist.[11]
3. *Minimal stimulation protocols:*[15] Mild stimulation is defined as "FSH or hMG administered at lower doses and/or for a shorter duration in a GnRH antagonist co-treated cycle, or when oral compounds are used alone or with gonadotropins". Ovulation induction with hCG or alternative medications, and luteal phase support is part of the protocol.
   a. *Short antagonist protocol with low-dose FSH:* Stimulation with low-dose gonadotropins FSH/hMG (150 IU/day) is delayed until the mid-follicular phase on day-5. A GnRH antagonist injection is added from when the follicle grows up to 14 mm. The induction of final maturation is with hCG 10,000 IU when the leading follicle is 18 mm

or more, and at least one additional follicle ≥ 15 mm.

b. *Clomiphene citrate + FSH protocol:* In this antagonist protocol, an initial 5 days of clomiphene citrate (100 mg/day) from day 2 of the cycle, is followed by continuous FSH/hMG at a fixed dose of 150 IU/day from day 9 onwards, until the ovulation induction trigger injection is to be given. A GnRH antagonist injection is added from when the follicle grows up to 13 mm.

c. *Late follicular phase hCG/LH protocol:* A stimulation protocol with late follicular-phase replacement of FSH administration by LH has recently been proposed as an alternative mild stimulation approach.

4. *Drugs used:* Costs of treatment are largely fixed costs (staff, facilities), but drugs, mainly gonadotropins, make up most of the total IVF fresh cycle costs. HP-hMG and rFSH have been found to be almost equally efficient despite the much lower costs of HP-hMG.[10]

5. *Prevention of OHSS:*
   - The protocol and the stimulatory agents have an important role and hence tailored protocols for every individual patient should be the norm.
   - Use of the antagonist protocol.
   - Replacing hCG as the trigger with recombinant LH or GnRH agonists (in an antagonist protocol cycle).
   - Prophylactic use of colloidal agents to prevent OHSS.

IVF LABORATORY

The IVF lab is what should be highly well-equipped and maintained in an area of low-resource settings. Since in such a scenario, the patient cannot afford to spend excessively on the IVF, the setup should be such that optimal results are assured and offered. It is the responsibility of the IVF specialist team to use the low-cost protocols prudently, in a so called 'bigger' setup, so as to minimize the chances of a repeat attempt and hence lessen the patient stress and financial burden.

Laboratory Setup

Ideally, the IVF laboratory should be located next to the oocyte collection and embryo transfer room. It should be seamless, with concealed wiring, stainless steel roof and walls and it should be fitted with air handling Units that can run 24/7. The temperature in the laboratory should be in the region of 26°C. The lab should have a minimum of two incubators. Higher the number of incubators in the laboratory better are the results. Some of the newer labs have one incubator per patient. However, this may not be possible in a low resource setting. Minimal opening of the incubators will result in better outcomes.

Intracytoplasmic Sperm Injection and Intracytoplasmic Morphologically Selected Sperm Injection

Intracytoplasmic sperm injection (ICSI) has been effectively used in patients in whom there is a male factor infertility. Normally, ICSI is performed at magnifications of 200 times. A new computer-based enhancing program called Intracytoplasmic Morphologically Selected Sperm (IMSI) can achieve magnifications of 7000 times. This higher magnification results in higher pregnancy rates especially in cases with a high degree of DNA-fragmentation. Also the early spontaneous miscarriage rate is reduced.

PICSI

Using the Hyaluronan-Bonding-Test, sperm cells get selected due to specific membrane-bonding characteristics. The PICSI Sperm Selection Device is a sterile, plastic culture dish with three microdots of hyaluronan hydrogel attached to the bottom interior of the dish. Mature human sperm attach themselves to the hyaluronan through specific receptors found on the sperm plasma membrane. These sperm exhibit no progressive movement, although their tails beat and they are capable of motility. They are easily selected and removed from the hyaluronan by a micropipette. Being mature the selected sperm do not show any DNA-degradation, and can be used for ICSI, with good outcomes.

In Vitro Maturation

In Vitro Maturation (IVM) as an alternative laboratory procedure applicable for young patients with normal menstrual cycles who would prefer lower stimulation, patients of PCOS where OHSS is to be avoided, and to salvage immature eggs collected during a standard IVF cycles, and in the poor responder patient.[19] IVM in the low-resource settings is applicable since lower doses and duration of the stimulation injections, and monitoring would cut down the basic costs to some extent.

Laser Hatching

Laser assisted hatching of the zona is done to aid the breaching of the zona pellucida and assist in the natural process of hatching. Most often the zona is not completely breached, but thinned from one side from where it cracks when the blastocyst is ready to hatch. The procedure is done to improve pregnancy rates. The indications for assisted laser hatching include, oocytes from a patient over 35 years of age, zona thickness >15 microns, previous IVF failures, post thaw embryo transfer, and prior to PGD.

According to a Cochrane review,[18] despite significantly improved odds of clinical pregnancy, there is insufficient evidence to determine any effect of assisted hatching on live birth rates. The increased multiple pregnancy rate is of concern although it likely that with a policy of single embryo transfer this may be lowered. Assisted hatching in the low-resource settings is applicable in general in an attempt to improve pregnancy rates, and especially in the younger patients where single embryo transfer is contemplated, to avoid multiple embryo pregnancies.

Blastocyst Culture

A day-5 embryo, i.e. the blastocyst, in the low-resource setting would be advantageous because of:

- Reduced number of embryos transferred, hence helps eliminate high order multiple gestations and the associated complications and increased costs.
- Better implantation rates.
- Avoids exposure to OHSS.
- Cryopreservation of embryos at blastocyst is more successful than earlier stages. Time for diagnosis if PGD done.
- Reduced pregnancy loss.
- Assessment of development and viability.

INVO Vaginal Culture

In this technique, after injection of the eggs with sperms, the eggs are placed in a specialized plastic container. This container is properly sealed and placed in a diaphragm. This diaphragm is inserted in the vagina of the patient, for 48 hours. After 48 hours, the eggs are assessed for fertilization and cleavage. The cleaved embryos are transferred back into the womb.[20] This is a very good technique in low resource area, as it eliminates the dependency on incubators and protects against electrical fluctuations/breakdown.

Embryo Cryopreservation

Embryo cryopreservation can be done by two methods; slow freezing, a traditional and time tested method, and vitrification, which is a relatively new technique. Vitrification is an advanced technique over slow freezing. It does not require any sophisticated instrumentation, is very quick and is known to give high (95%) survival of embryos as compared to slow freezing. In many units, the pregnancy rate following thaw of vitrified embryos is double that of slow freeze/thawed embryos.

Semen and Oocyte Banking

The techniques of freezing or vitrification have also been used for preservation of oocytes and sperm in cases of pre-therapy preservation, prior to cancer treatment, esp. chemo- and radiation therapy, and for oocyte preservation for reasons like procrastination of conception.

Human Embryo Selection — based on Morphology/Metabolism/ Genetics

The new science of selecting good quality embryos for transfer is called Omics. Omics enhances pregnancy rates and can also help decrease multiple pregnancy rates by enabling us to transfer fewer embryos back into the womb, without compromising results. This technique to rank and select the embryos that will be transferred into the uterus helps in improving the implantation rates. In metabolomics, the concentration of glucose and pyruvates in the culture medium surrounding the embryos is analyzed. Base on the levels, one can select a good quality embryo. One can also use high definition time lapse photography of the embryo development within the incubator using new systems such as Primovision or embryoscope. By comparing the morphological appearance of different embryos, the best embryo can be selected for transfer. The use of Genomics or preimplantation genetic diagnosis (PGD) should ideally be offered to all patients when indicated. PGD is especially important for aneuploidy screening, and in cases of familial genetic disorders, and clinically in cases of recurrent early pregnancy loss.

Luteal Phase Support

The natural cycle IVF does not require luteal phase support (LPS). Although debatable in the antagonist protocol, most prefer to support the luteal phase. The GnRH agonist protocol will always need LPS, since downregulated cycles are generally associated with luteal phase defect. The earlier use of hCG for LPS is now discouraged because of the associated risk of hyperstimulation. Progestogens and progesterone are the drugs of choice. The preferred routes of progesterone administration are oral, vaginal or intramuscular. Also, estradiol supplementation is added in most cases, for optimum results.

REFERENCES

1. Vayena E, Rowe P, Griffin PD, (Eds). Current practices and controversies in assisted reproduction: Report of a World Health Organization meeting. Geneva: World Health Organization, 2002.
2. Effy Vayena, Herbert B Peterson, David Adamson, Karl-G. Nygren. Assisted reproductive technologies in developing countries: are we caring yet? Fertility and Sterility July 2002;78(1):13-15.
3. David V Gardner, Botros RMB Rizk, Tommaso Falcone. Human Assisted Reproductive Technology – Future trends in Laboratory and Clinical practice. Cambridge University Press, 2011.
4. Vimercati A, Scioscia M, Lorusso F, Laera AF, et al. Do uterine fibroids affect IVF outcomes? Reprod Biomed Online. 2007;15(6):686-91.
5. Opøien HK, Fedorcsak P, Byholm T, Tanbo T. Complete surgical removal of minimal and mild endometriosis improves outcome of subsequent IVF/ICSI treatment. Reprod Biomed Online. 2011 Jun 15.
6. Bongioanni F, Revelli A, Gennarelli G, Guidetti D, et al. Ovarian endometriomas and IVF: a retrospective case-control study. Reprod Biol Endocrinol. 2011; 17(9):81.

7. Johnson N, van Voorst S, Sowter MC, Strandell A, et al. Surgical treatment for tubal disease in women due to undergo in vitro fertilisation. Cochrane Database Syst Rev. 2010;20(1):CD002125.
8. Gab Kovacs. How to Improve Your ART Success Rates: An Evidence-Based Review of Adjuncts to IVF. Cambridge University Press, 2011.
9. Tso LO, Costello MF, Albuquerque LE, Andriolo RB, et al. Metformin treatment before and during IVF or ICSI in women with polycystic ovary syndrome. Cochrane Database Syst Rev. 2009;15(2):CD006105.
10. Jaroslaw Wechowski, Mark Connolly, Dirk Schneider, Philip McEwan, et al. Cost-Richard Kennedy saving treatment strategies in *in vitro* fertilization: a combined economic evaluation of two large randomized clinical trials comparing highly purified human menopausal gonadotropin and recombinant follicle-stimulating hormone alpha. Fertility and Sterility April 2009;91(4):1067-76.
11. Al-Inany HG, Abou-Setta AM, Aboulghar M. Gonadotrophin-releasing hormone antagonists for assisted conception: a Cochrane review. Reprod Biomed Online. 2007;14(5):640-9.
12. Pelinck MJ, Knol HM, Vogel NE, Arts EG, Simons AH, Heineman MJ, Hoek A. Cumulative pregnancy rates after sequential treatment with modified natural cycle IVF followed by IVF with controlled ovarian stimulation. Hum Reprod. 2008;23(8):1808-14.
13. Nargund G, Frydman R. Towards a more physiological approach to IVF. Reprod Biomed Online. 2007; 14(5):550-2.
14. www.ismaar.org
15. Revelli A, Casano S, Salvagno F, Delle Piane L. Milder is better? Advantages and disadvantages of "mild" ovarian stimulation for human in vitro fertilization. Reprod Biol Endocrinol. 2011; 16(9):25.
16. Ombelet W, Campo R. Affordable IVF for developing countries. Reprod Biomed Online. 2007;15(3):257-65.
17. Sharma S, Mittal S, Aggarwal P. Management of infertility in low resource countries. BJOG. 2009;116 (Suppl 1):77-83.
18. Seif MM, Edi-Osagie EC, Farquhar C, Hooper L, et al. Assisted hatching on assisted conception (IVF and ICSI). Cochrane Database Syst Rev. 2006;25(1): CD001894.
19. Li J, Xu Y, Zhou G, Guo J, et al. Natural cycle IVF/IVM may be more desirable for poor responder patients after failure of stimulated cycles. J Assist Reprod Genet. 2011 Jun 22.
20. Lucena EE, Saa AM, Navarro DE, Pulido CA, et al. The new era in ART: INVO. Fertility and Sterility Vol. 94, Issue 4, S36. September 2010.

Chapter 18

The Art and Science of Embryo Transfer

Derek F Lok, Priya Sivadas

Embryo transfer is the final step in the process of *in vitro* fertilization (IVF). To most clinicians embryo transfer (ET) is a simple procedure and only means the simple task of inserting the embryo transfer catheter into the uterine cavity and ejecting the embryos. But it has been demonstrated that there is significant difference in pregnancy rates with different individuals performing the procedure within the same IVF unit.[1] The technique of embryo transfer needs to be standardized and this is regarded as the most important factor influencing the success rate in IVF in a survey of 80 IVF practitioners.[2] This final step in the whole process of assisted reproduction will determine the fate of a long process and great effort, from ovulation induction and oocyte retrieval, to the tedious lab procedures.

FACTORS AFFECTING THE ET SUCCESS

In natural conception, developing embryo enter uterine cavity from fallopian tube at morula or blastocyst stage, coordinated by the changing estrogen and progesterone levels after ovulation. Embryo transfer, on the other hand, involves transfer of either cleavage stage embryos or blastocyst into uterine cavity by blind introduction of foreign body from contaminated environment through the cervical canal. These artificial steps introduce deviations from the natural process and potentially compromise implantation. These may include timing of embryo arrival into uterine cavity, introduction of foreign materials which may negatively impact on endometrial environment, cause endometrial disruption or undesirable myometrial activities leading to displacement of transferred embryo, or misplacement of the embryo.

Timing or Stage of Embryo Transfer

In mammalian species, embryo undergoes cleavage and developments in fallopian tubes and enters uterine cavity at morula or blastocyst stages,[3] which equates to Day 4 – 5 of *in vitro* culture. The uterus provides a different nutritional environment from the oviduct during this early stage, particularly when subjected to superovulation with high levels of estrogen,[4] which can be toxic to early development of embryo in some species such as rabbit. While early arrival into uterine environment before compaction in other mammalian species mostly leads to poor pregnancy rates, this appears to be less crucial in human.[5] However, there are many physiological and theoretical advantages for later stage transfers, including:

1. Better uterine and embryonic synchronicity
2. Shortened period in uterine cavity before implantation which may reduce the risks of displacement, this together with
3. The larger size of the embryo at later stage of development may associate with reduced risks of ectopic pregnancy
4. The higher progesterone/estrogen ratio improve uterine myometrial quiescence hence lessen contraction, the latter an important factor in embryo transfer success.

A meta-analysis of 8 randomized trials selected from 282 studies showed blastocyst stage transfers resulted in higher implantation rates, clinical pregnancy and live birth rates than when embryos were transferred at cleavage stage.[6] The higher pregnancy rates with blastocyst transfer compared to cleavage stage were also demonstrated in an earlier Cochrane review,[7] with half the 18 studies included in the analysis showed higher implantation rates with blastocyst transfer, while the rest (apart from three showed lower) showed no differences. It is not certain how much of the higher implantation rates can be attributed to the timing of the transfer or higher viability of the embryos after self-selection in extended culture. However, it is noted that pregnancy rates per stimulated cycle were not higher in blastocyst transfer group despite higher implantation rates per transfer, likely due to higher cancellation rates (no blastocyst for transfer) especially in earlier studies when extended blastocyst culture laboratory conditions are less well developed or deficient. This highlight the importance of the tailoring of transfer strategies to local laboratory conditions, as the gain in more physiological stage of transfer may be offset by the compromise of the embryo wellbeing as a result of deficient *in vitro* conditions for embryo development available in the specific laboratory.

Introduction of Foreign Body (transfer catheter) into Endometrial Cavity

The insertion of embryo transfer catheter into uterine cavity can introduce undesirable materials into the uterine cavity including mucus and bacteria.

Cervical mucus can plug the catheter tip and affect the delivery of the embryos, especially as small volume of culture media is used to inject the embryos. This can lead to embryo retention, embryo damage and improper embryo placement.[8] It had been shown that the embryos were most likely to be retained when the catheter was contaminated with mucus and blood.[9] There is also the possibility of embryos sticking to the mucus around the catheter tip being dragged outside during the withdrawal of the catheter. Implantation may be affected if the mucus is pushed or injected higher into the uterus.[10]

Introduction of bacteria with embryos into endometrial cavity through contamination of the catheter tip occur in up to 49 percent of cases in one study,[11] and this lead to poorer pregnancy rates.[11-13] Use of antibiotics before embryo transfer has not been shown to improve pregnancy rates[14] and may disrupt the normal cervical bacterial flora hence is not recommended.

Removing the cervical mucus was associated with increased clinical pregnancy rates in one prospective control trial,[15] but vigorous flushing of the cervical canal is not necessary.[16,17] Gentle cleaning of vagina and cervix with sterile cotton ball or gauze soaked in saline or transfer medium will be sufficient to remove the cervical mucus and reduce bacterial contamination, the use of antiseptics for cleansing is not advisable due to toxicity to embryos.

Double lumen catheter (such as Cook Sydney IVF or Wallace ET catheters) with firmer outer sheath which is introduced up to the internal os, protecting the inner soft catheter from vaginal or cervical contact may reduce the problem of mucus and bacterial contamination, and may partly attribute to the higher success rates generally observed with these type of catheters.

Endometrial Trauma from Embryo Transfer Catheters

Traumatic or difficult transfers not only disrupt the endometrium affecting implantation, but also lead to undesirable myometrial activities which may displace the transferred embryos, resulting in poor outcomes.[18] Softer types of transfer catheters are less likely to dissect its way subendometrially compared to stiffer catheters, leading to endometrial damages when examined with ultrasound[19] and micro-hysteroscopy.[20] The use of soft catheters has also been shown in meta-analyses of 10 randomized controlled trials to improve pregnancy rates when compared to firm catheters.[21,22]

Embryo Misplacement, Displacement and Uterine Contractions

In human studies, up to 16 percent of the transferred embryos could be found after transfer from the external os, catheter tip or vaginal speculum.[23,24]

The quantity of fluid used for ET and the loading technique significantly affects the pregnancy outcome.[25] The amount of fluid used for transfer should be kept as small as possible to prevent embryos flowing out of the cervical canal or into the tubes.[23,26] However, volume less than 10 μL may negatively affect implantation rates.[27] Typically 20 μL of transfer medium surrounding the embryo is loaded. The presence of air bubbles before and after the medium containing the embryos marks the position of the embryos inside the catheter, protects against the loss or entanglement with cervical mucus and clings in the catheter, and also permits easier visualization under ultrasound.

The embryo transfer procedure would be a failure if the catheter does not pass through the internal os and enter the uterine cavity. This could happen with soft catheters, when the catheter tip curls inside the cervical canal and travel towards cervix unnoticed, not uncommonly seen when the transfer is performed under ultrasound control. The failure of the catheter to pass the internal os could also occur due to lack of alignment between the catheter and the utero cervical angle. This could be due to multiple reasons including anatomical distortion of the cervix from previous surgery, fibroids, congenital anomalies, scarring of the lower uterine segment and distorted endometrial cavity.[28] The use double lumen catheters with firmer malleable outer sheath (such as the Cook or Wallace Catheter) facilitates the passage through the often tortuous and rugged cervical canal and provide protection of the inner soft catheter. The advancement of the outer catheter is ceased at or just pass internal os, with the soft catheter then advanced into endometrial cavity.

Initiation of uterine contractions may lead to immediate or delayed expulsion of embryos in assisted reproduction. The pregnancy and implantation rates had been observed to decrease as the frequency of uterine contractions increased.[29]

Touching the uterine fundus with transfer catheter generated strong random waves of contraction from fundus to cervix, which relocated transfer fluid. Patients often experience immediate discomfort followed by suprapubic pain and heaviness due to initiation of uterine contractions when this occurs. Touching the fundus and the initiated contraction resulted in lower success rates and increased incidence of ectopic gestation.[30,31] It is generally recognized that avoiding the catheter tip touching the fundus was an important prognostic factor for the success of embryo transfers.[32]

Uterine contractions in the early luteal phase are generally cervicofundal in origin, this may account for some of the ectopic pregnancies seen after IVF.[33] Serum progesterone levels on the day of embryo transfer correlated with the frequency of uterine contractions. As progesterone levels increased, uterine contractions decreased. Uterine junctional zone contractions progressively decrease with progression into the luteal phase, and this may be a contributing factor in the success of day 5 blastocyst-stage embryo transfer.[34]

Contraction occurs more often in difficult embryo transfers,[35] when cervical or endometrial trauma or irritations occur such as when tenaculum is applied to cervix.[36] Difficult transfers were associated with lower pregnancy rates when 10 controlled trials were analysed (meta-analysis OR 0.73, 95% CI 0.63-085).[18]

Earlier studies have employed trial or dummy embryo transfer to diminish the incidence of difficult transfer.[8,9] However, uterine and cervical canal positions often changed when actual procedure takes place, such approaches are mostly not necessary particularly with the advent of ultrasound guidance which will be far superior in guiding the direction of the transfer catheter and accurate positioning of the tip for the embryo transfer.

Ultrasound Guidance and Depositing Embryo

When observed under ultrasound, the jet of transfer fluid often seen travel far beyond the catheter tip. Depositing the embryos too near to the fundus has negative effects on the outcomes of IVF. Implantation, pregnancy and birth rates improves when transfer catheter tip is positioned in lower uterine segment with embryos deposited in the mid to low uterine cavity,[37-39] at least 15-20 mm away from the fundus (Fig. 18.1).[40,41] Lower incidences of ectopic pregnancies were also observed when embryos were deposited away from the fundus.[31,41]

Ultrasound guidance is increasing used to facilitate atraumatic insertion of catheter, accurate positioning of the catheter tip within the uterine cavity, and visualization of the bubble and fluid transferred. The full bladder required for abdominal ultrasound also helps to straighten the cervicouterine angle and facilitate entry of catheter,[42] and provides superior visualization even with retroverted uterus.

Several meta-analysis of randomized studies over the years have consistently demonstrated that abdominal ultrasound-guided embryo transfer increased the clinical and ongoing pregnancy rates significantly when compared with the 'clinical touch' method,[43-45] including the recently updated Cochrane review (441/1254 vs 350/1218, OR 1.38, 95% CI 1.16-1.64, p<0.0003).[46]

EMBRYO TRANSFER

Currently at Sydney IVF where authors practise, over 90 percent of the embryo transfers are day-5 and mostly with single blastocyst, using Cook

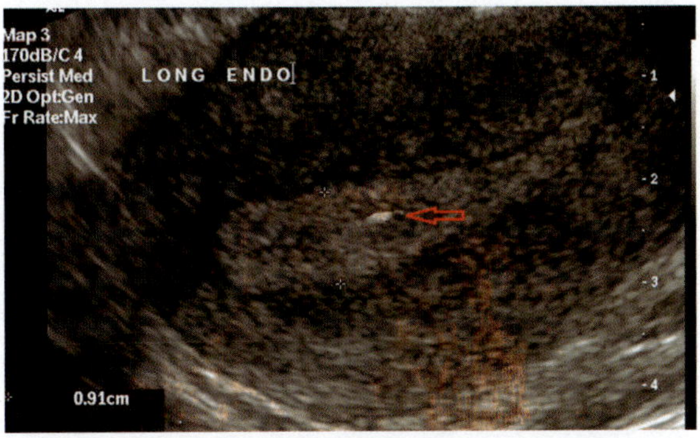

Fig. 18.1: Location of the air bubble seen with transvaginal ultrasound after embryo transfer aiming at mid cavity around 1.5-2 cm from the fundus

double lumen Sydney IVF embryo transfer catheter set which contains a firmer outer malleable cannula with round bulb head and a soft inner catheter.

1. Patients are advised not to empty but keep semi-full bladder prior to the procedure.
2. Patients are positioned in dorsal lithotomy position, knee-chest position is not necessary.[47]
3. A prewarmed, suitable sized sterile speculum is inserted into the vagina and positioned to clearly visualize the cervix. The cervix os is wiped with clean gauze saturated with normal saline with mucus removed from the cervical opening.
4. The procedures are performed under transabdominal ultrasound guidance. After ultrasound assessment of the cervicouterine axis, the curve of the malleable outer catheter can be adjusted. The "bulb-tipped" outer catheter with inner soft catheter loaded inside then is advanced gently through the cervical canal and through the point of resistance that marks the internal os but no further (clinical touch). The tip of the soft catheter is aimed at mid or just below the mid endometrial cavity at least 1.5-2 cm below the fundus under ultrasound guidance. This in most cases can be sufficiently visualized particularly with the enhancement of the air bubbles flanking the transfer medium.
5. In case visualization is not possible, then "clinical touch" method is practised. The Cook outer cannula has "bulb-tipped", which should be passed through the point of resistance that marks the internal os but no further (clinical touch), and a soft inner catheter, which can be passed a further 2 cm with care taken to avoid touching the fundus.
6. Gentle push of the plunger to allow slow movement of the fluid just beyond the catheter tip, brisk or jerky injection should be avoided as this lead to undesirable shear stress[48] negatively impacting on the transferred embryo.[49]
7. The catheter can be withdrawn slowly; delay of the catheter withdrawal did not increase pregnancy rates[50] but may have undesirable foreign body effects leading to uterine irritation or activities.
8. After the transfer, the catheter is flushed and inspected for retained embryo by the embryologist. Any retained embryos can be reloaded and transfer, with minimal impact on pregnancy outcomes.[51]
9. The patients can then be ambulated and empty their bladder, bed rest is not required.[52,53]
10. Patients are instructed to avoid extreme exercise or exertion but encouraged to continue normal daily activities. Bed rest[52,53] or avoidance of sexual activities[54] is not necessary as these have not been shown to affect the pregnancy rates.

DIFFICULT TRANSFERS

With the ultrasound guidance and using double lumen embryo transfer catheter, many difficult transfers due to malalignment of the advancing catheter through cervical canal and the cervico-uterine axis (ante or retroflexion) can be avoided. However, resistances at internal os often are encountered, but mostly can be negotiated by adjusting the angle of the outer catheter guided by the ultrasound. If resistance continues to be experienced, the small inner soft catheter often will negotiate its way through the internal os. However, the tip should be carefully observed with the ultrasound, as it is not uncommon for the soft tip to curl back to cervical canal and give the false sense of advancement. If good visualization cannot be achieved, it would be prudent to withdraw the soft catheter slowly while pressing the outer catheter, resistance will be experienced if the soft catheter is actually curled back and pressed at the bent. This is particularly important in women with previous history of cesarean sections; the soft catheter may curl within the lower segment defect which is present in significant proportion of these patients. It is in this specific group of the patients that the outer catheter tip should be advanced further into the lower segment once passed the internal os, to reduce such problem.

If desirable angle cannot be obtained at the cervicouterine junction, the soft catheter can be replaced with a metal stylette (available both to Cook's or Wallace set) which will toughen the outer catheter with desirable bent. With or without gentle pulling with tenaculum applied to the anterior or posterior cervical lip to straighten the uterus, the catheter can be manipulated as uterine sound to gently enter the internal os. Once internal os has been entered, the stylette can then be withdrawn while the outer catheter stays in position, and the soft inner catheter then introduced.

In a small number of patients small uterine dilators may be needed to negotiate the direction and dilate the internal os sufficiently to permit the entry of the outer catheter. If such attempts remain unsuccessful, the procedure should be temporarily abandoned and patient allowed to ambulate. A different operator can be called upon and transmyometrial embryo transfer needle and catheter can be prepared with transvaginal ultrasound guide setup. Transabdominal ultrasound guided procedure can be reattempted, often after 30 minutes' rest and repositioning, the right cervical passage can be identified with embryo transferred performed in the usual way.

Despite all the above efforts, some embryo transfers remain intractably difficult with catheter failed to be introduced into uterine cavity. Transmyometrial embryo transfer can be an alternative. A special transmyometrial embryo transfer needle (Towako Needle, Cook Australia) with stylette attached can be introduced with vaginal ultrasound guidance in the similar way as performing oocyte retrieval through myometrium into endometrial cavity. The transfer catheter loaded with embryo can be introduced after the stylette is removed.[55,56] Compatible pregnancy rates to conventional embryo transfer had been reported.[55,56]

If the transmyometrial transfer is not an option, embryos can be cryopreserved with frozen embryo transfer performed 1-3 months after cervical dilation. This mostly leads to easier procedures and improved outcomes.[57] In the intractable cases, laparoscopic zygote intrafallopian tubal transfer (ZIFT) will be the remaining option.

REFERENCES

1. Karande VC, Morris R, Chapman C, Rinhart J, Gleicher N. Impact of the physician factor on the pregnancy rates in a large assisted reproductive technology program: Do too many cooks spoil the broth? Fertil Steril 1999;71:1001.
2. Salha OH, Lamb VK, Balen AH. A postal survey of embryo transfer practice in the UK. Hum Reprod 2001;4:68.
3. Croxatto HB, Fuentaealba B, Diaz S, Pastene L, Tatum HJ. A simple non-surgical technique to obtain unimplanted eggs from human uteri. Am J Obstet Gynecol 1972;112:662-8.
4. Valbuena D, Martin J, dePablo J, Remohi J, Pellicer A, Simon C. Increasing levels of estradiol are deleterious to embryonic implantation because they affect the embryo. Fertil Steril 2001;76:962-8.
5. Imbar T, Hurwitz A. Synchronization between endometrial and embryonic age is not absolutely crucial for implantation. Fertil Steril 2004; 82:472-74.
6. Papanikolaou EG, Kolibianakis EM, Tournaye H, Venetis CA, Fatemi H, Tarlatzis B, Devroey P. Live birth rates after transfer of equal number of blastocysts or cleavage-stage embryos in IVF. A systematic review and meta-analysis. Hum Reprod. 2008; 23:91-9.

7. Blake D, Farquhar C, Johnson N, Proctor M. Cleavage stage versus blastocyst stage embryo transfer in assisted reproductive technology. Cochrane Database of Systematic Reviews 2007, Issue 4.
8. Schoolcraft WB, Surrey ES, Gardner DK. Embryo transfer: Techniques and variables affecting success. Fertl Steril 2001; 5:863.
9. Mansour R, Aboulgar M, Serour G. Dummy embryo transfer: A technique that minimises the problems of embryo transfer and improves the pregnancy rate in human *in vitro* fertilization. Fertil Steril 1990; 54:678.
10. Garcia J. Conceptus transfer. Jones G, Hodgen G, Rosen-Waks Z (eds). *In vitro* fertilization. Norfolk, Baltimore: Williams and Wilkins 1986;215.
11. Egbase PE, al-Sharhan M, al-Othman S, et al. Incidence of microbial growth from the tip of the embryo transfer catheter after embryo transfer in relation to clinical pregnancy rate following *in vitro* fertilization and embryo transfer. Hum Reprod. 1996; 11:1687-9.
12. Fanchin R, Harmas A, Benaoudia F, Lundkvist U, Olivennes F, Frydman R. Microbial flora of the cervix assessed at the time of embryo transfer adversely affects *in vitro* fertilization outcome. Fertil Steril 1998; 70:866.
13. Moore DE, Soules MR, Klein NA, Fujimoto VY, Agnew KJ, Eschenbach DA. Bacteria in the transfer catheter tip influence the live-birth rate after *in vitro* fertilization. Fertil Steril 2000; 74:1118-24.
14. Brook N, Khalaf Y, Coomarasamy A, Edgeworth J, Braude P. A randomized controlled trial of prophylactic antibiotics (co-amoxiclav) prior to embryo transfer. Hum Reprod 2006;21:2911-5.
15. Eskandar MA, Abou-setta AM, El-Amin M, Almushait MA, Sobande AA. Removal of cervical mucus prior to embryo transfer improves pregnancy rates in women undergoing assisted reproduction. Reprod Biomed Online 2007;14: 308-13.
16. Glass KB, Green CA, Fluker MR, et al. Multicenter randomized trial of cervical irrigation at the time of embryo transfer [Abstract]. Fertil Steril 2000;74 (suppl 1): S31.
17. Sallam HN, Farrag, Ezzeldin F, Agameya A, Sallam AN. The importance of flushing the cervical canal with culture medium prior tp embryo transfer. Fertil Steril 2000;74:31.
18. Sallam HN. Embryo transfer: Factors involved in optimizing the success. Curr Opin Obstet Gynecol 2005;17:289-98.
19. Lavie O, Margalioth EJ, Geva-Eldar T, Ben-Chetrit A. Ultrasonographic endometrial changes after intrauterine insemination: A comparison of two catheters. Fertil Steril 1997;68:731-4.
20. Marconi G, Vilela M, Bello J, et al. Endometrial lesions caused by catheters used for embryo transfers: A preliminary report. Fertil Steril 2003;80:363-7.
21. Abou-Setta AM, Al-Inany HG, Mansour RT, Serour GI, Aboulgar MA. Soft vs.firm embryo transfer catheters for assisted reproduction: A systematic review and meta-analysis. Hum Reprod 2005;11:3114.
22. Buckett W. A review and meta-analysis of prospective trials comparing different catheters used for embryo transfer. Fertil Steril 2006;85:728-34.
23. Poindexter AN, Thompson DJ, Gibbons WE, Findley WE, Dodson MG, Young RL. Residual embryos in failed embryo transfer. Fertil Steril 1986;46:262-7.
24. Ghazzawi IM, Al-Hasani S, Karaki R, et al. Transfer technique and catheter choice influence the incidence of transcervical embryo expulsion and the outcome of IVF. Hum Reprod 1999;14:677-82.
25. Diedrich K, Van der Ven H, Al-Hasani S, Krebs D. Establishment of pregnancy related to embryo transfer techniques after *in vitro* fertilization. Hum Reprod 1989;4:111.
26. Karaki R, Samarraie S, Younis N, Lahloub T, Ibrahim M. Blasotocyst culture and transfer: A step toward improved *in vitro* fertilisation outcome. Fertil Steril 2002;77(1):114.
27. Ebner T, Yaman C, Moser M, Sommergruber M, Polz W, Tews G. The ineffective loading process of the embryo transfer catheter alters implantation and pregnancy rates. Fertil Steril 2001;76:630-2.
28. Mansour RT, Aboulghar MA. Optimising the embryo transfer technique. Hum Reprod 2002;17:1149.
29. Fanchin R, Righini C, Olivennes F, Taylor S, de Ziegler D, Frydman R. Uterine contractions at time of embryo transfer alter pregnancy rates after *in vitro* fertilization. Hum Reprod 1998;13:1968-74.
30. Yovich JL, Turner SR, Murphy AJ. Embryo transfer technique as a cause of ectopic pregnancies in *in vitro* fertilization. Fertil Steril 1985;44:318-21.
31. Nazari A, Askari HA, Check JH, O'Shaughnessy A. Embryo transfer technique as a cause of ectopic pregnancy in *in vitro* fertilization. Fertil Steril 1993; 60:919-21.
32. Kovacs GT. What factors are Important for successful embryo transfer after *in vitro* fertilization? Hum Reprod 1999;14:590.

33. Lesny P, Killick SR, Robinson J, Maguiness SD. Transcervical embryo transfer as a risk factor for ectopic pregnancy. Fertil Steril 1999;72: 305-9.
34. Schoolcraft WB, Surrey ES, Gardner DK. Embryo transfer: Techniques and variables affecting success. Fertl Steril 2001; 5:863.
35. Lesny P, Killick SR, Tetlow RL, Robinson J, Maguiness SD. Embryo transfer–can we learn anything from the observation of junctional zone contractions? Hum Reprod 1998;13:1540-6.
36. Lesny P, Killick SR, Robinson J, Raven G, Maguiness SD. Junctional zone contractions and embryo transfer: Is it safe to use a tenaculum? Hum Rerod 1999; 14:2367.
37. Waterstone J, Curson R, Parsono J. Embryo transfer to lower uterine cavity. Lancet 1991;337:1413.
38. Frankfurter D, Trimarchi JB, Silva CP, Keefe DL. Middle to lower uterine segment embryo transfer improves implantation and pregnancy rates compared with fundal embryo transfer. Fertil Steril 2004;5:1273.
39. Oliveira JB, Martins AM, Baruffi RL, et al. Increased implantation and pregnancy rates obtained by placing the tip of the transfer catheter in the central area of the endometrial cavity. Reprod Biomed Online 2004; 9:435-41.
40. Coroleu B, Barri PN, Carreras O, Martinez F, Parriego M, Mereter L, et al. The influence of the depth of the embryo replacement into the uterine cavity on implantation rates after IVF: A controlled, ultrasound guided study. Hum Reprod 2002;17:341-6.
41. Pope CS, Cook EK, Arny M, et al. Influence of embryo transfer depth on *in vitro* fertilization and embryo transfer outcomes. Fertil Steril 2004; 81:51-8.
42. Oorusso F, Depalo R, Bettocchi S, Vacca M, Vimercati A, Selvaggi L. Outcome of *in vitro* fertilization after transabdominal ultrasound-assisted embryo transfer with a full or empty bladder. Fertil Steril 2005;84: 1046-8.
43. Sallam HN, Sadek SS. Ultrasound-guided embryo transfer: A meta-analysis of randomized controlled trials. Fertil Steril 2003; 80:1042-6.
44. Buckett WM. A meta-analysis of ultrasound-guided versus clinical touch embryo transfer. Fertil Steril 2003; 80:1037-41.
45. Abou-Setta AM, Mansour RT, Al-Inany HG, Aboulghar MM, Aboulghar MA, Serour GI. Among women undergoing embryo transfer, is the probability of pregnancy and live birth improved with ultrasound guidance over clinical touch alone? A systemic review and meta-analysis of prospective randomized trials. Fertil Steril 2007;88:333-41.
46. Brown J, Buckingham K, Abou-Setta AM, Buckett W. Ultrasound versus 'clinical touch' for catheter guidance during embryo transfer in women. Cochrane Database of Systematic Reviews 2010, Issue 1.
47. Englert Y, Puissant F, Camus M, Van Hoeck J, Leroy F. Clinical study on embryo transfer after human *in vitro* fertilization. J *In Vitro* Fert Embryo Transf 1986; 3:243-6.
48. Grygoruk C, Ratomski K, Kolodziejczyk M, Gagan J, Modlinski JA, Gajda B, Pietrewicz P, Mrugacz G. Fluid Dynamics during embryo transfer. Fertil Steril 2011;96:324-7.
49. Grygoruk C, Sieczynski P, Modlinski JA, Gajda B, Greda P, Grad I, et al. Influence of embryo transfer on blastocyst viability. Fertil Steril 2011;95:1458-61.
50. Martinez F, Coroleu B, Parriego M, Carreras O, Belil I, Parera N, et al. Ultrasound-guided embryo transfer: immediate withdrawal of the catheter versus a 30 second wait. Hum Reprod 2001;16:871-4.
51. Nabi A, Awonuga A, Birch H, Barlow S, Stewart B. Multiple attempts at embryo transfer: Does this affect *in vitro* fertilization treatment outcome? Hum Reprod 1997;12:1188-90.
52. Amarin ZO, Obeidat BR. Bed rest versus free mobilisation following embryo transfer: A prospective randomised study. BJOG Int J Obstet Gynaecol 2004; 111:1273-6.
53. Bar-Hava I, Kerner R, Yoeli R, Ashkenazi J, Shalev Y, Orvieto R. Immediate ambulation after embryo transfer: A prospective study. Fertil Steril 2005; 83(3):594-7.
54. Tremellen KP, Valbuena D, Landeras J, Ballesteros A, Martinez J, Mendoza S, et al. The effect of intercourse on pregnancy rates during assisted human reproduction. Hum Reprod 2000;15:2653-8.
55. Kato O, Takatsuka R, Asch RH. Transvaginal transmyometrial embryo transfer: The Towako method; experiences of 104 cases. Fertil Steril 1993;59:51-3.
56. Sharif K, Kato O. Technique of transmyometrial embryo transfer. Middle East Fertil Society Journal 1998;3:124-9.
57. Prapas N, Prapas Y, Panagiotidis Y, et al. Cervical dilatation has a positive impact on the outcome of IVF in randomly assigned cases having two previous difficult embryo transfers. Hum Reprod 2004; 19:1791-5.

Chapter 19

Third Party Reproduction: Techniques, Ethics and Economics

Nandita Palshetkar, Hrishikesh Pai, Shivanand Sakhare, Nandan Roongta

Every couple has the right to procreate. And if the desire to do so also exists, it is appropriate to use medical technology to help them achieve their goals as far as appropriately possible. As per the World Health Organization, approximately 8 to 10 percent of couples experience some form of infertility. Also, today as women worldover, are delaying childbearing, their needs with regards to assisted reproduction and further third party reproduction, continue to grow.

"Third Party Reproduction," according to the American Society for Reproductive Medicine, refers to the use of eggs, sperm or embryos that have been donated by a third person (donor) to enable an infertile individual or couple to achieve parenthood. The use of donor eggs, sperm or embryos can then be used in ART (Assisted Reproductive Technology) procedures such as IUI and IVF. The term also encompasses surrogacy (gestational carrier) and traditional surrogacy arrangements. Third party reproduction is a complex process requiring consideration of social, ethical and legal issues, in addition to the medical and emotional needs of the patient. A compassionate and sensitive approach on the part of the IVF specialist and staff involved is essential. This chapter will be discussing the various aspects of oocyte donation, embryo donation and surrogacy.

OOCYTE DONATION

Oocyte donation is an important option for many patients, and is recommended for women who have age-related infertility, poor egg quality, premature menopause, diminished ovarian reserve, gonadal dysgenesis, iatrogenic ovarian failure due to ovarian surgery or radiation, or chemical castration, and women who are carriers of autosomal recessive disorders. The oocyte donation makes pregnancy feasible in virtually any woman with a normal uterus, regardless of age.[1-3] A woman's reproductive age was the dictate of nature, but now it has been artificially extended and women of menopausal age can also give birth by using donor oocytes using IVF.

Selection and Screening of Oocyte Donor

- Donors should be healthy and give no history to suggest hereditary disease.
- A complete personal and sexual history should be obtained to exclude individuals who might be at high risk STIs.
- Psychological evaluation and counseling by a qualified professional is recommended for the oocyte donor and her partner as well as for the recipient and her partner. It is also recommended in circumstances involving known donors.

- The donor is well informed about the procedure, possible complications and their anonymity.
- The relevant information in respect to the donor, such as age, height, weight, the family background, educational qualifications, profession, color of the skin and the eyes must be recorded and can be conveyed to the recipient without disclosing the identity of the donor.

According to ICMR (Indian Council of Medical Research):

- The donor should be anonymous.
- The donor should be in the age group of 21 to 35 years.
- The donor should be tested for Blood group, HIV, HBsAg, HCV and VDRL.
- In our clinic we also evaluate for thalassemia and do peripheral blood karyotype to rule out numerical chromosomal anamolies.
- The recipient should be well counseled, and medically fit to carry the pregnancy.
- The uterine cavity is evaluated by HSG or hysteroscopy.

Donor Stimulation

In our clinic donor stimulation consists of oral contraceptive pills in a previous cycle, with overlapping long leuprolide acetate protocol starting two days before stopping pills. Gonadotropins (FSH or HMG) starting dose 150 IU per day for the day 2 of cycle, with adjustments of the dose according to the ovarian response, measured by ultrasound and estradiol levels. The criteria for hCG administration (10,000 IU) is at least three follicles of 17 mm with a normal rising estradiol levels. Cycle cancellation is done if their is inadequate response on day 5 of stimulation, i.e. estradiol levels <150 pg/ml, less than 6 follicles measuring smaller than 9 mm. Cancellation rates in our clinic are 5 to 7 percent. Coasting is done if estradiol levels on the day of hCG are above 2000 pg/ml. Alternatively antagonist stimulation protocol is used if donor reports on day 2 or 3 of cycle.

Recipient Preparation

Preparation of recipients in our clinic includes confirmation of a normal uterine cavity by means of hysteroscopy, hysterosalpingogram or saline infusion ultrasound. The recipient cycle is matched with donor cycle using standard oral contraceptive pills. For hormonal synchronization, the recipients should be down-regulated with GnRH agonist daily/depot from midluteal phase of previous cycle (leuprolide acetate, 1 mg sc per day or leuprolide depot 3.75 mg single shot) to achieve pituitary suppression if there is evidence of spontaneous ovarian function. Measurement of estradiol levels (<30 pg/ml) and endometrial thickness (<6 mm) assessed by ultrasonography, is required to confirm pituitary downregulation on day 2 of menstrual cycle or day 7 to 10 of GnRH analogue in case there are no menses. On day 2 of menstrual cycle the estrogen supplementation is started as oral estradiol valerate tablets 2 mg three times a day. On day 10 of estradiol valerate a Applebaum scoring (Uterine Biophysical Profile) is performed and if the score is more than 17, the progesterone supplementation is started matching with oocyte retrieval. For day 3 transfer, four days of progesterone supplement is ideal. Progesterone is used either vaginally or intramuscularly. The embryo transfer can also be performed in natural cycle, provided that exact timing of endogenous LH surge is documented.

Intrafamilial Donation: Ethical Issues

Some couples prefer to involve the family members in the arrangement. This may occur *intra-generationally* between siblings or cousins of similar ages, or it may also occur *inter-*

generationally, as when a mother gestates her daughter's embryos. Familial collaboration offers many advantages, but it may present unique problems arising from the familial closeness, like issues of consanguinity, undue influence for donor or surrogate to participate, uncertainty about lineage and parenting relations and confused parentage for the resulting children.[4-8] In many cases it is ethically acceptable and satisfying for the participants, but that some cases it might raise serious problems. But there is no way to judge the seriousness of these problems.

Shared Oocyte Donation: Economical in a Low-Resource Setting

Difficulties involved with oocyte donor recruitment:

- Due to imbalance between need of recipients and availability of donors, recipients often waits longer until a matched donor is available.
- The time wasted, efforts involved, the commitment, discomfort, and minor risks involved with ovarian stimulation and oocyte retrieval continue to limit donor availability.[9-11]
- Donor recruitment is a difficult task considering that a considerable number of potential donors may have a positive finding on medical, genetic, or psychological testing during the recruitment that prohibits donation.
- There is still no concluding proof, about the association between ovarian stimulation and epithelial ovarian carcinoma,[12-16] but the theoretical risk is a concern. The conservative limit on total number of oocyte donation cycles per donor can be set to reduce exposure of multiple ovarian stimulation.
- Providing oocyte to two recipients from a single donor has the theoretical advantage of permitting two fresh ETs from a single donor.

Shared oocyte donation has hence emerged as a more efficient use of precious human oocytes. By using shared oocyte donation, there is a decrease in the population of donors exposed to ovarian stimulation for a given population of recipients. Historically, shared donation involved ART patients willing to donate extra oocytes to the recipient, with reduction in treatment cost.[9,10] The cost reduction with this form of treatment is obvious. The costs of shared oocyte donation are 40 percent lower than unshared donation, while avoiding medical risks for the donor group. The inadvertent consanguinity brought about by the use of shared oocyte donation is of concern.

In a study by Moomjy et al,[17] in a shared oocyte donation, clinical pregnancy rate per recipient fresh ET was 56.8 percent, with ongoing pregnancy and delivery rate of 49.7 percent. The implantation rates was 31.8 percent and the miscarriage rate was 12.4 percent.

Oocyte Donation in Postmenopausal Women: Ethical Issues

Arguments in favor of oocyte donation for postmenopausal women:

- Right to procreate: According to the social norm of gender equality and reproductive freedom, every women has a right to procreate. Our society respects the rights of individuals to make reproductive choices regardless of age or life expectancy.

Arguments against oocyte donation for postmenopausal women:

- One major argument against oocyte donation to postmenopausal women is that there is a "natural" limit in reproductive capacity in humans and to cross this limit is "unnatural."
- Parenting is both an emotionally stressful and physically demanding experience. Older couple

would not be able to meet the needs of a growing children.

- In elderly women, in pregnancy there is increased medical risk of hypertension, diabetes, multiple gestation, preterm labor, pre-eclampsia, and other gestational complications.
- There also is the possibility of multiple gestation, which has its own risks and risk of fetal reduction.[8]
- When the male partner is more than 50 years of age, there is minor genetic risks associated with conception.

The central ethical issue is whether the interests of couple and children are served by this technology. Parents and physician have a moral responsibility to ensure that third party reproduction is protective of both the well-being and welfare of resulting children. These interests can be served when the desire for a child and the ultimate bearing and rearing of a child contribute to mutual well-being.[9]

Oocyte Donation: Emotional Aspects

The couples are upset and grieved of not having a child, the traditional way. They are shocked when their doctors begins to discuss the option of oocyte donation. Taking the time to get over all these emotional disturbances, sets the foundation for moving forward in a well-informed manner. Couples will want to discuss about physical characteristics, the background, educational status, professional background and risk of transmission of STDs. Some couples are obsessed on finding the perfect donor who looks most like the recipient, but it is the combination of genes that will express themselves in the child. There are worries about being able to bond with the child, feelings related to the loss of the genetic connection may occur.

Whether to share this information with your child is the common question in the mind of couples. Some couples are fearful that, it would disturb or harm the parent-child bonding. Some couples want to protect the child from the pain or mental disturbances caused by the knowledge of oocyte donation. Sharing this information with born child will further cause the bonding and it gives affirming message about your desire to have this child.

EMBRYO DONATION

The use of donor embryos provides couples, the opportunity to become pregnant with embryos donated by patients who have extra embryos either fresh or frozen. Most commonly embryo donors have completed their family and have cryopreserved embryos that they wish to donate to other infertile couple. This is also resorted to whom the male partner of a couple requiring oocyte donation has indications such as primary germ cell failure and inheritable genetic disorder. ICMR encourages embryo donation.

In our clinic, we use frozen embryos for transfer in monetarily poor patients. We have 47 percent pregnancy rates and 12 percent miscarriage rates in over 300 cycles performed in last two years.

Recipient preparation and investigation on the donor couple are same as quoted in oocyte donation program.

GESTATIONAL SURROGACY

A surrogate or gestational carrier is a woman who carries a pregnancy for another couple or woman. There are two types of surrogacy arrangements. In traditional surrogacy, the surrogate is inseminated with sperm from the male partner of the intended parent couple. ICMR does not allow traditional surrogacy in India. In gestational surrogacy, the surrogate is transferred with embryos created with the sperm and egg of the intended parents (or donors) and carries a pregnancy. Use of a gestational carrier is indicated for a woman who lacks a uterus secondary to surgery, damaged uterus due to severe Asherman's syndrome, recurrent implantation failure, recurrent miscarriage and absent or congenitally abnormal uterus. Gestational surrogacy is also needed for women with a medical contraindication to pregnancy such as severe diabetes, heart or kidney disease. Gestational surrogates can be relatives or friends of the intended parents who volunteer to carry a pregnancy for them. Alternatively, gestational surrogates can be identified through agencies that specialize in recruiting women to become surrogates. According to ICMR regulations, commercial surrogacy is permitted in India.

Selection and Screening of Surrogate

- Surrogate should be healthy.
- The surrogate undergoes extensive medical testing and a thorough medical history and physical exam is performed.
- A complete personal and sexual history should be recorded to exclude individuals who might be at high risk for STIs.
- Psychological evaluation and counseling by a qualified professional is recommended for the surrogacy and her partner.
- The donor is well-informed about the procedure, possible complications.

According to ICMR (Indian Council of Medical Research):

- The surrogate should be in the age group of 21 to 45 years.
- The surrogate should be tested for Blood group, HIV, HBsAg, HCV and VDRL.

Gestational Surrogacy: ICMR Code of Practice, Ethical Considerations[18]

1. A child born through surrogacy must be adopted by the genetic (biological) parents unless they can establish through genetic (DNA) fingerprinting (of which the records will be maintained in the clinic) that the child is theirs.
2. Surrogacy by assisted conception should normally be considered only for patients for whom it would be physically or medically impossible/undesirable to carry a baby to term.
3. Payments to surrogate mothers should cover all genuine expenses associated with the pregnancy. Documentary evidence of the financial arrangement for surrogacy must be available. The ART center should not be involved in this monetary aspect.
4. Advertisements regarding surrogacy should not be made by the ART clinic. The responsibility of finding a surrogate mother, through advertisement or otherwise, should rest with the couple, or a semen bank.
5. A surrogate mother should not be over 45 years of age. Before accepting a woman as a possible surrogate for a particular couple's child, the ART clinic must ensure (and put on record) that the woman satisfies all the testable criteria to go through a successful full-term pregnancy.
6. A relative, a known person, as well as a person unknown to the couple may act as a surrogate mother for the couple. In the case of a relative acting as a surrogate, the relative should belong to the same generation as the women desiring the surrogate.
7. A prospective surrogate mother must be tested for HIV and shown to be seronegative for this virus just before embryo transfer. She must also provide a written certificate that: (a) she has not had a drug intravenously administered into her through a shared syringe, (b) she has not undergone blood transfusion, and (c) she and her husband (to the best of her/his knowledge) has had no

extramarital relationship in the last six months (This is to ensure that the person would not come up with symptoms of HIV infection during the period of surrogacy). The prospective surrogate mother must also declare that she will not use drugs intravenously, and not undergo blood transfusion excepting of blood obtained through a certified blood bank.

8. No woman may act as a surrogate more than thrice in her lifetime.
9. A surrogate mother carrying a child biologically unrelated to her must register as a patient in her own name. The birth certificate shall be in the name of the genetic parents. All the expenses of the surrogate mother during the period of pregnancy and postnatal care relating to pregnancy should be borne by the couple seeking surrogacy. The surrogate mother would also be entitled to a monetary compensation from the couple for agreeing to act as a surrogate. The exact value of this compensation should be decided by discussion between the couple and the proposed surrogate mother.
10. The surrogate mother must relinquish in writing all parental rights concerning the offspring and vice versa.
11. No ART procedure shall be done without the spouse's consent.
12. Sex selection at any stage after fertilization, or abortion of fetus of any particular sex should not be permitted, except to avoid the risk of transmission of a genetic abnormality assessed through genetic testing of biological parents or through preimplantation genetic diagnosis (PGD).
13. Law firms and semen banks will be encouraged to obtain and maintain information on possible oocyte donors and surrogate mothers. The above organizations may appropriately charge the couple for providing an oocyte or a surrogate mother. The oocyte donor may be compensated suitably (e.g. financially) by the law firm or semen bank when the oocyte is donated. However, negotiations between a couple and the surrogate mother must be conducted independently between them.
14. Advertisements regarding surrogacy should not be made by the ART clinic. The responsibility of finding a surrogate mother, through advertisement or otherwise, should rest with the couple, or a semen bank.

Unanswered Ethical Issues

- Should the surrogate be paid? Would this lead to commercialization of surrogacy and expose the surrogate mother to possible exploitation?
- Will surrogate arrangements be used not only by infertile couples but also for the sake of convenience, or by single men or women?
- Are surrogacy contracts enforceable? Are they illegal?
- What if there is a desire on the part of the child to know his/her gestational mother?
- What are the possible adverse psychological effects on the child?
- What happens when no one wants a handicapped newborn ?
- What if the surrogate and the spouse violate the abstention clause?
- What if the surrogate decides to keep the baby?
- Is handing over a child after delivery for a fee "baby-selling"?

Intrafamilial Surrogacy: Economical Option

According to the Ethics Committee, American Society for Reproductive Medicine, use of family members as surrogates is ethically acceptable. ICMR does not allow intergenerational surrogacy. Intergenerational surrogacy is especially challenging. Counseling is encouraged for all parties including the commissioning couple and the surrogate. Till date intrafamilial surrogacy in the form of sister-for-sister, sister-for-brother and mother-for-daughter have been reported. The main reason why the family member may be selected as a surrogate, is to speed the process and to reduce the expensive costs associated with commercial surrogacy. The family member involvement may result in significant financial savings and enable the couple to have a procedure that otherwise would not be available to them. A major concern in intrafamilial collaboration is protecting the autonomy of the surrogate from manipulative or undue influences by family members.

REFERENCES

1. Sureau C, Shenfield F. Oocyte donation by a daughter. Hum Reprod 1995;10:1334.
2. Marshall LA. Intergenerational gamete donation: ethical and societal implications. Am J Obstet Gynecol 1998;178:1171-6.
3. Sauer MV, Paulson RJ, Lobo RA. A preliminary report on oocyte donation extending reproductive potential to women over 40. N Engl J Med 1990;323:1157-60.
4. Sauer MV, Paulson RJ, Lobo RA. Pregnancy after 50: application of oocyte donation to women after natural menopause. Lancet 1993;341:321-45.
5. Sauer MV, Paulson R, Lobo R. Pregnancy in women 50 or more years of age: outcomes of 22 consecutively established pregnancies for oocyte donation. Fertil Steril 1995;64:111-5.1.
6. Andrews B, Tiefel HO. When baby's mother is also grandma—and sister. Hastings Center Report 1985;15:29-31.
7. Pierce J, Reitmeier PJ, Jameton A, Maclin VM, DeJonge CJ. Should gamete donation between family members be restricted? The case of a 16-year-old donor. Hum Reprod 1995;10:1330-2.
8. Schenker JG. Oocyte donation by a minor to her mother. Hum Reprod 1995;10:1332.
9. Ahuja KK, Mostyn BJ, Simons EG. Egg sharing and egg donation: attitudes of British egg donors and recipients. Hum Reprod 1997;12:2845-52.
10. Ahuja KK, Simons EG, Fiamanya W, Dalton M, Armar NA, Kirkpatrick P, et al. Egg-sharing in assisted conception: ethical and practical considerations. Hum Reprod 1996;11:1126-31.
11. Englert Y, Govaerts I. Oocyte donation: particular technical and ethical aspects. Hum Reprod 1998;13 (Supp 2):90-7.
12. Rossing MA, Daling JR, Weiss NS, Moore DE, Self SG. Ovarian tumors in a cohort of infertile women. N Engl J Med 1994;331:771-6.
13. Shushan A, Paltiel O, Iscovich J, Elchalal U, Peretz T, Schenker JG. Human menopausal gonadotropin and the risk of epithelial ovarian cancer. Fertil Steril 1996;65:13-8.
14. Mosgaard BJ, Lidegaard O, Kruger Kjaer S, Schou G, Nyboe Andersen A. Infertility, fertility drugs, and invasive ovarian cancer: a case-control study. Fertil Steril 1997;67:1005-11.
15. Parazzini F, Negri E, La Vecchia C, Moroni S, Franceschi S, Crosignani PG. Treatment for infertility and risk of invasive epithelial ovarian cancer. Hum Reprod 1997;12:2159-61.
16. Mosgaard BJ, Lidegaard O, Nyboe Andersen A. The impact of parity, infertility and treatment with fertility drugs on the risk of ovariancancer. Acta Obstet Gynecol Scand 1997;76:89-95.
17. Maureen Moomjy, Robin Mangieri, Fernando Beltramone. Shared oocyte donation: society's benefits. Fertility Sterility 2000;73:(6).
18. Indian Council of Medical Research (ICMR) ART (Regulation) Bill on Surrogacy, 2010.

Chapter

20

In Vitro Fertilization on the Move

Jaideep Malhotra, Rageshwar Jyoti

Infertility is ever increasing, more so in the developing countries. Studies show that 6-30 percent of the world's population suffers from infertility and childlessness which is on higher side in the developing world.[1] It has deep negative impact on the physical, mental, social, psychological and financial conditions of the suffering family.[2] The irony is that in the developing countries almost 70 percent of the couples have no access to the treatments available and those who have access almost 70 percent cannot afford them because of financial or other logistic reasons.

Infertility treatment is neither a one time nor a one step treatment; it needs many visits to the clinic starting right from, initial consultation, diagnosis, monitoring and management. Couples undergoing infertility treatment have to battle through all kinds of circumstances, and abide by the various protocols and visits to clinic.[3] It is not an easy task by any means and many will not be able to juggle through the days and the dates and the dropouts for this reason only are many.[4] Moreover, it needs a constant support and coordination with each other, with the medical and paramedical staff of the clinic and with the workplace and family. Only the ones who are very strongly motivated and determined are able to start the treatment though still not many are able to stick to the treatment protocols.

Of the many problems which come in the way of these couples in the developing countries,most important one is that infertility services are not easily accessible to them.[4] Sometimes they have to travel long distances for just a consultation and frequent visits to these clinics may not be logistically possible for them. Taking long holidays from work and home very often also become increasingly difficult. Based on all these problems, the idea of having ART on the move is being considered and practiced in many countries and by various tertiary centers, which seems to be a viable alternative. There has been a lot of hue and cry regarding the governments' involvement in providing ART services; it is needless to say that the governments in the developing countries are still struggling to take measures to reduce maternal and neonatal mortality and reproductive health services are not their top priority. Though I must admit that Indian government lately has started setting up ART units in prime medical educational institutions so as to make the treatment available to lower socio-economic status population and also train our young medical professionals. Till date, the majority of ART services in developing countries are under the umbrella of private sector because of which it is difficult to curb the cost of these services, hence are beyond the reach of common man.

On the other hand, in setting up an ART clinic and maintaining a trained staff is challenging and also leads to a significant expenditure. Another major hurdle in these clinics in developing countries is the cost of salaries of trained personnel and also retaining them. Once these personnel are trained, they tend to move onto bigger setups and higher pay brackets.[4] Setting up and maintenance of equipments is also no mean task, especially in smaller towns or rural setups.

The need of the hour is to setup low cost ART service centers, that provide safe, effective, acceptable and affordable treatment for all the underprivileged and the options available are:

1. The first option is for a fully equipped and functional tertiary center, have a few satellite centers where the medical personnel and staff can be trained for consultation and initial work-up of patient along with the availability of primary investigations, monitoring and management (Fig. 20.1). These satellite centers will screen patients who require ART services. They can prepare them till the stage of ovum pick-up and once ready, refer them to tertiary center for ovum pick-up to embryo transfer. This referral process, if streamlined can reduce the movement and number of visits and number of days outside their home for the couple along with the availability of good facilities of tertiary center. But still these couples have to move to a new environment and relate to new people and also stay away from home for at least a week. Follow-up of complications also becomes a problem with this kind of movement, who to manage and where? It is not very encouraging for the couples to be on the move and many are daily wages earners. Also many may not be able to come out for treatment for social reasons as almost 50 percent of the couples do not reveal at home and to friends that they are undergoing such a treatment. But, this kind of setup has many benefits too, that these satellite centers can make the local public aware of the magnitude of the problem and the treatment modalities available. These centers can also cater, non IVF treatments like IUI and basic infertility investigations and endoscopy facilities which is beneficial to the patients and tertiary centers too as they decrease workload on the tertiary centers and offer easy and accessible treatment to majority.
2. The second option is, that around a tertiary center, build-up facilities capable of providing ART services (Fig. 20.2). These setups can have medical and technical staff capable of screening and preparing patients for ART with the availability of adequate equipments to carry out various basic procedures of ART. A day before the ovum pick-up, a team of trained laboratory personnel and clinician can move to this satellite center, perform pick-ups to embryo transfers and go back. This option seems to be quite appealing to the technical and clinical staff and also to the patients. The patients stay in their own environment, procedures are done at same place as day care, while technical and the clinical staff works in tertiary center, only to move to the satellite center for a short time. The satellite center can invest in setting up a basic infrastructure and equipments while rest of the things which are not in common use,or are needed for backup, can be transported from tertiary center like centrifuge, suction pump, laser hatching unit, cryopreservation unit, and even bench top incubators. Provision of this kind of setup may increase the initial cost of infrastructure and equipment but if we calculate it according to the cost of providing services per patient, this might turn out to be much more efficient and accessible. Also it will slowly help staff at satellite center to be trained

in due course of time and become self sufficient in the long run. Needless to say these satellite centers can perfom all basic investigations, surgeries and non ART procedures themselves on a daily basis which forms the major chunk of infertility management. The staff at satellite center can also be trained with time and can become self sufficient. Quality control and trouble shooting can be challenging in these centers. Disadvantages of this option can be that a small number of early or late responders can fall out of the batch and may be compromised. Though we still feel that this small number, if detected early, can be counseled and moved to tertiary center for management to reduce compromise. Another problem in these centers may be the management of complications, the number of complications are extremely low, with proper patient selection and protocol monitoring and can be either managed at the satellite center or moved to tertiary centers.

3. Third option is transport IVF where the assessment, drug therapy, monitoring and ovum pick up is done at the transport center but the embryology and embryo transfer takes place at the tertiary center (Fig. 20.3). Advantages of this type of setup are that patients get advanced management and has to stay for a lesser number of days outside their familiar environment. Disadvantage is that facilities at the transport center have to be more, i.e. for ovum pick up and anesthesia, etc. which increase the cost of the setup and still

Option I	
Pros	*Cons*
• Semi facilities at door step though still have to move to tertiary center. • Less number of days absence from workplace • Low cost setup at satellite centers • No need of specialist team at all satellite centers • One specialist team can cater to more than one satellite centers at the same time • New technology and advances only to be introduced at the teritary center • Non-IVF procedures like IUI can be done here.	• Patients have to move a new unfamiliar surroundings for at least one week • Follow-up is a problem • Complication management is difficult • More financial loss to the patients for loss of days at work • Staff at satellite centers is dependent on higher center • Troubleshooting is challenging.

Option II	
Pros	*Cons*
• More patient friendly as all the services are at door steps in a familiar environment • Specialist team can enjoy the living of bigger town and still serve the people of underpriveleged areas • Satellite center staff can be trained in due course of time • Awareness regarding the treatment modalities available can be spread in remote areas.	• More costly for the satellite center to set-up and maintenance of more procedures and lab equipments • Difficulty in keeping a check on more number of ART centers • Back up is required • Some poor responders who are not ready for OPU on the day of planned visit may still have to move to higher center for further treatment.

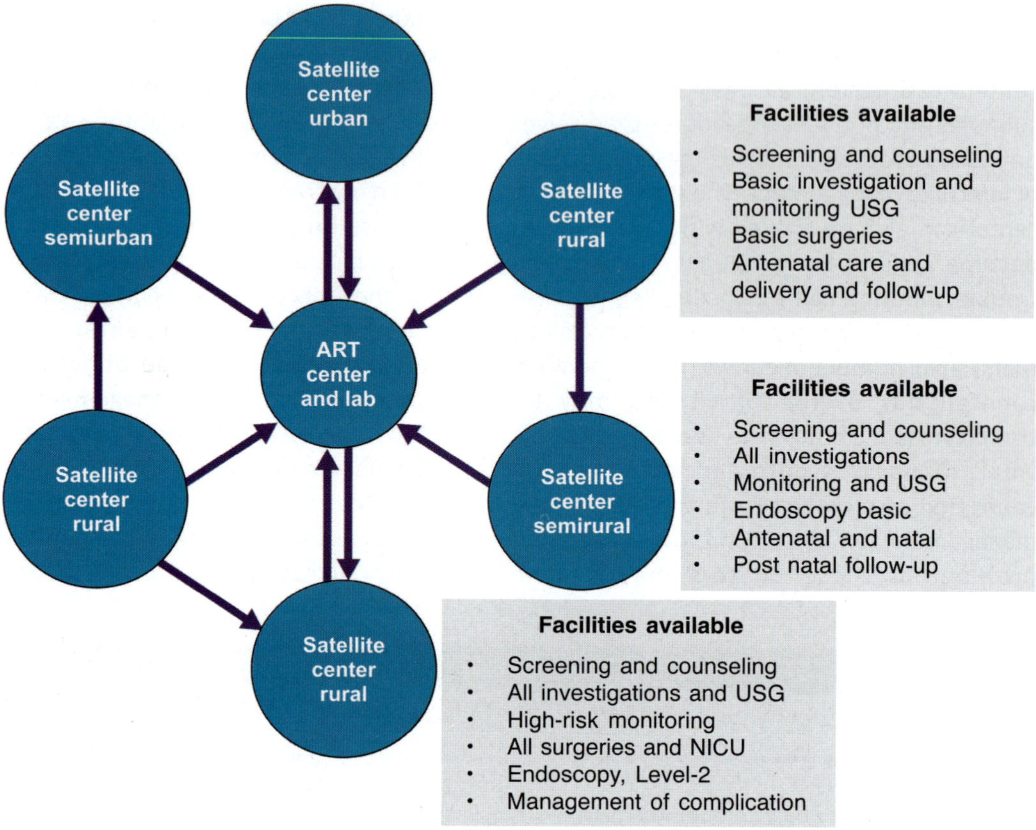

Fig. 20.1: Option 1 — Fully equipped and functional tertiary center

the patient has to move to the tertiary center. Facilities for transport of gametes are also needed, and transport of gametes should ideally not take more than two hours.[5,6] There is always a chance of some problem happening to the gametes on the way to tertiary center. Similar is the problem with management of complications.

All these three options have their own advantages and disadvantages. It is felt that in the second option lesser number of people's movement is happening and the patients are more comfortable in their own home atmosphere and the extra stress of taking too many holidays for the sake of treatment again and again is reduced, which is one of the major reasons for treatment drop outs. Though the responsibilities and involvement of the core team will remain quite high for the first few years and troubleshooting can also be very time consuming, but slowly it will settle down. Having enough experience of running this kind of setup, I can safely say that it is definitely a very viable, patient friendly and satellite center educating option. Also the satellite center staff can be trained in due course of time at their own setup and a slow and steady up gradation of the clinic and laboratory can be done. Though when it comes to weighing the pros and cons of cost benefit analysis, it might prove to be a little more expensive, than option one as all centers have to invest in the equipment and minimal trained staff, but when it comes to assessing it from patient point

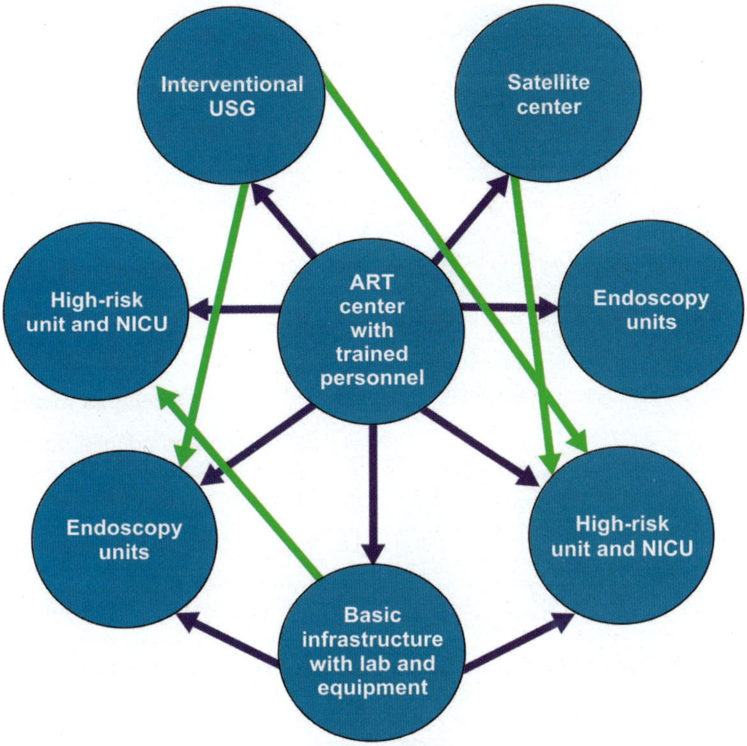

Facilities available

- Screening and counseling facilities
- Monitoring of cycles
- Post follow-up
- Antenatal and natal
- Postpartum follow-up and neonatal care

Fig. 20.2: Option 2 — Tertiary center providing ART services

of view it is a very successful experiment and more numbers can be treated. What really helps in these clinics is to train staff to be multitasking to reduce the cost of trained personnel and also helps in keeping these units small and under control. Of course in the long run, the satellite centers can become self sufficient and they can still keep on tagging with the primary for up gradation and new technology and advancement.

Problem which could arise from this is the mushrooming of centers doing ART and keeping a check on the ethical aspect of ART and could lead to exploitation of the couples and medical personnel. This could be an issue anywhere and the national guidelines and laws can take care of them as they do for other issues. I feel that this should not be a reason of depriving infertile couples or physicians from low resource setups and

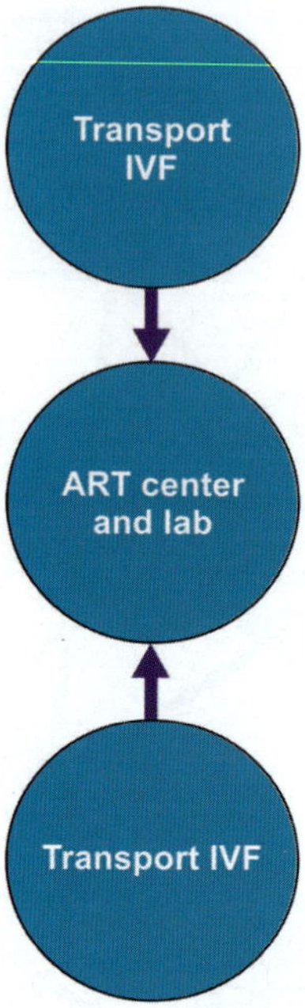

Facilities available

- Screening and counseling
- All investigation and USG
- High-risk monitoring
- All surgeries and NICU
- Endoscopy Level-2
- Ovum pick-up
- Management of complication

Fig. 20.3: Transport IVF (Embryo transfer takes place at the tertiary center)

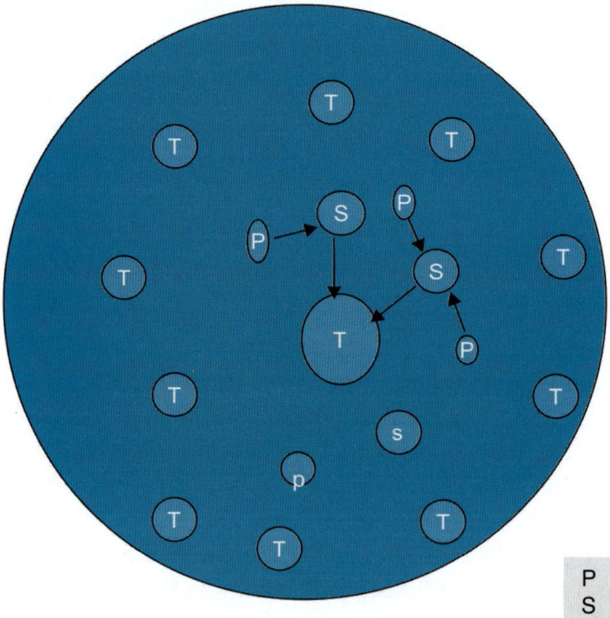

P Primary
S Secondary
T Tertiary centers for ART

Fig. 20.4: Centers for ART (Primary, Secondary and Tertiary)

challenging circumstances from getting ART services or providing them.

Ideally in the developing countries like India, Africa, tertiary ART centers should be scattered, equidistant about 300-400 km distance so that they can cater a 200 km radius maximally (Fig. 20.4). Patients can reach their nearest tertiary center within 3 to 4 hours so that they can reach home on the same day after consultation and follow-up. This will also prevent the mushrooming of ART centers and the overall cost to the country will also be less than what it is in present scenario. If budget is a problem to the government, then public private partnership is another option.

To conclude, infertility is a common problem all over the world. Assisted reproductive technologies have revolutionised the possibilities for childless couples. But the use of this technology for the underprivileged and in the developing countries has been limited by high cost of treatment. Even in developed countries, cost is a limiting factor, wherever these treatments are not state sponsored or covered under insurance. A number of low cost facilities and regimens have been developed, none with distinct advantage over other, we are still searching an ideal protocol with a low cost and low complication rate. Time has come to give adequate attention to the issue of infertility in developing countries also, so that more and more underprivileged population is able to have access to these facilities where ever and whenever required.

REFERENCES

1. Ombelet Willen, Cooke ian, Dyer Silke, Serour Gamel, Paul Devroy. Infertility and the provision of infertility medical services in developing countries. Human reproduction update 2008;14(6):605-21.
2. Daar AS, Merali Z. Infertility and social suffering: the case of ART in developing countries. In: Vayena E, Rowe PJ, Griffin PD (Eds). Current Practices and Controversies in Assisted Reproduction. Geneva, Switzerland: World Health Organization 2002;15-21.
3. Lisa C. Ikemoto. Reproduction tourism; Equality concerns in the global market for fertility services. A Journal of theory and Practice 2009;277.
4. Hovalle O, Cooke I. Cost effective approaches to *in vitro* fertilization: Means to improve access. International Journal of Gynecology and Obstetrics 2006.
5. Miller R. Difficulties in providing fertility treatment for rural women. O and G magazine 2010;12(3): 26-27.
6. *In Vitro* Fertilization by Kay Elder, Brian Dale, Joyce Harper, John Huntriss page 182 3rd edn.

Chapter

21

Minimizing Risks and Complication of ART in Restricted Resource Setup

Jaideep Malhotra, Jaydeep D Tank, Bhavna Sharma

Recent times have seen a rapid surge in the number of ART procedures all over the world and it is estimated that almost 2 percent of these have complications varying from mild to severe and some can be life-threatening too.[1] Ovarian hyperstimulation syndrome (OHSS) and multi-fetal pregnancies are the two major issues. Majority of the other complications are either related to the procedure of ultrasound guided oocyte pickup such as hemorrhage, pelvic infections or could be ectopic pregnancies, ovarian torsion, etc. Under any circumstances, the best strategy would be to avoid these complications in the first place, more so in countries with low resources need special consideration especially where facilities and finances are both lacking. The protocols in such set-ups need to be slightly biased towards staying away from any such possible complications. And the irony is that most of these complications are actually preventable.

OVARIAN HYPERSTIMULATION SYNDROME (OHSS)

Ovarian hyperstimulation syndrome (OHSS) is a potentially lethal condition and accounts for almost 1 percent of these get hospitalized in the western world. It is characterized by a massive extravascular accumulation associated with depletion in the intravascular volume, and, consequently hemo-concentration with its attendant complications.

This syndrome is probably the only serious complication of ovarian stimulation. Mild OHSS is seen in 8 to 23 percent of stimulation cycles, moderate in about 0.005 to 7 percent and severe in about 0.008 to 1.8 percent.

Classification

Mild Hyperstimulation

Grade I: Abdominal distention and discomfort.

Grade II: Features of grade I with gastrointestinal symptoms (nausea, vomiting, diarrhea); ovaries are enlarged up to 5 to 12 cm (Fig. 21.1).

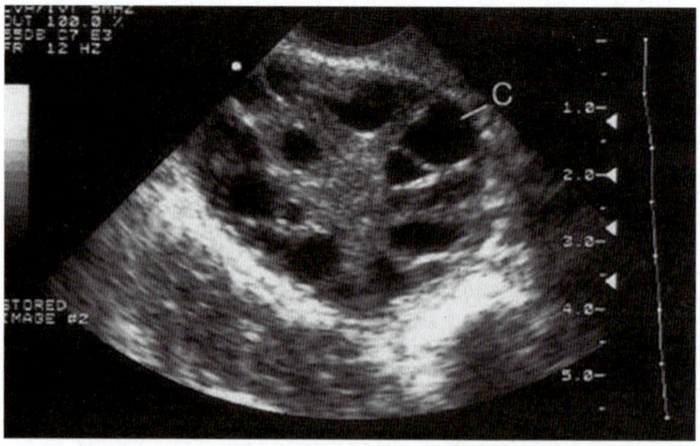

Fig. 21.1: Hyperstimulated enlarged ovary

Moderate Hyperstimulation

Grade III: Features of mild hyperstimulation with ultrasonic evidence of ascites.

Severe Hyperstimulation

Grade IV: Features of moderate hyperstimulation with clinical ascites and/or hydrothorax and respiratory difficulties.

Grade V: All of the above with change in the blood volume, increased blood viscosity due to hemoconcentration, coagulation defects and diminished renal perfusion.

The current hypothesis indicates that the initiating event is an increased capillary permeability in the enlarged ovaries, leading to extravasations of fluid into the peritoneal cavity. Accumulation of fluid in the peritoneal cavity leads to the formation of ascites, depletion of the intravascular volume, hypotension and renal sodium and water retention.

Vascular complications include hemoconcentration, high hematocrit, increased levels of factor V, platelets, fibrinogen, profibrinolysin, fibrinolytic inhibitors and thromboplastin generators. This can lead to cerebrovascular and cardiovascular embolic phenomenon.

Venous compression due to the pressure exerted by the ovaries and ascites can also lead to thromboembolism.

Liver dysfunction is manifested as deranged liver functions and the structure remains essentially unchanged. Any ultrastructural changes seen are a compensatory response to the increase in demand on liver enzymes.

Respiratory complications are now seen more commonly since the use of cabergoline for OHSS has increased though there has been no documented association between the two. This can manifest as pleural effusion, respiratory distress secondary to ascites, hydrothorax or rarely adult respiratory distress syndrome.

Renal complications as prerenal failure or hydroureter and gastrointestinal complications nausea, vomiting, diarrhea or pain abdomen are associated with the condition.

Adnexal torsion due to enlarged ovaries has been seen. They need to be treated on the regular lines of ovarian torsion.

Prevention

Prevention is probably the most important aspect, since apart from a few empirical therapies; there is no definitive treatment for OHSS. The presence of various risk factors should be looked for to isolate the ones who are more prone to land in OHSS.

Thin and young patients (<35 yrs) and those having polycystic ovarian disease are more prone to OHSS. Oligomenorrhoic anovulation should also raise the level of suspicion. Ultrasonography appearance of the developing follicles on the day of hCG administration. Mild OHSS is common when there are more numbers of intermediate follicles (9–15 mm) and severe OHSS when there are small follicles (5–8 mm). OHSS is usually seen when estradiol levels are > / = 2500 pg/ml and is rare when the concentration is < / = 1000 pg/ml on the day of hCG administration, however, serial monitoring of E2 levels has not proven to be infallible, since OHSS has also been reported with levels of < / = 1500 pg/ml. An important factor to be considered here is the slope or rate of rise in E2 concentrations—risk of OHSS is higher, if the values of E2 are more than doubling. OHSS has been noted to be more frequent in conception cycles.

One important step towards prevention of OHSS is the choice of stimulation protocols along with the patient profile. Mild stimulation protocols are the dictum and can almost avoid OHSS along with proper monitoring.

Chronic low-dose regimen is more likely to result in a quasifollicular response and therefore a significantly lower rate of OHSS. Similarly, unlike a step-up protocol, a step-down protocol will allow more follicles to undergo atresia, thus reducing the overall number of follicles capable of secretory activity by the time hCG is administered, naturally translating into a reduction in the rate of OHSS.

An extension of the step-down concept is 'coasting' or 'controlled drift' may work to prevent or reduce the severity of OHSS by altering the capacity of the granulosa cells to produce VEGF.[2] However, there are diminished oocyte collection rates and implantation and pregnancy rates when coasting is prolonged particularly > 3 days. The use of GnRH-a in conjunction with COH, either as a 'long' or 'short' protocol, profoundly affects the risk of OHSS. Gonadotropin-releasing hormone agonists play a paradoxical role in OHSS abolishing the midcycle luteinizing hormone (LH) surge. This suppression of the LH surge allows continued stimulation by gonadotropins, which in turn will drive more follicles to maturation, with a consequent rise in serum E2 values and a markedly increased risk of OHSS.

In contrast, during cycles without GnRH-agonist suppression, either a significant LH surge or at least marked luteinization will limit continued gonadotropin stimulation and thus lead to a concomitantly lesser risk of OHSS. However, the suppressive effect of GnRH-a on ovarian function can be utilized as continuing GnRH-a administration for 1 week following hCG administration in GnRH-a down-regulation cycles where all embryos are electively cryopreserved because of a high-risk of OHSS. This strategy can be extended easily to oocyte donation cycles.

Avoidance of hCG or substitution by a low-affinity, shorter-acting compound is the main-stay for the prevention of OHSS. Indeed, the acknowledgment of the role of hCG in OHSS has led to complete discontinuation of hCG administration for luteal supplementation. Use of rLH may be safer than hCG as far as OHSS is concerned.

The rLH newly used probably has a relatively long half-life compared with native LH. Alternatively, it is possible that a single peak of rLH is sufficient to induce final oocyte maturation, as opposed to the 24-hour-long naturally occurring LH surge.

There is decreased incidence of OHSS with GnRH-agonist compared with hCG as the triggering agent for ovulation. Most importantly, there have been no reports of severe or critical OHSS after triggering ovulation with midcycle GnRH-a. But, it must be realized that because of pituitary desensitization, GnRH-agonist cannot be used as an ovulation trigger for cycles in which GnRH-agonist was previously used for down-regulation. If a patient at high-risk for OHSS is identified and GnRH-a triggering is contemplated, a GnRH-antagonist protocol, rather than a long-GnRH-a protocol, should be used for suppression of the endogenous midcycle LH surge. GnRH antagonists seem to be associated with a decreased risk of OHSS compared with the GnRH-agonist long protocol in patients undergoing IVF.

Liberal application of embryo cryopreservation for patients showing early signs of hyperstimulation can be an important safety net in guarding against severe OHSS. With routine culture of embryos to the blastocyst stage, it is possible to accurately assess the degree of OHSS prior to embryo transfer; because blastocyst transfer takes place on the seventh day after hCG, absence of even a moderate degree of OHSS is reassuring, and one may safely proceed with embryo transfer. The higher implantation rates associated with blastocyst transfer have led some to employ single blastocyst transfer in patients at risk of developing severe OHSS. Such a strategy results in a negligible multiple gestation rates, which purportedly is associated with more severe OHSS, presumably secondary to higher hCG levels. Improvements in *in vitro* maturation of immature oocytes might also enable women, particularly those with polycystic ovary syndrome (PCOS) who are at greatest risk of OHSS, to undergo assisted reproduction using minimal if any gonadotropin stimulation. This may dramatically reduce or eliminate the risk of OHSS.

Transvaginal ultrasound guided follicle aspiration will empty the follicles of fluid and granulosa cells—thus protecting against the development of OHSS. But intrafollicular hemorrhage may occur which can adversely affect follicular function at a later date.

Twenty percent human albumin (50 gms) administered IV at the time of oocyte recovery may prevent OHSS. This not only maintains the intravascular volume, but also sequesters the vasoactive substances released by the corpora lutea. The only complication associated with intravenous albumin is the occasional manifestation of serum sickness as flu like syndrome.

Glucocorticoids: 100 mg hydrocortisone IV at the time of oocyte recovery has also been tried as a preventive measure, however, it is not of any proven scientific benefit. Use of dexamethasone (0.5 mg daily orally) along with hMG/FSH in the step up (titrated) protocol for controlled ovarian hyperstimulation in PCOS has also been found to reduce the incidence of OHSS.

Treatment

There is no definitive treatment for OHSS. Most of what is advised is basically supportive therapy, to maintain the intravascular volume and avoid the complications associated with hypercoaguability.

Mild OHSS requires no hospitalization, only regular follow-up and close observation for any worsening. This usually resolves spontaneously within 2 to 3 weeks.

Moderate and severe degrees of OHSS require immediate hospitalization for close monitoring and supportive therapy.

Monitoring protocols in these patients will include regular assessment of vital signs (TPR / BP), daily weight recording, daily abdomen girth measurement, input and output charting, plasma and urine osmolarity, blood urea, serum electrolytes, coagulation profile, liver function tests, ultrasonography—pelvis/abdomen and X-ray of the chest.

Ultrasonography is the most important monitoring modality, since it helps to evaluate the severity, as well as whether the condition is under progression or regression (Fig. 21.2).

Dramatic clinical deterioration is most likely to manifest 8 to 9 days after hCG administration, when endogenous pregnancy derived hCG becomes perceptible. The single most important variable that indicates the severity of the OHSS is hemoconcentration, reflected in the hematocrit. Any increase in the hematocrit as it approaches 45 percent underestimates the magnitude of plasma volume depletion and thus the seriousness of the patient's condition. An additional measure of hemoconcentration is the magnitude of leukocytosis; white blood cell (WBC) counts higher than 25000/mm^3, largely reflecting a

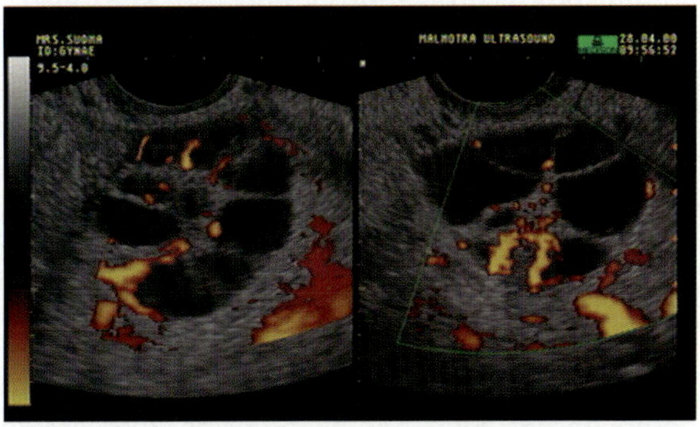

Fig. 21.2: Color Doppler in mild hyperstimulated ovary

granulocytosis, may be seen. This massive neutrophilia may be attributed to hemoconcentration and generalized stress reaction. When oral isotonic fluid intake is insufficient to maintain plasma volume, intravenous fluid therapy becomes mandatory. Because of the tendency for hyponatremia, sodium chloride with or without glucose is the crystalloid of choice. The daily volume infused may vary from 1.5 L to > 3.0 L.

Although some advocate fluid restriction to minimize the accumulation of ascites, one should rather deal with the discomfort of ascites than face the consequences of hemoconcentration with the attendant risks of thromboembolism and renal shutdown. In order to maintain fluid balance, the patient's urine output, oral and intravenous fluid intake, body weight, abdominal girth, hematocrit, and serum electrolytes must be monitored. In addition, coagulation parameters and liver enzymes should be periodically assessed. Intravenous volume replacement should aim to improve renal perfusion before fluid escapes into the peritoneal and/or pleural cavities; this transient hemodilution is achieved at the expense of increased third spacing and increased total body water. Albumin is the main protein lost in OHSS. Human albumin is physiological and thus the colloid of choice. Albumin at doses of 50 to 100 g at 25 percent concentration should be administered intravenously and repeated every 2 to 12 hours until the hematocrit falls below 45 percent and urine output increases. When oliguria persists despite evidence of adequate hemodilution, intravenous furosemide at a 10 to 20 mg dose is often beneficial. In practice, an albumin-furosemide chase protocol seems to yield the best results. Two units of albumin, 50 g each, followed immediately by intravenous furosemide, will often result in diuresis. In states of volume contraction, hemoconcentration, and hypotension, furosemide should be strictly avoided. In this precarious stage of OHSS with impending renal failure, a renal-dose of dopamine drip should be used for renal rescue. The single most important treatment modality in life-threatening OHSS that cannot be controlled by medical therapy is paracentesis. The indications for paracentesis include the need for symptomatic relief, tense ascites, oliguria, rising serum creatinine concentration or falling creatinine clearance and hemoconcentration unresponsive to medical treatment. Paracentesis should be performed aseptically under ultrasound guidance.

Prophylactic treatment of women with OHSS with unfractionated or low-molecular-weight heparin is of some theoretical value. Rarely, as a last resort, when the critical stage of OHSS is complicated by renal failure, thromboembolism, acute respiratory distress syndrome and multiorgan failure, there is no choice but to perform a potentially lifesaving termination of pregnancy.

Newer therapies include Tab Cabgolin 0.5 mg twice a day. This is hypothesized to act on the VEGF2 receptors which are responsible for the increased vascular permeability responsible for OHSS. Calcium infusion has also been proposed as a membrane stabilizer and initial studies seem promising. Intravenous calcium gluconate injection effectively arrests development of clinical symptoms in mild and moderate OHSS and may improve blood clotting parameters such as hematocrit. No negative influence of this treatment is seen in case of clinical pregnancy.[3]

Calcium gluconate 10 percent, 10 ml dissolved in 200 ml of normal saline given at rate of 90 drops per minute. It is given for three consecutive days starting from the day of oocyte retrieval, next day and the day of embryo transfer.[4]

MULTIPLE PREGNANCIES

Multiple pregnancies remain the most common complication of ART as transferring multiple embryos which is a common practice. Most of them are dizygotic twins, related to excess number of embryos transferred to increase the results.

In the last decade, the significant increase in the incidence of multiple births may be attributed to the increased use of ARTs. The incidence of twins with the use of clomiphene citrate is 10 percent and triplets or other higher order multiples approximately 1 percent. Treatment with gonadotropins increases the percent (17% twins and 3 to 6% higher—order multiples). With ARTs there is 30% multiple—pregnancy rate (24% twins and 6% higher—order multiples).

With an increase in the incidence of multiple pregnancies, there is an increase in maternal and perinatal morbidity and mortality.[5] The most common perinatal complication is prematurity, whereas the most common maternal complication is maternal hypertension in patients with multiple gestation. Other maternal complications include iron deficiency, increased operative delivery, uterine rupture, and preterm labor. In terms of neonatal morbidity, there is an increase in intrauterine growth retardation, and prematurity with multiple pregnancies as compared with singletons. There is also increase in the admissions to ICU and NICU, which is not acceptable especially in developing countries and in many areas; these facilities may not be available. So the best way of preventing these complications would be to transfer not more than two embryos at a time (Fig. 21.3).

Reducing the number of embryos transferred would tremendously decrease multiple pregnancy.[6] With a good freezing program, the cumulative pregnancy rate in single or two embryo transfer are similar to more than two embryos transferred. Embryo reduction can be done especially in cases of triplets and higher maternal age but not without its related complications.

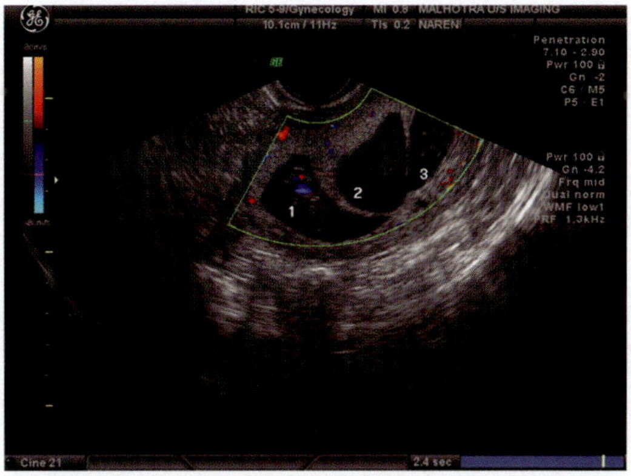

Fig. 21.3: Triplets

Elective single embryo transfer vs double embryo transfer may improve the odds of delivering a term singleton live birth by nearly 5 fold in good prognosis patients in fresh cycles and in frozen/thawed cycles too. In addition to lowering the risk of preterm birth, also appeared to lower the risk of delivering LBW baby by 3 fold and also avoids the increased risk of multiple pregnancies and its complications to mother as well as fetus.[7]

There are also financial and emotional costs to undergo a procedure twice as there is always a risk for failure. Overall, it depends on how much the patient is willing to pay for one extra pregnancy, whether one cyclesingle embryo transfer (SET) or one cycle double embryo transfer (DET) is preferred from a cost or increased pregnancy point of view, not to forget the complications associated with multiples. So SET is definitely the future but not for everybody. The better we get at selecting which embryos have higher potential of implantation, the better we can opt for eSET.

COMPLICATIONS OF OOCYTE PICK-UP

Vaginal puncture hemorrhage may result in 1 percent of the patients after the needle is removed.

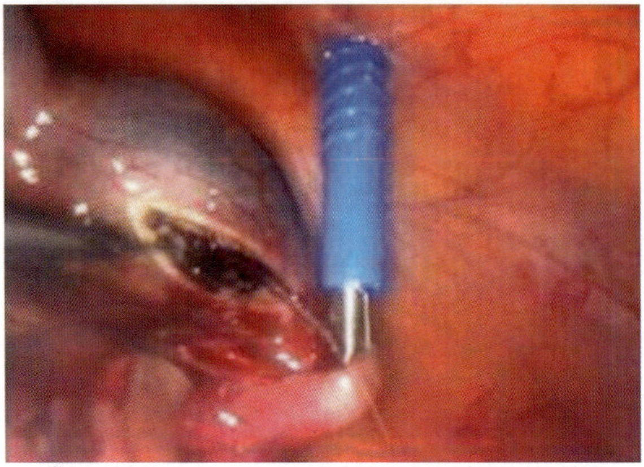

Fig. 21.4: Salpingostomy for ectopic pregnancy

Usually vaginal packing and direct pressure upon the puncture site stems the flow and nothing else seems to be necessary.

Hemorrhage within the pelvis and or ovarian follicles may be detected by postprocedural ultrasound.[8] However, small surface bleed is often seen and needs careful postpickup monitoring.

A vascular injury as internal iliac vessel puncture is a major complication and laparotomy may have to be done to arrest the hemorrhage.

Pelvic infections can occur in 0.4 to 1.3 percent even after the administration of antibiotics.[9]

Ectopic pregnancies (Fig. 21.4) can occur in almost 4 percent of all ART pregnancies, especially in developing countries, attributable to increasing incidence of tubal factor.[10] It is estimated that the ectopic pregnancy rates will decrease with a reduction in number of embryos transferred.

Ovarian torsion complicates about 0.1 percent of all patients undergoing ART and this incidence increases with OHSS.[9]

CONCLUSION

Identifying the patients prone for such complications need to be isolated and the protocols modified to avoid such complications is the key to management in restricted resource IVF cycles. Soft protocols, step-down, coasting and if required abandoning the cycle and cryofreezing need to be slighty higher on the list as the resources might not support the costly and prolonged management which follows.

REFERENCES

1. El-Shawarby SA, Margara RA, Trew GH, Lavery SA. A review of complications following transvaginal oocyte retrieval for in vitro fertilization. Hum Fertil 2004;7:127-33.
2. Sher G, Zouves C, Feinman M, Maassarani G. 'Prolonged coasting': an effective method for preventing severe ovarian hyperstimulation syndrome in patients undergoing in vitro fertilization. Hum Reprod 1995;10:3107-9.
3 Yakovenko SA, Sivozhalozov VS, Zorina IV. Prevention of OHSS by intravenous calcium. Abstract of 25th annual meeting of ESHRE, Amsterdum, the Netherlands, 28 June-1 July, 2009.
4. Gurjan T, Demirol A, Guvan S. Intravenous calcium infusion as a novel preventive therapy of ovarian hyperstimulation syndrome for patients with Polycystic ovarian syndrome. Fertility and sterility, May 2011.
5. Wennerholm UB, Bergh C. Obstetric outcome and follow-up of children born after *in vitro* fertilisation (IVF). Hum Fertil (Camb) 2000;3:52-64.
6. Gerris J, De Neubourg D, Mangelschots K, Van Royen E, Vercruyssen M, Barudy-Vasquez J, Valkenburg M, Ryckaert G. Elective single day-3 embryo transfer halves the twinning rate without decrease in the ongoing pregnancy rate of an IVF/ICSI programme. Hum Reprod 2002;17:2621-6.
7. Fiddles AAA, Severens JL, Dirksen CD. Economic evaluation of single versus double embryo transfers in IVF. Human Reproduction Update 2007;13(1):5-13.
8. Dicker D, Ashkenazi J, Feldberg D, Levy T, Dekel A, Ben-Rafael Z. Severe abdominal complications after transvaginal ultrasonographically guided retrieval of oocytes for in vitro fertilization and embryo transfer. Fertil Steril 1993;59:1313-5.
9. Tureck RW, Garcia CR, Blasco L, Mastroianna L Jr. Perioperative complications arising after transvaginal oocyte retrieval. Obstet Gynecol 1993;81:590-3.
10. Strandell A, Thorburn J, Hamberger L. Risk factors for ectopic pregnancy in assisted reproduction. Fertil Steril 1999;71:282-6.

Chapter

22

Cryopreservation: A Frozen Life

Ivan Rizal Sini

Assisted reproductive treatment has been strongly associated with hormonal intervention, which may be resulted in disruption of physiological pelvic and reproductive environment for an embryo to result in a healthy pregnancy. The move towards more natural approach has been postulated to improve and more healthier endometrium for embryo implantation. In a controlled hyperstimulation (COH) regimen often many oocytes would be forced to grow with a potential alteration to vascularization of endometrium spiral arteries. This may not only to have consequences in a short-term possibility of implantation failure but also in a long-term possibility with risks early pregnancy loss and poorer obstetrics outcome.

In obtaining better result in an assisted reproductive program, a clinician must pay an attention to how to put an embryo in the most suitable environment. Inevitably this will closely linked to freezing embryos when situation does not permit one in transferring them during the stimulated cycle. Unfortunately there have been many skeptical and rather pessimistic views in frozen thawed cycles. This particularly the case in newly started program where the concentration is to achieve the best pregnancy rate in a fresh cycle. Ultimately in a responsible IVF clinic both fresh and frozen thawed program should have been address equally and maintained consistent results.

Development in IVF protocols creates more demand to preserve gametes and embryos. Ministimulation and *in vitro* maturation program are examples of increasing needs to sustain a successful outcome. Since further improvement in freezing and thawing technique has given an opportunity to cancel a fresh cycle with preserving the embryos should there is any concern.

SLOW FREEZING VS VITRIFICATION

Methodology of embryo freezing technique has developed quite rapidly, in which slow freezing technique is still the most commonly used protocol. Major injuries to ice crystal formation is one of the main concerns with slow freezing technique. Vitrification can eliminate this potentially hazardous environment to the embryos although the technique and handling can be difficult and quite challenging. But recently the improved methodology in vitrification and warming embryos are becoming increasingly popular and from the view point of minimal cost IVF this technique provides much efficient and effectiveness economically. This also would allow eliminating the use of expensive programmable freezing equipments. However due to skill dependency IVF laboratory needs to adjust carefully in shifting from previous slow freezing technique to vitrification without disturbing overall clinical performance. We will be discussing more on vitrification in this chapter and view the benefit and the drawbacks of this technique.

As early as 1985, ice-free cryopreservation of mouse embryos at –196 °C by vitrification was reported (Rall and Fahy, 1985) as a possible alternative approach to cryostorage. Vitrification is an ultra-rapid method of cryopreservation whereby the embryo is transitioned from 37 °C to –196 °C in <1 s, resulting in extremely fast rates of cooling (>10 000 °C/ min). High concentrations of cryoprotectants together with rapid cooling rates are essential to cryopreserve embryos in a vitrified, glass-like state (Vajta and Kuwayama, 2005).

Vitrification appears to be more attractive than slow freezing, because it does not require expensive equipment, uses small amount of liquid nitrogen, and is not time consuming. Another practical advantage of vitrification is that the speed of the process minimizes the period the embryos outside of the incubator. Vitrification requires minimal set-up time, being performed as needed during the course of the day. The main concern, however, is the need for using high concentrations of cryoprotective solutions that might lead to osmotic shock, affecting embryo survival and potentially disturbing meotic spindle hence DNA damage to the cell.

To achieve optimal vitrification a radical increase of both cooling rates and the cryoprotectant concentration is required. Unfortunately with the use of higher concentration of cryoprotectants with relatively ultrarapid rates of temperature changes in vitrification, this would expose the embryos to potentially toxic and osmotic injuries. Few strategies have been developed to maintain the high level of cryoprotectants concentration tolerated by embryos and oocytes, but still the best approach is to increase cooling and warming rates.

To facilitate rapid heat transfer, minimal volumes are used in vitrification, facilitated through the use of minute tools as carriers. The carrier systems that have been developed for the vitrification procedure include the electron microscope grid (Park et al. 2000; Son et al. 2002), pulled and hemi-straws (El-Danasouri and Selman, 2001; Vanderzwalmen et al. 2002, 2003), flexipipet (Liebermann and Tucker, 2002), cryotop and cryotip (Kuwayama, 2007) and the cryoloop (Lane et al. 1999; Mukaida et al. 2001, 2003a, b; Reed et al. 2002; Rama Raju et al. 2005). The use of each technique has recently been reviewed (Chen and Yang, 2007).

Different cryoprotectant solutions also have been developed. Ali and Shelton investigated various combinations of cryoprotectant solutions. They developed an ethylene glycol (EG)- based solution consisting 5.5 mol/L EG and 1.0 mol/L sucrose. EG is an important component of vitrification solution with features of low toxicity and rapid permeation of the cell. Some other investigators have combined with other permeating agents such as dymethylsulfoxide (DMSO) or 1-2. Propanediol (PROH) to reduce toxicity of singular cryoprotectant.

For warming technique, typical process would be as follows. Carrier are unloaded into warming solution 1 (0.65 M sucrose dilution in HEPES buffered supplemented with 12 mg/ml HAS), embryos then will fall off the carrier and then moved to warming solution 1 for 30s, and then moved to warming solution 2 (0.325 M sucrose) for 1 min, warming solution 3 (0.125 M sucrose) for 2 min and then located to usual culture media prior to embryo transfer.

Some of other known disadvantages of vitrification includes high requirement in delicate handling particularly during cooling, warming and storing the embryos. And also potentially high concentration toxic cryoprotectants is still relatively unknown. Liquid Nitrogen is also linked with viral, fungi and microorganism pathogens with potential contamination or cross contamination. Therefore direct plunge into liquid nitrogen has been considered not acceptable in most European countries.

Recently many meta-analysis and systematic reviews have been published to support the role of vitrification in freezing embryo program. Loutradi et al 2008 showed that post thawing survival rate of cleavage stage embryos or blastocysts is significantly higher after vitrification as compared with slow freezing. From the 90 potential studies, only 4 were deemed suitable for analysis. Two of these studies reported a direct comparison of day 3 cryopreservation with slow freezing and vitrification (Rama Raju et al. 2005; Zheng et al. 2005). Zheng et al. used abnormal, patient donated, research embryos, which underwent subsequent biopsy, and demonstrated significant improvement of embryo survival following vitrification compared with slow freezing. However, there was no statistical difference between the groups for embryo development to the blastocyst stage. In the larger clinical study, Rama Raju et al. cryopreserved approximately 120 embryos using slow freezing or vitrification. Significantly better survival and implantation rates were achieved following vitrification. Thus, vitrification appears to offer improved survival rates over slow freezing, but further studies are required to determine the most efficient cryopreser vation method.

In evaluating long-term impact of vitrification Wikland et al. 2010 reported obsterics outcome of vitrified blastocysts, fresh blastocysts and slow-frozen early cleavage stage embryos. 321 vitrified blastocyst transfers, 563 fresh blastocyst transfers and 871 transfers of slow-frozen/thawed early cleavage stage embryos were performed resulting in 172, 296 and 309 pregnancies which led to 103 (1d4106 children), 203 (1d4207 children) and 200 (1d4206 children) deliveries, respectively. Embryo survival rate was 81.4 percent in the vitrified blastocyst group and 80.8 percent in the slow-frozen early cleavage stage group. Preterm birth (<37 weeks) occurred in 6.9, 7.0 and 4.6 percent of the vitrified, fresh blastocyst and slow-frozen early cleavage stage embryo groups, respective. The rate of post-term birth was significantly higher in the vitrified blastocyst group.

No statistically significant difference was found for the rate of birth defects between the vitrified and fresh blastocyst groups or between the vitrified and slow-frozen groups. Birth defects were found in 1 percent of the children in the vitrified blastocyst group (one child with branchial cleft cyst), in 2.0 percent of the children in the fresh blastocyst group (three children with unilateral cryptorchidism and one child with bilateral pes equinovarus) and in 4.1 percent of the children in the slow-frozen early cleavage stage embryo groups (one child with bilateral syndactyly of digits 2 and 3, one child with exstrophy of the urinary bladder and anal atresia, one child with a persistent ductus arteriosus, one child with a small ventricular septum defect, one child with hydrocele testis, one child with unilateral cryptorchidism and one child with unilateral hip instability).

VITRIFICATION OF OOCYTES

Embryo freezing has been implemented very successfully in assited reproductive technique (ART) and now allows supernumerary embryos generated through *in vitro* fertilization (IVF) to be routinely frozen and stored. However, the oocyte has proved to be far more troublesome (Coticchio et al. 2004). Chen (1986) reported the first pregnancy following IVF of a cryopreserved human oocyte. Together with the fact that the number of births per number of oocytes frozen thawed program is typically no greater than 3 percent. The difference between the success of oocyte and embryo cryopreservation has yet to be strictly explained, but differences in cell size and membrane permeability have been proposed (Stachecki and Cohen 2004). The oocyte is unique in that the maternal DNA is held suspended in the cytoplasm on the meiotic spindle and not within the protective confines of the nuclear membrane, as it is for the majority of the time during subsequent preimplantation development. Damage to the DNA and/or microtubules could explain the limited success of oocyte cryopreservation. However, a further consideration is that the oocyte is arrested in a state primed for activation and changes in its environment can cause pathogenetic activation.

Recently many development has taken place in strategy to cryopreserve oocytes that is through the ultrarapid cooling or vitrification which is proven to be more promising then the earlier method. This technology has been widely used in animals but only recently has been studied in humans (Feichtinger et al. 1991; Mukaida et al. 1998; Vajta et al. 1998; Mauri et al. 1999; Vanderzwalmen et al. 2002; Son et al. 2003; Chian et al. 2005; Huang et al. 2007). The first birth after human oocyte vitrification was recorded in 1999 with a standardized protocol used on animals (Kuleshova et al. 1999).

Cao et al 2009 reported there was a statistically significant difference in oocyte survival rates of after thawing between the slow-freezing group (75 out of 123, 61.0%) and vitrification group (268 out of 292, 91.8%). Vitrification also has been associated with superior survival particularly to meotic spindle (MS) changes after warming when compared to frozen thawed oocytes. Disruption of the MS results in disorganization of the maternal chromosomes and, once fertilized, a higher risk for aneuploidy in the resulting embryo.

Recently, Chian et al 2008 reported a large series of obstetric and perinatal outcomes in infants conceived from vitrified oocytes in which the mean birth weight and the incidence of congenital anomalies were comparable to spontaneous conceptions in fertile women or infertile women undergoing *in vitro* fertilization (IVF) treatment.

ASSISTED HATCHING IN CRYOPRESERVATION

It has been suggested, but not reliably well documented, in the literature that the process of embryo cryopreservation may affect the physicochemical characteristics of the zona pellucida (ZP) causing its hardening and apparently impairing blastocyst hatching. Larman et al 2006 showed that cryoprotectant exposure alone causes zona hardening. Since introduction of the calcium chelating agent, prevents zona hardening, it appears that the cryoprotectants used increase intracellular calcium to levels sufficient to induce cortical granule release and subsequent zona hardening. Removing calcium during vitrification significantly reduces the degree of zona hardening, which dramatically improves fertilization and development to the two-cell stage. It has also been theorized that creating an artificial opening or assisted hatching (AH) in the ZP allows the embryo to hatch after blastocyst formation. Some older studies have demonstrated that the use of AH for thawed human embryos can improve pregnancy and implantations rates (Check et al. 1996; Lee et al. 1999). However, AH has been carried out using various methods whose clinical relevance in a cryopreservation program remains controversial and undefined.

The assisted hatching procedure is generally performed on the day after warming procedure has complete using various methods. These include the creation of an opening in the zona either by drilling with acidified Tyrode's solution, PZD with a glass microneedle, laser photoablation, or use of a piezomicromanipulator. The ZP can be artificially thinned without breaching its integrity with proteolytic enzymes, acidified Tyrode's solution, or laser.

ENDOMETRIUM PREPARATION

In a frozen thawed cycle synchronization of endometrium and embryo is very critical. Still debatable whether any endometrium preparation regimen is better than others. Many studies failed to confirm which protocol is the most superior. In most cases these are very subjective to clinicians preference.

Hormone replacement therapy regimen is quite simple yet can be time and cost consuming. Hills et at reviewed 1391 natural vs HRT supplemented frozen thawed cycle and showed that HRT protocols associated with higher liver birth. This has been challenged in other studies. In anovulatory or women over the age of 40, HRT can be a more suitable option. Protocol usually started with or without downregulating ovarian activities on the preceding cycle. Estrogen supplementation then commenced with a target to reach endometrial thickness of 8 mm and full appearance of trilaminar on ultrasound scan. Dosage increment regimen or fixed dose of 6 mg of estradiol valerate throughout the initial phase is not clear to which one is the better option. Progesterone supplementation then added to start a calculating the timing of embryo transfer. Most centers would follow 2 days of once daily progesterone supplementation which then start calculating the embryos age when progresterone has been added to twice daily. This regimen usually is continued until 3 months pregnancy.

In efforts to reduce the cost and inconvenience natural cycle seems to be more sensible. There has been also numerous clinical advantages in allowing an embryo to implant into a naturally developing endometrium. Studies in endometrium have considerably significant in showing potential changes to endometrial vascular architecture which may lead to improper implantation (Salamonsen et al. 2009). The inconvenience of natural cycle is related to close monitoring of ovulation which may require frequent clinical visits and blood tests. To overcome this often a strategy which a use of artificial LH surge may be an option. There has been some concern over the change of window of implantation by using this method.

FUTURE

Gamete and embryo freezing thawing/warming process will be an area where IVF cycles are leading towards more natural and simpler to clinicians and patients. The cost efficiency which can be obtained by stimulating ovaries with cheaper stimulation regimen and utilizing freezing and thawing embryos in subsequent natural cycles. Vitrification technique has allowed us to have more efficient and effective program, and this will continue to evolve.

With much improved oocytes vitrification technique, there will be more options to diverse range of fertility or infertility clients. Oocyte banking for social need although still very much in the early stages will continue subjected to a challenging ethical dilemma and debates.

52 publications have been published from 2004-2010 in regards to whole or some part of ovarian tissue cryopreservation. Although still in its premature stage this could also be an attractive solution a certain medical conditions such as premature ovarian failure.

BIBLIOGRAPHY

1. Ali J, Shelton JN. Vitrification of preimplantation stages of mouse embryos. Reprod Fertil 1993;98:459-65.
2. Cao YX, Xing Q, Zhang ZG, Wei ZL, Zhou P, Cong L. Cryopreservation of immature and *in vitro* matured

human oocytes by vitrification. Reproductive Biomedicine Online, 2009;19:369-73.
3. Chian RC, Son WY, Huang JY, et al. High survival rates and pregnancies of human oocytes following vitrification: preliminary report. Fertility and Sterility 2005;80 (Suppl. 1): S36.
4. Chian RC, Huang JYJ, Tan SL, et al. Obstetric and perinatal outcome in 200 infants conceived from vitrified oocytes. Reproductive Biomedicine Online 2008;16:608-10.
5. Check JH, Hoover L, Nazari A, et al. The effect of assisted hatching on pregnancy rates after frozen embryo transfer. Fertil Steril, 1996;69:254-7.
6. Chen SU, Yang YS. Vitrification of oocytes; various procedures. In: Tucker MJ, Libermann J (Eds), vitrification in assisted reproduction: A User's Manual and Troubleshooting Guide. Informa Healthcare, 2007. pp.129-44.
7. Chen C. Pregnancy after human oocyte cryopreservation. Lancet 1986;1:884-6.
8. Coticchio G, Bonu MA, Sciajno R et al. Truths and myths of oocyte sensitivity to controlled rate freezing. Reproductive Biomedicine Online 2007;15: 24-30.
9. El-Danasouri I, Selman H. Successful pregnancies and deliveries after a simple vitrification protocol for day 3 human embryos. Fertil Steril 2001;76:400-2.
10. Feichtinger W, Hochfellner C, Ferstl U. Clinical experience with ultrarapid freezing of embryos. Human Reproduction 1991;6:735-6.
11. Hill MJ, Miller KA, Frattarelli JL. A GnRH agonist and exogenous hormone stimulation protocol has a higher live-birth rate than a natural endogenous hormone protocol for frozen-thawed blastocyst-stage embryo transfer cycles: an analysis of 1391 cycles. Fertil Steril 2010;93:416-22.
12. Huang JYJ, Chen HY, Tan SL, Chian RC. Comparison of spindle and chromosome configuration in in vitro and in vivo-matured mouse oocytes after vitrification. Fertility and Sterility 2007;90 (Suppl. 4): 1424-32.
13. Kuleshova L, Gianaroli L, Magli C, et al. Birth following vitrification of a small number of human oocytes: case report. Human Reproduction 1999;14:3077-9.
14. Kuwayama M, Vajta G, Kato O, Leibo SP. Highly efficient vitrification method for cryopreservation of human oocytes. Reproductive BioMedicine Online 2005;11:300-8.
15. Kuwayama M. Highly efficient vitrification for cryopreservation of human oocytes and embryos: the Cryotop method. Theriogenology 2007;67:73-80.
16. Lane M, Schoolcraft WB, Gardner DK. Vitrification of mouse and human blastocysts using a novel cryoloop container-less technique. Fertil Steril 1999;72:1073-8.
17. Larman MG, Sheehan CB, Gardner DK. Calcium-free vitrification reduces cryoprotectant-induced zona pellucida hardening and increases fertilization rates in mouse oocytes. Reproduction. 2009;131:53-61.
18. Liebermann J, Tucker MJ. Effect of carrier system on the yield of human oocytes and embryos as assessed by survival and developmental potential after vitrification. Reproduction 2002;124:483-9.
19. Loutradi KE, Kolibianakis EM, Venetis CA, Papanikolaou EG, Pados G, Bontis I, Tarlatzis BC. Cryopreservation of human embryos by vitrification or slow freezing: a systematic review and meta-analysis. Fertil Steril. 2008, in press.
20. Mauri AL, Petersen CG, Baruffi RLR, et al. Clinical experience with ultrarapid cryopreservation of human embryos resulting from intracytoplasmic sperm injection. Human Reproduction 1999;14: 2362-66.
21. Mukaida T, Nakamura S, Tomiyama T, Wada S, Kasai M, Takahashi K. Successful birth after transfer of vitrified human blastocysts with use of a cryoloop containerless technique. Fertil Steril 2001;76:618-20.
22. Park SP, Kim EY, Oh JH, Nam HK, Lee KS, Park SY, Park EM, Yoon SH, Chung KS, Lim JH. Ultra-rapid freezing of human multipronuclear zygotes using electron microscope grids. Hum Reprod 2000;15:1787-90.
23. Rall WF, Fahy GM. Ice-free cryopreservation of mouse embryos at –196 °C by vitrification. Nature 1985;313: 573-5.
24. Rama Raju GA, Haranath GB, Krishna KM, Prakash GJ, Madan K. Vitrification of human 8-cell embryos, a modified protocol for better pregnancy rates. Reprod Biomed Online 2005;11:434-7.
25. Reed ML, Lane M, Gardner DK, Jensen NL, Thompson J. Vitrification of human blastocysts using the cryoloop method: successful clinical application and birth offspring. JAssist Reprod Genet 2002;19:304-6.
26. Salamonsen LA, Nie G, Hannan NJ, Dimitriadis E. Society for Reproductive Biology Founders Lecture. Preparing fertile soil: The importance of endometrial receptivity. Reproduction, Fertililty and Development 2009;21:923-4.
27. Son WY, Yoon SH, Park SJ, Yoon HJ, Lee WD, Lim JH. Ongoing twin pregnancy after vitrification of blastocysts produced by in vitro matured oocytes retrieved from a woman with polycystic ovary

syndrome: case report. Hum Reprod 2002;17: 2963-6.

28. Son WY, Yoon SH, Yoon HJ. Pregnancy outcome following transfer of human blastocysts vitrified on electron microscopy grids after induced collapse of the blastocoele. Human Reproduction 2003;18: 137-9.
29. The Practice Committee of the Society for Assisted Reproductive Technology and the Practice Committee of the American Society for Reproductive Medicine. The role of assisted hatching in in vitro fertilization: A review of the literature. A Committee opinion, Fertil Steril 2008;90:S196-8.
30. Vajta G, Nagy ZP. Are programmable freezers still needed in the embryo laboratory? Review on vitrification. Reproductive Biomedicine Online 2006;12:779-96.
31. Vanderzwalmen P, Bertin G, Debauche C. Births after vitrification at morula and blastocyst stages: effect of artificial reduction of the blastocoelic cavity before vitrification. Human Reproduction 2002;17:744-51.
32. Vanderzwalmen P, Bertin G, Debauche C, Standaert V, van Roosendaal E, et al. Births after vitrification at morula and blastocyst stages: effect of artificial reduction of the blastocoelic cavity before vitrification. Hum Reprod 2002;17:744-51.
33. Vanderzwalmen P, Bertin G, Debauche C, Standaert V, Bollen N, et al. Vitrification of human blastocysts with the hemi-straw carrier: application of assisted hatching after thawing. Hum Reprod 2003;18:1504-11.
34. Wikland M, Hardarson T, Hillensjo T, Westin C, Westlander G, Wood M, Wennerholm UB. Obstetric outcomes after transfer of vitrified blastocysts Hum Reprod 2010;25:1699-1707.
35. Zheng WT, Zhuang GL, Zhou CQ, Fang C, Ou JP, Li T, Zhang MF, Liang XY. Comparison of the survival of human biopsied embryos after cryopreservation with four different methods using non-transferable embryos. Hum Reprod 2005;20:1615-8.

Chapter 23

The Law and Assisted Reproductive Technology

Sanjay Gupte

INTRODUCTION

Recent advances in the field of genetics have opened up unlimited possibilities for treatment of infertility. Infertility causes a lot of personal and emotional trauma to the couple especially due to the social setting in this country. Infertility therefore, has been seen as a problem which merits treatment. However, every society in the world has shown varying degree of reluctance to assisted reproductive techniques.

In India, in order to regulate and supervise the ART clinics, the indian council of medical research (ICMR) and national academy of medical sciences (NAMS) have devised National Guidelines for Accreditation, Supervision and Regulation of ART Clinics in India. These Guidelines have been designed to ensure safe and ethical services to needy couples and help in regulating and supervising the functioning of ART clinics.

WHAT IS ASSISTED REPRODUCTIVE TECHNOLOGY?

All treatments or procedures that include the *in vitro* handling of human oocytes and human sperm or embryos for the purpose of establishing a pregnancy are termed as assisted reproductive technology (ART). These include *in vitro* fertilization and transcervical embryo transfer, gamete intra-fallopian transfer, zygote intrafallopian transfer, tubal embryo transfer, gamete and embryo cryopreservation, oocyte and embryo donation, gestational surrogacy.

THE LAW AND ART

Infertility of any kind should ideally merit assisted reproduction. However, societies remain polarized about gay couples, lesbian couples, menopausal women, and HIV-positive individuals. Advancements in eugenics also make it possible to 'customize' the fetus, making it extremely controversial. Specifications about donor eggs or donor sperm, criteria for lineage, genetic pedigree, religion or aesthetic aspects and commercialization of the process have resulted in severe conflagrations against exploitation of science. Germ line alterations have so far been the most important cause for denial of assisted reproduction techniques.

While genetic advancements have thrilled those aspiring to become parents, they have also created huge moral panic. No society has been neutral about assisted reproduction. Those with pro-natalist attitudes have seen red on issues such as separation of sex from reproduction, involvement of third party in procreation, same sex couples aspiring parenthood and unnatural means of reproduction. The overall strategy of doctors playing God to help in reproduction induces various reactions in civilian society, ranging from fears arising from cultural adherence, to morally and ethically challenging debates to downright categorization as 'unnatural and hence antisocial'.

The practitioners of ART also face unprecedented challenges in treating infertile couples. Here in India, reproductive failure may lead to isolation of the couple and even social ostracism in some cultures. Having a child, a legacy bearer or an heir, slowly and naturally becomes a force which can drive the needy couple to any extent. But ART is not so advanced as to guarantee cent percent positive results. The ART practitioner has to select the correct type of treatment for the couple, knowing fully well that it may not bear results. There is also an added responsibility to make the couple aware and convince them of the techniques and the time required.

Protecting the interests of the needy couple and simultaneously guiding ART clinics towards safe and ethical practice is the need of the hour. While some countries like Australia, UK, France and Germany already have legislation in place defining laws for assisted reproductive technologies, many others have guidelines to deal with medicolegal issues arising from these procedures. With rapid developments and pioneering advances in the treatment of infertility, there is growing need for every country to define fair and just procedures ensuring safety of all stakeholders.

LAWS AND GUIDELINES REGARDING ASSISTED REPRODUCTION

Every country in the world prohibits germ line modification, reproductive cloning, commercial trading of human eggs, sperm and embryos and commercial surrogacy, creation of hybrid embryos, transfer of nonhuman embryos to humans or human embryos to nonhumans, nonmedical sex selection (Kirsten Riggan, 10/01/2010).

Following are laws and/or guidelines from nations who are forerunners in assisted reproductive techniques.

AUSTRALIA

Legislation governs the practice and provision of assisted reproductive treatment (ART) in South Australia in parts. Concrete laws concerning ART exist in New South Wales, Victoria and Western Australia. There is no common legislation applicable to all of Australia. States and territories without specific legislation rely on the Reproductive Technology Accreditation Committee accreditation scheme which sets standards for practice and requires compliance with the National Health and Medical Research Council's ethical guidelines on the use of assisted reproductive technology in clinical practice and research. A person is authorized to provide assisted reproductive treatment if the person holds a current RTAC license. (Assisted Reproductive treatment legislation, 2011).

There are two main acts with respect to ART. Previously known as 'Reproductive Technology (Clinical Practices) Act 1988 (SA)', the Act is now known as the 'Assisted Reproductive Treatment Act 1988 (SA)', which operates in conjunction with the 'Assisted Reproductive Treatment Regulations 2010'. Many aspects of clinical practice in ART raise ethical issues. The ART Guidelines cover activities including:

- Posthumous use of gametes
- Surrogacy
- Sex selection
- Preimplantation genetic diagnosis (PGD).

The *Involving Human Embryos Act 2002* and the *Prohibition of Human Cloning for Reproduction Act 2002* permit research on excess ART embryos, including those that are unsuitable for implantation, and embryos created by means other than by fertilization of a human egg and human sperm. Consent from the donor must also be sought prior to use of excess ART embryos for research. Reproductive cloning is entirely banned.

It is lawfully mandated that incidence of ovarian hyperstimulation syndrome (OHSS) should be monitored and corrected in all treatment cycles, including artificial insemination and ovulation induction (CODE OF PRACTICE FOR ASSISTED, 2010). Patients must receive information on the risks, symptoms and management of OHSS. No more than 1 embryo or oocyte can be transferred in a single reproductive cycle in women aged below 35 years and no more than 2 embryos or oocytes in women aged below 40 years. In case of oocyte donation, it must be ensured that these are collected from healthy women aged less than 40 years at the time of collection.

The country recently faced a huge social outcry regarding destruction of unused embryos. The donors were contacted and cryopreservation was offered for an extended period until their decision was made. Most donors opted to give up their embryos for research.

Only noncommercial or altruistic forms of surrogacy are allowed in Australia.

BELGIUM

ART is legally allowed in Belgium. ART is completely covered by the national health coverage plan. The law on Medically Assisted Reproduction and Disposition of Supernumerary Embryos and Gametes was passed in 2007. It is adjuvant to the Law on Research into Embryos *in vitro* (2002). No governing body exists to oversee ART activities. (Kirsten Riggan, 10/01/2010).

Both reproductive and research cloning are banned under these laws. The country has strict policies in terms of creation and transfer of embryos. Only 2 can be transferred in women less than 36 years of age and up to 3 can be transferred in women up to 42 years of age. A maximum of 6 cycles in women under the age of 42 years can be attempted under the national health coverage.

CANADA

In Canada, ART is practices under the aegis of assisted human reproduction agency of Canada (AHRAC). AHRAC is the authority that monitors clinics, sets up standardization and provides clear guidelines on proper and improper usage of genetic material. The Assisted Human Reproduction Act of 2004 is said to be the most significant piece of legislation focusing on human genetic and reproductive technologies. The AHRA provides for a legislative review after three years. This provision enabled many who were not completely satisfied with the measure to support it nonetheless (Assisted Human Reproduction Act, SC 2004, c 2, 2007).

The following are absolutely banned:

- The creation of human embryos solely for research
- Germ line engineering (i.e. inheritable genetic modification)
- The creation of human/nonhuman hybrids and chimeras
- All use of somatic cell nuclear transfer (cloning), whether for research or reproduction
- Sex selection except to prevent, diagnose or treat a sex-linked disorder or disease
- Commercial surrogate motherhood contracts and the sale of sperm, eggs and embryos.

Research involving human embryos, including embryonic stem cell research, is permitted; using embryos created but not used during *in vitro* fertilization procedures. ART is offered to everyone irrespective of sexual orientation or marital status. The AHRA agency calls for absolute due diligence for the safety of mother and child during and after ART.

FRANCE

In France, French Biomedicine Agency, which is under the supervision of the Minister of Health, is responsible for quality assurance and ensuring ethical practices in biomedical research. Particular to cell and gene therapy research, the Biomedicine Agency collaborates with the French Health Products Safety Agency, which has the mandate to authorize and control the preparation, transformation, and use of human tissues and cells. The main law regarding ART here is the Law no. 94-654 governing the donation and use of elements and products of the human body, medically assisted reproduction, and prenatal diagnosis (1994), which was been amended in 2004 by the Bioethics Law no. 2004-800, regulates gene therapy and gene therapy products (Genetics and Policy Center, 2010).

France practices conservation Catholicism and ART has been subject to intense scrutiny. All assisted reproductive technologies are only accessible to heterosexual couples who are of age to procreate and are married or have lived together for at least two years prior to the reproductive procedure. The national health plan provides complete coverage to such couples.

The bioethics law explicitly prohibits germ line therapy and considers eugenic practices to be a crime against the human species. Furthermore, in order to protect biotechnology an intervention, French law provides that processes of modification of the human genetic identity cannot be patented (Article 17).

Preimplantation genetic diagnosis is permitted in France for the selection of healthy embryos when a parent or other close relative has a serious genetic disease. It is also allowed for HLA tissue matching. However, PGD for sex selection is only allowed for medical reasons and prohibited for cultural reasons or for family balancing (Genetics and Policy Center, 2010).

GERMANY

With a long and glorious history of scientific innovations, Germany also has its share of moral disgrace. The collective memories of extremities of eugenics resulting in holocaust have shaped the nation's conservative approach towards reproductive technology. Germany's key laws and guidelines pertaining to ART include the *Federal Embryo Protection Law 1990,* the *Adoption Brokerage Law 2006,* and the *Guideline of the German Federal Medical Chamber 2006*. Due to the restrictive nature of these laws, no governing agency is required to monitor ART.

The distinguishing feature of the German reproductive policy landscape is its strong formal protection of fetuses and embryos. In Germany, implanted embryos and fetuses are constitutionally protected by the Basic Law, and are thus entitled to the same right to life and dignity that all persons have (Robertson, 2004).

The Federal Embryo Protection Act is highly protective of embryos as incipient forms of human life. Its definition of embryo chooses the point after fertilization at which nuclear fusion, or syngamy, occurs (ordinarily about twenty hours after insemination).

The Act makes it a crime punishable by three years in prison:

- To fertilize more eggs that have attained syngamy than can be transferred to a woman in one cycle
- To transfer more than three embryos to the uterus
- To engage in egg donation and gestational surrogacy, or to create embryos for research
- Also prohibits nonmedical sex selection
- Posthumous *in vitro* fertilization.

German fertility doctors practice ovarian hyper-stimulation albeit with smaller amounts of drugs and retrieve fewer eggs. The common practice is to inseminate with a single sperm (ICSI).

Somatic cell transfer (cloning) is prohibited for both research and reproductive purposes. Cryopreservation of embryos is banned. However, since the Act restricts itself to protection of embryos "after fusion or syngamy", it allows freezing of zygotes or pronuclear embryos prior to syngamy. All forms of surrogacy are prohibited. Preimplantation genetic diagnosis is banned. However, sperm sorting is allowed for prevention of sex-lined genetic disorders.

ITALY

After several failed bills catering to different schools of thought, finally, ART is regulated under the *Medically Assisted Procreation Law* (2004) in Italy. There are strict and remarkable restrictions on various aspects of practice of ART. Most prominent are the intervention of the legislature to protect the child born through the use of ART, by establishing his legal status (Art 8), and prohibiting the disownment of paternity and the mother's anonymity (Art 9). ART guidelines are subject to review every three years. A national register has been established (Art 11) by the Istituto Superiore di Sanità (National Institute of Health) to monitor ART activities, number of embryos created, number of children born this way and quality checks. No authoritative agency exits solely for ART. Italy extends ART only to heterogenous couples who live together, are of reproductive age, with documented infertility and who have been offered adoption (Kirsten Riggan, 10/01/2010).

The Medically Assisted Procreation law prohibits:

- Cryopreservation of embryos
- Limiting to three the number of embryos that can be implanted in each single cycle
- Forbids assisted reproduction using a third party in any way
- Access to reproductive technology for couples who carry genetic diseases with risk of transmission.

The law details every ART related procedure minutely and defines stepwise approach to technical instructions to the medical staff of every center authorized to conduct ART. Reproductive and research related cloning is banned. Cryopreservation of fertilized eggs is banned, with the exception of severe injury/illness preventing embryo transfer. Sex selection is only permitted through sperm sorting for sex-lined genetic diseases. All forms of surrogacy are prohibited. Pre-implantation genetic diagnosis for the selection of embryos is prohibited, but can be allowed on a case-by-case basis.

INDIA

There is no specific legislation in India governing human genetic modification. Under authority from indian council of medical research (ICMR), national academy of medical sciences (NAMS) and the Ministry of Science and Technology, detailed guidelines to establishing, regulating and monitoring ART facilities have been devised. They prohibit:

- Reproductive cloning
- Germline modification
- Prenatal Genetic Diagnosis, except for detecting specific genetic and chromosomal abnormalities or for sex-linked genetic disorders
- Sex selection "at any stage of fertilization, except to avoid the risk of transmission of a genetic abnormality assessed through PGD" is banned
- More than 3 oocytes or embryos in one reproductive cycle, except for elderly women, poor implantation, adenomyosis, or poor embryo quality
- Transfer of gametes or embryos of more than one man or woman at one cycle
- Placing human embryos in animals
- Research on embryos beyond 14 days of gestation

Identity of the donor cannot be disclosed to the offspring. ART can be availed irrespective of gender or marital status. Cryopreservation of embryos is allowed for 5 years. Posthumous usage of husband's stored sperms has been encouraged, although the law is yet to be modified accordingly.

ICMR Guidelines for Setting up ART Clinics

The Indian Council of Medical Research clearly defines guidelines for setting up primary, secondary and tertiary ART clinics. The document is a detailed hand book of rules and regulations for practitioners of ART. The online version can be found here -http://www.icmr.nic.in/art/art_clinics.htm

- All ART clinics are expected to be registered with and supervised by the State Accreditation Authority/State Appropriate Authorities
- All clinics are expected to comply with the mandatory code of practice as defined in the ICMR guidelines, failure of which can lead to prosecution or suspension of the clinic's registration
- Space requirements, staff requirements, equipment and methodology used, issues regarding sterility and safety are well defined in the ICMR guidelines. Strict adherence of these rules is expected.

Primary (Level 1A) Infertility Care Units

These would be clinics where preliminary investigations are carried out and type and cause of infertility diagnosed. Primary infertility care unit or clinic could be a doctor's consulting room, such as a gynecologist's or a physician's consulting room, or even a general hospital. Depending on the severity of infertility, the couple could be treated at the Level 1A clinic or referred to a specialty (Level 1B, Level 2 or Level 3) clinic.

Investigations into the cause of infertility by diligent history taking, physical examination and a simple semen analysis that can detect cases of azoospermia, can determine if the cause of infertility is related to the female or the male or to both the partners. Multifactorial or unexplainable cases should be referred to specialty secondary (Level 2) or tertiary (Level 3) infertility care units.

In case a Level 1A clinic is engaged in AIH and IUI it must maintain records of the use of the requisitioned semen and of all AIH and IUI done, appropriately and confidentially; these records will be liable to inspection by an appropriate Review Committee. A Level 1A infertility care unit will not require an accreditation under these guidelines.

Primary (Level 1B) Infertility Care Units Engaging in IUI

These units would be required to have, in addition to what has been stated in ICMR guidelines, the facilities mentioned in the following two subsections—appropriate facilities for investigation and for treatment. The facilities for investigation and for sperm preparation mentioned above could be shared with another accredited infertility clinic or semen bank.

Infertility clinics falling into this category like those of Level 2 and Level 3 (see the following sections) shall need accreditation. The IUI in such clinics must be done under the supervision of a gynecologist with a postgraduate degree.

Secondary (Level 2) Infertility Care Units

These units must have infrastructure for further in-depth investigation and extended treatment of infertility except where oocytes are handled outside the body.

Facilities for investigations:

i. Immunological tests for infertility, sperm cervical mucous penetration test (SCMPT), sperm cervical mucous test (SCMT), and tests for antibodies (IgG, IgA) against sperm antigen in cervical mucous.

ii. Sperm function tests like hypo-osmotic swelling test (HOST), and assessment of the improvement of sperm motility potential with pentoxifylline co-culture.

iii. Assessment of follicular growth and ovulation by serial transvaginal sonography (TVS).

iv. Hysteroscopy, laparoscopy and transvaginal sonography.

Treatment facilities:

i. Facilities for semen preparation and intrauterine insemination (IUI).

ii. Provision for semen collection in men with a vibrator or an electroejaculator in functional erectile and ejaculatory problems.

iii. Conservative surgery either through a laparoscope, hysteroscope or via laparotomy. It should be possible to perform hysteroscopic cannulation of blocked tubes, and resection of submucous myoma or uterine septum.

iv. Combined medical-surgical therapy by a co-ordinated team as in endometriosis or in some cases of polycystic ovaries (ovarian drilling).

v. Provision for extended treatment of infertility except for oocyte pick up and IVF, ICSI, etc.

Tertiary (Level 3) Infertility Care Units

Such units will have three functions to perform, viz. diagnostic and therapeutic at the highest level of specialization and with the best of facilities, and research. If any of the facilities mentioned below does not exist in the clinic, the clinic should have access to such a facility in another appropriately accredited clinic, semen bank, or laboratory.

Diagnostic procedures for male infertility:

i. Endocrine assay.

ii. Further tests for sperm function and integrity such as acrosome reaction and sperm-oocyte interaction *in vitro*.

iii. Assessment of cell contaminants, debris and infection.

iv. Karyotyping when sperm density, morphology and motility are abnormal.

v. Assessment of seminal plasma for viscosity, thinness, blood contamination and biochemical constituents.

Diagnostic procedures for female infertility:

i. Endocrine assay.

ii. Karyotyping in premature ovarian failure in Kallman's syndrome.

iii. Color Doppler for checking growing follicles, functional integrity of corpus luteum, and developing endometrium in stimulated or unstimulated cycle.

iv. GnRH challenge test in nonovulation due to hypothalamic pituitary failure.

v. Clomiphene challenge tests to ascertain ovarian reserves before ovulation induction or controlled ovarian hyperstimulation.

Therapeutic procedures:

i. Induction of ovulation in refractory non-ovulation due to PCO down regulation with a GnRH-agonist followed by induction with gonadotropin.

ii. All varieties of assisted reproductive technologies, including ICSI, mentioned earlier.

iii. Procedures for IUI using split ejaculate, pooled ejaculate or sperm recovered from postcoital specimen of urine in retrograde ejaculation.

iv. Embryo freezing.

Surrogacy in India

It is only in the last 20 years that surrogate motherhood has increasingly become an issue of national and international public debate. Although there has been much publicity surrounding the practice of surrogacy the incidence of surrogate motherhood in India is not known at present.

The Ministry of Women and Child Development is examining the issue of 'surrogate motherhood' in India for bringing up a comprehensive legislation. But surrogate motherhood—as an arrangement, in which a woman carries and bears a child for another person or persons, but takes no ownership of the child born—has also raised moral, ethical and social and legal questions about both—the woman and the 'commissioned baby'.

ICMR clearly states that surrogate mother should mention her name, declare her surrogacy status and provide details of the genetic parents at hospital registration. The birth certificate issued should bear the name of commissioning parents and they are legally bound to accept the custody of the baby irrespective of any abnormality in the child.

Finances Involved in Surrogacy

Surrogate mothers are entitled to monetary compensation. The financial aspect of the process has to be decided upon independently by the woman and the couple. The ART center can in no way become involved in the money that the surrogate mother receives. As agreed upon, the couple should make their payment to the surrogate mother at the right time (immediately after delivery). It is necessary to keep all these dealings on paper as per the contract, and it is also necessary to preserve these documents.

The entire cost of care during pregnancy and rearing of the child should rest with the couple seeking surrogacy. There should not be a scenario where unfavorable allocation of financial burden in the event of a medical emergency during pregnancy, rests on the surrogate.

Surrogate Mother Criteria

The surrogate mother should be of 21 to 45 years of age. The responsibility to certify that her womb is capable of child bearing rests on the ART center. A relative or an unknown woman can become a surrogate mother. If a relative of the couple chooses to become the surrogate mother, and then she should be of about the same age as the couple is.

It is compulsory for the woman who wants to be a surrogate mother to furnish proof of her diagnosis to ensure that she is healthy. If a surrogate is married, the consent of her spouse shall be required before she may act as such surrogate. A woman cannot become a surrogate mother more than three times. A surrogate mother shall not act as an oocyte donor for the couple or individual.

Commercialization

The ART center **should not advertise** its surrogacy services in any way. No ART clinic shall provide information on or about surrogate mothers or potential surrogate mothers to any person. For this, the needy couples and the semen bank have been given certain stipulations.

Cheap availability of surrogacy has been attracting a lot of interest. ICMR advises foreigners or a nonresident Indians to appoint a local guardian who will be legally responsible for taking care of the surrogate during and after the pregnancy till the child is delivered to the foreigner or nonresident couple or the local guardian. Proper documentation should be made to take the child outside of India to the country of the party's origin or residence. A couple or an individual shall not have the service of more than one surrogate at any given time. A couple shall not have simultaneous transfer of embryos in the woman and in a surrogate.

Rights of the Child Born Via Surrogacy

A child can, at age of 18, apply for any information, excluding personal identification, relating to his/her genetic parent or parents or surrogate mother.

Risks in Being a Surrogate

It has been observed that usually most of surrogates come from lower socio-economic strata with little knowledge of legalities involved. Surrogates should be legally represented by lawyers from ART clinics. They must be protected from getting into unfair legal contracts such as a candidate surrogate persuaded to sign a contract reserving the right of the intended parents to refuse custody or parental rights of the resulting infant for any reason.

Potential areas for exploitation in surrogacy contracts include certain risky medical protocols, such as fertility treatment and multiple embryo transfer. There is always a risk of being left with complete responsibility of child, if intended parents back out. There is a dire need for stricter rules protecting rights of surrogates.

JAPAN

The law related to ART in Japan is the *Law Concerning Regulation Relating to Human Cloning Techniques and Other Similar Techniques* (June 2001). ART related activities are voluntarily monitored by the Japan Society of Obstetrics and Gynecology (Kirsten Riggan, 10/01/2010).

This law prohibits:

- Reproductive cloning
- Germline modification
- The transfer of human/animal hybrid embryos to either a human or animal.

SINGAPORE

Human Cloning and Other Prohibited Practices Act is the main legislative piece governing ART procedures in Singapore. It was passed by Parliament in September, 2004 and came into effect on 1 October, 2004. (Ministry of Health, Singapore, 2007). A human embryo is defined as having "been developing for less than 8 weeks since the appearance of 2 pronuclei or the initiation of its development by other means".

The law prohibits:

- Reproductive cloning activities
- Developing human embryo outside for more than 14 days
- Removal of human embryos from a woman to obtain viable human embryos
- Placing a human embryo in a body of a human or an animal
- Import or export of any human embryo in or out of Singapore
- Commercial trading of egg, sperm and embryo.

The bioethics advisory committee (BAC) is a governmental advisory body formed in the year 2000 that published its report entitled *Ethical, Legal and Social Issues in Human Stem Cell Research, Reproductive and Therapeutic Cloning* (Genetics and Public Policy Center, 2010). It seeks a complete ban on reproductive cloning practices but supports the special status of the human embryo. It has recommended the formation of a legislative and regulatory body to license and monitor ART services. This body has supported therapeutic cloning, provided there is scientific merit from such research and with approval from a statutory body.

UNITED KINGDOM

In UK, IVF and embryo research are regulated by the human fertilization and embryology authority (HFEA). Three main laws are Surrogacy Arrangement Act of 1990; Human Embryology and Fertilization Act and Human Reproductive Cloning Act (Kirsten Riggan, 10/01/2010).

The Surrogacy Act prohibits all kinds of commercial surrogacy. Other prohibitions for ART:

- Reproductive cloning
- Cloning for research
- More than 1-2 embryos transferred per cycle in women under 40 years old
- Maximum up to 3 embryos transferred per cycle in women above 40 years old.

UNITED STATES OF AMERICA

The USA does not enforce strict legislation over individuals but closely monitors ART clinics. Only Pennsylvania State actively regulates and monitors its ART clinics. Standards of care are monitored and ART clinics submit their statistics to the state authority. Although comprehensive legislation is absent, legal matters are subject to state level jurisdiction. The Fertility Clinic Success Rate and Certification Act 1992 remains the most important law with respect to ART (Kirsten Riggan, 10/01/ 2010).

Both reproductive and research cloning is banned in totally 7 American states. The other states either have no stand on the issue or have some degree of monitoring over the ART clinics. Commercial surrogacy is regulated in some states while others completely ban this form of ART. Financial coverage for ART is strictly private (via private insurance).

BIBLIOGRAPHY

1. Assisted Human Reproduction Act, SC 2004, c 2. (2007, Dec 1). Retrieved May 28, 2011, from www.canlii.org: http://www.canlii.org/en/ca/laws/stat/sc-2004-c-2/latest/sc-2004-c-2.html
2. Assisted Reproductive treatment legislation. (2011, Mar 2). Retrieved May 23, 2011, from www.sahealth.sa.gov: http://www.sahealth.sa.gov.au/wps/wcm/connect/Public+Content/SA+Health+Internet/Health+services/Womens+health/Pregnancy+and+fertility/Fertility+treatment/ART+Legislation
3. CODE OF PRACTICE FOR ASSISTED. (2010, Oct). Retrieved May 28, 2011, from www.fertilitysociety.com: http://www.fertilitysociety.com.au/wp-content/uploads/201011201-final-rtac-cop.pdf
4. Genetics and Policy Center. (2010). Retrieved May 2011, from www.dnapolicy.org: http://www.dnapolicy.org/policy.international.php?action=detailandlaws_id=37
5. Genetics and Public Policy Center. (2010). Retrieved June 7, 2011, from www.dnapolicy.org: http://www.dnapolicy.org/policy.international.php?action=detail&laws_id=30
6. Kirsten Riggan, M. (10/01/2010, Jan 10). Retrieved May 25, 2011, from www.chbd.org: http://cbhd.org/content/g12-country-regulations-assisted-reproductive-technologies
7. Ministry of Health, Singapore. (2007). Retrieved June 7, 2011, from www.moh.gov.sg: http://www.moh.gov.sg/mohcorp/legislations.aspx?id=7084
8. Robertson JA. (2004, 2 12). Reproductive Technology in Germany and the United States. Retrieved May 2011, from www.utesxas.edu: http://www.utexas.edu/law/faculty/jrobertson/rt_germany_usa.pdf.

Chapter 24

Role of Alternative Therapies

Tomoko Inoue, Yoshiharu Morimoto

WHAT ARE ALTERNATIVE THERAPIES?

In the field of reproductive medicine, we have achieved astonishing technological advances such as *in vitro* fertilization and embryo culture. Couples with long-term infertility can increase their chances of having children through these new reproductive technologies, especially in developed countries. In contrast, many countries have very limited health resources; couples in these countries may try to conceive with the assistance of alternative health care. Including such basic methods as religious praying, meditation, and herbal medicine, there are plenty of alternative options for health promotion worldwide. Even in developed countries where people have easier access to sophisticated Western medicine, Eastern medicines or alternative methods have become increasingly popular among the general public. In the United States, a national survey reported that more than 42 percent of adult Americans had tried at least 1 of 16 types of complementary and alternative therapies in 1997,[1] a substantial increase over the 33.8 percent reported in 1990. The survey also estimated that out-of-pocket expenditures for alternative medicine professional services reached at least $21.2 billion in 1997, which is comparable to out-of-pocket expenditures for all US physician services in the same year.

Alternative medicine covers a broad range of healing philosophies, approaches, and therapies that are usually outside the mainstream of conventional modern medicine. While conventional medicine usually regards the human body as an integrated collection of cells that display physiological phenomena, the Eastern or holistic approach emphasizes the balance of mind and body. The later approach offers natural products and mental or physical techniques that are believed to have healing powers. Some of these therapies are closely tied to specific indigenous cultures, religions, regions, or ethnicities. The following are examples of major alternative treatments used worldwide.

Natural Products

- Herbal medicines
- Vitamins
- Minerals.

Mind-Body Therapies

- Meditation
- Yoga
- Autogenic training

- Hypnotherapy
- Deep-breathing exercises
- Progressive relaxation
- Guided imagery
- Qi Gong
- Tai chi
- Counseling.

Manipulation and Body-Based Practices

- Acupuncture
- Spinal manipulation
- Massage therapy
- Chiropractic
- Shiatsu
- Reiki.

Other Therapies

- Movement therapies
- Music therapies
- Color therapy
- Homeopathy
- Naturopathy
- Ayurveda
- Aromatherapy.

If any product or therapy listed above is used alone or instead of conventional medicine, it is considered an *alternative medicine*. If the therapy is provided in conjunction with conventional medicine, such as the use of deep breathing exercises in conjugation with standard care to help reduce physical pain, it is called *complementary medicine*. Recently, the concept of *integrated medicine* has come to our attention.[2] Integrated medicine focuses on health and healing rather than disease and treatment. It regards patients as whole entities with minds and spirits as well as bodies and includes these dimensions in diagnosis and treatment. Patients and doctors work together to maintain health by paying attention to lifestyle factors such as diet, exercise, quality of rest and sleep, and the nature of relationships.

People in different countries, cultures, religions, and circumstances may define health in different ways. The World Health Organization defines health as a complete state of physical, mental, and social well-being, not merely the absence of disease or infirmity.[3] Australian aboriginal people generally define health as follows: "Health does not just mean the physical well-being of the individual but refers to the social, emotional, spiritual, and cultural well-being of the whole community".[4] Both statements see human health not only as a physical aspect, but also as a union of body, mind, and spirit. In this century, we have an opportunity to expand the concept of conventional medicine as it was practiced in the last century; integration of conventional medicine with alternative therapies could provide the tools for achieving total health. When we considering reproductive health of infertile couples in a holistic manner, we should consider that their whole lifestyle influences their reproductive function. The task of a health specialist is to provide an overview of available therapies so that these couples can select the most appropriate therapies for their situation. In addition to the advanced conventional technologies, alternative therapies provide an opportunity for a deep healing of the body and mind.

In the next sections, we introduce some promising alternative therapies that are available in daily practice at modern reproductive clinics. All of these therapies are actually used as part of treatment for patients experiencing difficulty in conceiving.

HERBAL MEDICINES

Herbal medicine (Kampo in Japan) is an important part of traditional Chinese medicine. The roots, peels, or stalks of plants are the major ingredients of each prescription, and different types of plants are mixed together to produce synergic effects. In

Western conventional medicine, generally patients with the same diagnosis would have the same prescription, despite differences in personal characteristics. In contrast, traditional Chinese medicine has a different philosophy; the formula of herbal medicine for the treatment or prevention of disease is specific for each individual and thus would be different for two patients with the same diagnosis. The composition of each herbal medicine is primarily based on an examination and diagnostic process that includes observation of the tongue, assessment of the pulse on the wrist, and manipulation of the abdomen. Questionnaires can aid in further evaluation of the physical and/or emotional status of the patient. Patients are usually classified into three groups according to their physical characteristics, and the corresponding herbal medicine is prescribed. Additionally, herbal medicines could improve resistance to diseases. In relation to the reproductive system, we expect that Chinese herbal medicine would not only relieve physical symptoms or disorders but also gradually alter the patient's body to make it more suitable for conception. Infertile couples often suffer psychological and physical stress from the failure of conventional treatment; in this situation, Chinese medicine could benefit both mind and body. There are numerous studies about the effects of Chinese herbal medicines and their influence on infertility.

Improvement of Reproductive Function

Women with the medical diagnosis of unexpected infertility were recruited to evaluate the effectiveness of herbal medicines on reproductive factors such as endometrial thickness, basal follicle stimulating hormone (FSH) levels, number of follicles, size of dominant follicles, and pelvic blood flow, which were evaluated before and after the treatment.

The study demonstrated that women who took herbal medicines showed improvement in reproductive factors compared with the pre-treatment data. The effectiveness of herbal medicine appeared to be independent of patient age. There were no adverse effects from the treatment, and most importantly, 28 of 50 women conceived within 6 months of initiating treatment.[5] Although there were only 50 women in this study, this result suggests that herbal medicines improve a woman's chance of natural conception with few side effects.

Herbal Medicine for Polycystic Ovary Syndrome

Polycystic ovary syndrome (PCOS) is a complex reproductive endocrinology disease. PCOS may affect the ability of women to conceive, since irregular or anovulation is one of its characteristics. Chinese herbal medicines have been reported to be an alternative approach for subfertile women with PCOS. Four randomized controlled trials that used Chinese herbal medicine for the treatment of PCOS were identified and statistically analyzed. One report showed a statistically significant improvement in pregnancy rate (per woman) for women treated with Chinese herbal medicine plus clomiphene compared with clomiphene only; however, there was insufficient evidence to demonstrate the effectiveness and safety of Chinese herbal medicine in terms of live birth rate, pregnancy rate, ovulation rate and adverse events in subfertile women with PCOS.[6]

Hachimijiogan for Hyperprolactinemia and Male Infertility

Hachimijiogan, a Chinese herbal medicine used widely in Japan, has several effects on infertility. In a study reported in 1989, Hachimijiogan was shown to control the serum level of prolactin with a lower incidence of adverse effects, such as nausea, than bromocriptine. Once the hormone levels of women were normalized, many of them recovered from their previous anovulatory cycles, and some were able to conceive.[7] In a second study, men treated with *Hachimijiogan* showed improved spermatogenesis.[8]

Wen-Jing-Tang for Inducing Ovulation

Wen-Jing-Tang (Unkeito in Japan), another popular Chinese herbal medicine in Japan, was shown to induce ovulation in previously anovulatory patients when used in conjunction with clomiphene citrate. A previous study on rats has shown that Wen-Jing-Tang increases LH-RH release from the hypothalamus; a similar response in humans could explain the induction of ovulation in women who are resistant to clomiphene citrate treatment alone. Ovarian hyperstimulation syndrome did not develop in the women who took Wen-Jing-Tang. This study supports the use of Wen-Jing-Tang as a complementary treatment for women with ovulation failure before the use of gonadotropins.[9]

Other Herbal Medicines for Various Symptoms of Female Patients

Many Japanese doctors recognize Chinese herbal medicines as effective tools for health promotion in women, and some have used these medicines to treat reproductive disorders. In addition to Hachimijiogan or Wen-Jing-Tang, Toki-shakuyaku-san and Keishi-bukuryo-gan appear to be promising medicines for women with frequent anovulation or hypothalamic amenorrhea. One report showed that pregnancy rates were ranging from 31 percent to 65 percent with the use of one of these four medicines. This report also showed that in daily practice, 66.9 percent of Japanese gynecologists used Kampo medicine for disorders such as climacteric syndrome, ovarian deficiency syndrome, infertility, dysmenorrhea, failure of ovulation, complications of pregnancy, postoperative fatigue, benign tumors, malignant tumors, and infectious diseases.[10]

ACUPUNCTURE

Acupuncture uses needles or moxibustion at specific points on the body to activate circulation and regulate Qi and Blood in order to remove pathogenic factors and heal the body. This therapy is an important part of Chinese traditional medicine and has been popular in Japan and Korea for centuries. Recently, many Western countries have paid increased attention to acupuncture. The National Center for Complementary and Alternative Medicine (NCCAM), a center within the National Institutes for Health in the US, refers to acupuncture as one of key components of mind-body medicines.

Acupuncture is based on the theory that meridians, collaterals, and the Zang Fu organs are physiologically related to each other in human body and that the breakdown of this balance produces ill health. Meridians and collaterals are pathways through which Qi and Blood circulate and through which the exterior of the body connects with the interior. They are closely related to the Zang Fu organs. When a person becomes ill, the meridians and collaterals are affected first, and then the Zang Fu organs become involved; in other words, a blockage in the meridians and collaterals produces illness. Acupuncture removes the blockages in the meridians and collaterals, which restores the circulation of Qi and Blood and adjusts the Zang Fu organs; this restoration of balance promotes health.

Acupuncture has the power to strengthen the body's resistance and eliminate pathogenic factors. Diseases develop when the anti-pathogenic Qi is not strong enough to overcome pathogenic factors; strengthening the anti-pathogenic Qi enables the body to fight the pathogenic Qi and cure the illness.

If the anti-pathogenic Qi is not strengthened, the disease will progress.

Finally, another important function of acupuncture is the regulation of the balance between Yin and Yang. When Yin and Yang are balanced, the body is in a state of well-being; however, an imbalance between Yin and Yang may lead to illness. Yang syndrome is caused by an excess of Yin, and conversely, Yin syndrome is caused by an excess of Yang. Acupuncture therapy controls the balance between Yin and Yang through the use of reinforcing and reducing needle techniques on appropriate combinations of stimulation points. Acupuncture practitioners examine the patient by placing needles and moxibustion at diagnosis points and monitoring the response of the body. Based on this diagnostic observation, practitioners use acupuncture to regulate the patient's Qi and Blood to achieve a balance between Yin and Yang.[11]

For example, although male infertility is considered to result from a combined malfunction of the kidneys, heart, liver, and spleen, the main causes are insufficiency of kidney essence; stagnation of Qi and Blood; and downward flow of damp heat. On the basis of this theory, specific acupuncture points on the body are stimulated with needles or by other special manipulation techniques.

The NCCAM report states that acupuncture is useful for easing certain types of physical pain, such as headache, back pain, and tennis elbow, and that acupuncture can provide some relief from the pain accompanying menstruation.[12] The Cochrane Reviews also provide convincing evidence that acupuncture relieves dysmenorrhea.[13] Another Cochrane Review finds that acupuncture increases the live birth rate for *in vitro* fertilization (IVF) treatment performed around the time of embryo transfer; however, there is no benefit when acupuncture is performed 2 to 3 days after embryo transfer.[14] This report also recommends that acupuncture should not be performed during early pregnancy because of potential harmful effects. Although acupuncture has great potential in curing the body and mind when used as a complementary and alternative therapy, more well-designed studies are needed to further clarify the impact of acupuncture on the different aspects of fertility.

AUTOGENIC TRAINING

JH Schultz, a German psychiatrist, developed autogenic training (AT) in the 1920s. This self relaxation method is said to be especially effective for dealing with psychosomatic disorders or neurosis.[15] The practice of AT is designed to turn off the body's stressful "fight-flight" reaction and turn on the restorative rhythms associated with profound psychophysical relaxation. When practiced regularly, AT produces a mental state compatible to that achieved by Eastern meditation and a physical state comparable to the chemical and physiological changes associated with rigorous athletic training. AT appeals to people with a modern lifestyle; it can be practiced almost anywhere at any time. Once mastered, AT relaxes body muscles and dilates vessels. In addition, it can soothe an agitated mind and produce serenity. These physical and emotional changes have a synergistic effect on reducing stress produced from daily life activities or health problems. AT promotes recovery from fatigue, alleviates physical or emotional pain, reduces insomnia, decreases frustration, increases mental stability, improves operating efficacy, and stimulates one's spirit.

Stress and anxiety can be important contributory factors to infertility. For example, some couples manage to conceive soon after they adopt a child or have completely given up the idea of having their own children. This probably happens because anxiety is removed from the process of conceiving. AT has been primarily tried with couples who have no or mild physical problems causing infertility, but couples under medical treatment would also be candidates for this technique. The practice of AT is thought to reduce the stress that couples suffer when treatments for infertility are unsuccessful.

Precautions before starting the training:

1. If possible, learn AT from a qualified trainer; however, many instruction books are available. Read the instructions carefully and practice daily.
2. AT is not suitable for people with health issues such as heart disease, diabetes, glaucoma, schizophrenia, severe depression, alcoholism, or drug abuse.
3. Make sure that you are comfortable before starting the exercise. Do not start if you are very hungry or have the urge to defecate or urinate. Take off your shoes and loosen your clothing. The room should be warm, quiet, and dimly lit.
4. Set up training areas suitable for the exercise positions, such as the lying down position or the easy chair position.
5. Achieve passive concentration and scan your body before you start the exercise. Passive concentration, an unfamiliar concept to beginners, is an important step in AT. It is a state of being free from thought and emotion; you just sit and observe what happens to your body and mind.
6. Learn AT step by step.
7. Cancel AT properly at the end of each exercise. The cancellation steps are as follows: clench both fists tightly; bend your elbows briskly by stretching your arms out either in front of you or sideways; take a deep breath in; and finally, open your eyes and breathe out.

AT, in brief, consists of following six steps.

1. Feeling of heaviness in the limbs.
2. Feeling of warmth in the limbs.
3. Feeling of regular heart beat.
4. Feeling of easy breath.
5. Feeling of warmth in the stomach.
6. Feeling of coolness in the forehead.

Trainees should do these exercises repeatedly following the directions of the trainer or themselves. The instruction words should be simple, and the steps can be arranged according to the needs of the trainee. A calm mind is prerequisite for the exercise, though it can be difficult to achieve for the beginner.

SUPPLEMENTS

Antioxidant Supplements for Male Infertility

Oxidative stress could have an adverse effect on spermatogenesis. Sperm analysis of infertile men frequently shows an increased number of DNA-fragmented spermatozoa, which is known to compromise male fertility. The percentage of DNA-fragmented spermatozoa was markedly reduced after treatment with oral antioxidants. A 2-month administration of vitamin C (1g) and vitamin E (1g) was sufficient for improvement.[16]

Anti-aging Supplements for Female Infertility

The current trend for women, especially in developed countries, is to have a baby later in life; these older women often struggle with infertility. A woman's fertility decreases as she ages, and this significantly impacts a couple's ability to have children. Although there are several complementary and alternative anti-aging compounds, very few of them have been shown to have efficacy. Some of the compounds with potential anti-aging activity are vitamins, co-enzymes, minerals, amino acids, hormones, and placental extracts.

Melatonin

Melatonin reduces oxidative damage to cells by a number of methods. First, it works as a direct free radical scavenger. Second, it stimulates a production of antioxidative enzymes in the cell, and on the other hand, it inhibits a synthesis of oxidative enzymes. Finally, melatonin stabilizes cellular membranes, which may help cells become resistant to oxidative damage. Recently, melatonin has been used as a drug for neurological disorders that are thought to be caused by oxidative stress.

An investigation of oocytes and follicular fluids retrieved from ovaries during *in vitro* fertilization and embryo transfer (IVF-ET) found that in the follicular fluids aspirated with oocytes, the concentration of melatonin decreased significantly when the retrieved oocytes were damaged.[17] In contrast, 8-hydroxy-2'-deoxyguanosine (8-OHdG), a stress marker, was elevated in the follicular fluids when the quality of the oocyte was poor. The concentration of melatonin rises in inverse relation to the concentration of 8-OHdG; this implies that melatonin could help protect oocytes from oxidative stress. In fact, the women taking melatonin showed improvement in their fertilization rate compared to the women without melatonin treatment. The same study also found that melatonin enhanced the maturation of mice eggs from preovulatory follicles incubated in the presence of H_2O_2 for 12 hours. These studies support the theory that melatonin's anti-oxidative effects would help women, especially older women, conceive.

LIFESTYLE

Infertility may be caused by a large number of factors related to individuals, families, or the wider community. The chance of having a healthy, live birth may be influenced by factors such as weight, diet, smoking, substance abuse, environmental pollutants, infections, medical conditions, medications, and family medical history. Although there are no current guidelines regarding the preconception advice offered to people seeking infertility treatment, it is important to determine which advice would help couples make positive changes and improve their chance of conception and delivery of a healthy baby. A search of the Cochrane Reviews showed that no studies could have demonstrated the impact of preconception advice on infertility; therefore, further research into this important subject is required.[18]

Cessation of Smoking

Tobacco severely impacts health. The data from IVF-ET treatment or gamete intrafallopian tube transfer (GIFT) showed that the chance of pregnancy decreases when at least one member of the couple is a smoker.[19] Furthermore, the rate of treatment failure increased significantly according to the length of tobacco abuse. In preliminary observations with an electron microscope, we found that the intracellular organelles of oocytes retrieved from smoking women had an abnormal distribution of surface granules and deformed mitochondria. This finding suggests that cigarettes damage human gamete cells. Even after successful conception, smoking results in a higher prevalence of miscarriage or preterm birth. Both maternal and fetal morbidity are serious complications in smokers during pregnancy. Health impairments such as SIDS, bronchitis, growth deficiency, and various types of infantile diseases are reported to occur more often in families with a smoker; therefore, cessation of smoking is important for couples who are planning to become parents.[20]

Avoidance of Alcoholic Beverages and Recreational Drugs

The use of alcoholic beverages, marijuana, cocaine, morphine, heroin, and other stimulants can be dangerous for women who are planning to conceive because of the risk of serious physical and mental problems for themselves and their babies.

While the amount of damage from alcohol and drugs may vary from one person to person, in general, the larger the dose and the longer the period of use, the more severe is the impact. Once alcohol and drug addictions are established, it can be difficult to quit them.

Alternative therapies for the treatment of infertility are appealing to couples around the world, and many have found them to be effective. The approach of some of these therapies is different from that of conventional medicine when it comes to dealing with human health; these therapies emphasize the natural healing and recovery powers of the patient themselves. There is still room for further studies on these attractive approaches to the treatment of infertility.

REFERENCES

1. DM Eisenberg, et al. Trends in alternative medicine use in the United States, 1990-1997: Results of a follow-up national survey. JAMA 1998;280(18): 1569-75.
2. L Rees, A Weil. Integrated medicine imbues orthodox medicine with the values of complementary medicine. BMJ 2001;322(7279): 119-20.
3. WHO. Preamble to the Constitution of the World Health Organization as adopted by the International Health Conference, New York, 19-22 June 1946, and entered into force on 7 April 1948.
4. National Health and Medical Research Council. Promoting the health of Indigenous Australians. A review of infrastructure support for Aboriginal and Torres Strait Islander health advancement. Final report and recommendations. Canberra: NHMRC 1996;part 2: 4.
5. T Wing, E Sedlmeier. Measuring the effectiveness of Chinese herbal medicine in improving female fertility. J Chin Med 2006;80: 22-8.
6. J Zhang, et al. Chinese herbal medicine for subfertile women with polycystic ovarian syndrome. Cochrane Database of Systematic Reviews 2010, Issue 9. Art. No.: CD007535. DOI: 10.1002/14651858. CD007535. pub2
7. S Usuki, Y Usuki. Hachimijiogan treatment is effective in the management of infertile women with hyperprolactinemia or bromocriptine-resistant hyperprolactinemia. Am J Chin Med. 1989;17(3-4): 225-41.
8. S Usuki. Hachimijiogan changes serum hormonal circumstance and improves spermatogenesis in oligozoospermic men. Am J Chin Med. 1986;14: 37-45.
9. Y Yoshimoto, et al. Ovulation following combined therapy with Wen-Jing-Tang and clomiphene citrate therapy in anovulatory women. Am J Chin Med. 1989;17(3-4): 243-4.
10. M Igarashi. Effectiveness of Kampo medicine in obstetrical and gynecological diseases. Recent advances in the pharmacology of KAMPO (Japanese herbal) medicines. Excerpta Medica. 1988.
11. X Cheong, et al. Acupuncture therapeutics. People's Military Medical Press, 2011.
12. The National Center for Complementary and Alternative Medicine; Acupuncture for Pain. http://www.nccam.nih.gov/
13. CA Smith, et al. Acupuncture for primary dysmenorrhea. Cochrane Database of Systematic Reviews 2011, Issue 1. Art. No.: CD007854. DOI: 10.1002/14651858.CD007854.pub2
14. YC Cheong, et al. Acupuncture and assisted conception. Cochrane Database of Systematic Reviews 2008, Issue 4. Art. No.: CD006920. DOI: 10.1002/14651858.CD006920.pub2
15. K Kermani. Autogenic training; The effective holistic way to better health. Souvenir Press, 1996.
16. E Greco, et al. Reduction of the incidence of sperm DNA fragmentation by oral antioxidant treatment. J Androl 2005;26(3):349-53.
17. H Tamura, et al. Oxidative stress impairs oocyte quality and melatonin protects oocyte from free radical damage and impairs fertilization rate. J Pineal Res 2008;44(3): 280-87.
18. K Anderson, et al. Preconception lifestyle advice for people with subfertility. Cochrane Database of Systematic Reviews 2010, Issue 4. Art. No.: CD008189. DOI: 10.1002/14651858.CD008189.pub2
19. H Klonoff-Cohen, et al. Effects of female and male smoking on success rates of IVF and gamete intra-fallopian transfer. Hum Reprod 2001;16(7):1382-90.
20. J Britton. Passive smoking damages children's health. Practitioner 2010;254(1729): 27-30.

Chapter 25

Managing Failures—Troubleshooting and Patient Counseling

RJ Norman

INTRODUCTION

While patients and doctors are always good at dealing with positive news, we are not well trained in managing disappointments. While infertility can be managed and there are a large number of technologies available to allow infertile couples to have children, there will always be a significant minority who do not get pregnant despite the best advice and the best technologies available. These are often term 'failures' but this is a pejorative word to describe a disappointment. In developing countries, inability to have a child is clearly more than just a disappointment—it can be psychologically and socially disabling. It is clear that we must do the best we can to help the people who are not getting pregnant but it is a probability that there will be a substantial number of couples who will never achieve a child, despite what we do.

APPROACHES TO LACK OF SUCCESS IN INFERTILITY TREATMENT

The more experienced the doctor and the better the resources available, the more likely it is that a proper diagnosis and treatment will be made. It is always wise to review the history and to make sure that a wide range of male and female factors have been considered, including environmental exposures, genetic conditions and lifestyle habits. Some of these include:

1. *The role of weight and nutrition:* Both under and over nutrition have been shown to have significant effects on the ability to achieve a pregnancy and to carry it through to term, while traditionally under nourishment is the more common component in under resourced areas, obesity is becoming increasingly prevalent. Both of these extremes of weight and nutrition impact significantly on fertility and can be addressed by appropriate advice and resources.
2. *Cigarette smoking:* While cigarette smoking is reducing throughout the world in developed countries, it continues to increase in developing countries. Cigarette smoke is an anti-fertility agent for both men and women and advice needs to be given for patients to completely stop smoking.
3. *Knowledge about reproductive physiology:* Many women are unclear as to when they ovulate and have no idea of when it is most appropriate to have intercourse in order to conceive. Monitoring of the cycle, either through temperature or through a more complicated hormonal measurement, may be

illuminating to a woman and her partner or allow them to time intercourse more effectively.

4. *Environmental chemicals and other exposures:* For couples who live in an environment where there is a high prevalence of environmental chemicals such as pesticides, there is a strong likelihood of infertility or miscarriage but it is often not easy for a person to leave their job or to move to another geographical situation, though this maybe all that is required to improve fertility.
5. *General ill health:* This is detected by history and examination and adequate care by the medical services. Often a number of medications are used to control medical conditions and these may also have an anti-fertility potential.
6. *Age:* Extremes of age are also associated with infertility, being too young has high-risks of problems in pregnancy while waiting until later in reproductive life is associated with poor reproductive outcomes as well. General education needs to be available to young girls and older women about the optimal time for fertility. While the evidence is not as strong for men, evidence is approaching that a later age of paternity may be associated with a number of diseases including mental and behavioral.

Adequate Diagnosis

In countries where *in vitro* fertilization (IVF) is widely available the practice of making an adequate diagnosis is disappearing. Where simple and more sophisticated methods of fertility treatment have failed it is appropriate to revisit the diagnosis and causes behind infertility, further investigations may include:

1. *Laparoscopy to exclude endometriosis and pelvic disorders:* While there maybe no history to suggest endometriosis or pelvic infection it is often wise to perform a laparoscopy to adequately refute this. A hysteroscopy and tubal patency test can be done at the same time and if there are significant abdominal findings, these can be dealt with simultaneously.
2. *Hysterosalpingogram:* This is often a valuable substitute for tubal patency testing by laparoscopy or uterine normality by hysteroscopy. It does not require sophisticated equipment and is generally reasonably reliable.
3. *Other medical conditions:* Thyroid abnormalities are known to be involved with fertility problems and miscarriage, rarely adrenal disorders can lead to hyperandrogenism and antiphospholipid antibodies can lead to recurrent miscarriage. All of these should be adequately investigated in couples who are not becoming pregnant.
4. *Semen analysis:* In societies where the woman is often attributed to be the major cause of infertility, not a lot of attention is paid to the semen analysis. It is mandatory that the man is tested under ideal conditions through a laboratory with reliable criteria, including those of the World Health Organization (WHO).

Counseling

There are a number of areas in which the practitioner can make a significant difference in terms of counseling:

1. *Assessment of the emotional and psychological needs of the male and female:* Infertility is an extremely stressful position, particularly in societies where the role of motherhood is highly valued. While the necessary psychological counseling facilities may not be available, it is appropriate for the medical practitioner and their staff to provide some of this through reassurance and assistance. The reduction of stress may well improve the chance of getting pregnant spontaneously as

well as through assisted reproductive technologies, both male and female should be included and it is wise to see both together at every appointment rather just dealing with the woman.

2. *Role of the male:* Much attention is often paid to the female who cannot get pregnant but the secrets to unlocking the problem may lie with the male. Cigarette smoking, environmental exposure, malnutrition and obesity are all causes of impaired semen analysis. While the assessment of DNA fragmentation requires sophisticated methods, the advocation of a healthy diet with plenty of fruit and vegetables and antioxidants is a valuable addition. Alternatively, the use of added vitamin E, vitamin C and other antioxidants may improve DNA fragmentation and potentially natural fertility. There also needs to be an evaluation of whether there are ejaculatory problems or indeed whether the occupation of the male allows for infrequent intercourse, e.g. truck drivers and those employed in the mining industry.
3. *Attention to periconceptual health:* Appropriate use of folic acid, avoidance of environmental toxins and alcohol and other periconceptual considerations allow maximization of the health of any embryo conceived and therefore of any ongoing pregnancy.
4. *Detection of ovulation:* Many women are not aware of when they ovulate and it is appropriate, through the use of temperature charts, hormone measurements or urinary LH sticks, to help them determine when they ovulate, this will often educate a woman so she knows when she is at maximum fertility potential. A single progesterone in the luteal phase may also be helpful to ensure that there is no luteal phase defect.
5. *Advice on alternative medicines:* Alternative therapy is extremely common in developed countries and has been well established in developing countries for many years. Some of these may be beneficial but others may have adverse affects on fertility, a full history and evaluation of some of these products needs to be carried out. There is some evidence that acupuncture may be of value while others find benefit in massage and local herbs and potions.
6. *Adequate advice on Assisted Reproductive Technology (ART):* For many infertile couples, the dream of having an IVF cycle is out of their financial reach and yet they may be tempted to borrow or sell possessions to go through an IVF cycle. The doctor and staff have enormous responsibility to protect the patient from poor practices and unproven therapies in assisted reproductive technology and should act as a mentor and guide and not assist in exploitation of inappropriate therapies. In addition, they should only refer to clinics with excellent pregnancy rates and not use personal financial remuneration as a priority in advice.

ASSISTED REPRODUCTIVE TECHNOLOGY

If simple methods fail there is some value in contemplating the use of intrauterine insemination or IVF. This will depend on the availability of the therapy, whether there is any health funding from the state and the financial background of the patients concerned. Intrauterine insemination (IUI) particularly with clomiphene citrate, aromatase inhibitors or follicle stimulating hormones does improve fertility rates above the background and could be contemplated if relatively inexpensive. A low dose of any stimulating drug should be used to potentially achieve one or two follicles to allow conception of no more than twins. The practice of high dose follicle stimulating hormone (FSH) with a conception of multiple fetuses and subsequent fetal reduction is not one than should be favored. Increasingly it has been shown that intrauterine insemination for poor semen is not a good option and IUI should largely be kept for patients with unexplained infertility.

In Vitro Fertilization

IVF is a valuable addition for couples where there is unexplained infertility, semen problems or a tubal blockage, the use of ART has been extensively covered in previous chapters but good success can be obtained with relatively low doses of FSH, the use of clomiphene citrate or through a unit that is experienced in doing *in vitro* maturation.

Chapter 26

When to Call it a Day

Asma Munir

Assisted reproductive technology (ART) have provided many people suffering subfertility with the desired goal of a family – a fundamental human right even in these days of human overpopulation effects in finite resources, with ±16 percent of the world's population affected. The use of ART is expanding particularly in the developed world, e.g. in Denmark 6 percent of all births are the result of ART.

Denying the access of these services is considered to violate a basic human right, established in the UN Declaration of Human Rights Article 16.1: Xvi, which states "men and women of full age, without any limitation due to race, nationality or religion, have the right to marry and to found a family."

Although the science and technology of ART are far in advance of society's legal moral and ethical acceptance processes the procedure is not without disadvantages, with a take home baby rate approaching 50 percent in the most successful clinics. The dark obverse side of the picture is when to call a halt on medical, social, ethical, economic and biological grounds for an individual patient. This distressing professional duty must always be undertaken in the patient's best interest after a fill discussion and consideration of the alternatives as the acceptance of this advice is ultimately made by the patient and her husband. Some will accept any chance that is not zero, whereas other couples have a much higher outcome threshold before accepting further management. The doctor must be the honest broker of the couples best interests. The issues to be considered include:

- Biological factors inhibiting pregnancy and their progression
- Economic and financial implications
- Alternatives to ART in obtaining a family
- Religious cultural and ethical limitations on alternatives
- Implications of the extended family in Indo Pakistan.

BIOLOGICAL FACTORS INHIBITING PREGNANCY AND THEIR PROGRESSION

This is a moving target with technological and biological advances rapidly improving outcomes:

- *Age:* Few successful pregnancies occur in patients over 40 years of age and hence most ethical ART units prescribe further efforts in these patients. This advice must be qualified by the evaluation of biological as opposed to chronologically determined age. Biological youth has a genetic component so the patient's mother's reproductive history is important and confirmation of biological youth is shown in hemoglobin levels and subcutaneous atrophy leading to the well-known wrinkles. Make confirmation is best obtained by a combination of blood pressure and blood lipids. Although fathering a child has been reliably reported in to the 80s, it is becoming clear that the male factor of age requires consideration—a much ignored but highly important factor.

In counseling about this aspect, the outcomes achieved at a particular clinic require to be considered. In many developing world clinics, this aspect is ignored and world leading clinics outcomes are stated as relevant. This is a major ethical and moral issue, requiring national surveillance in the interests of patients to prevent overuse of this expensive suboptimal procedure. At one stage, less than ten years ago, only 5 out of 48 clinics in a major Indian city produced adequate statistics in the interests of patient protection.

Even the age barrier is under attack by advances in modern biology. At menopause, some 2000 primordial follicles are present in the ovaries. These are not defective and do not inter into the maturation cycle because of their aged microenvironment. As stimulation in androgen-dependent in the meiotic proteomics for up to 200 days to reach the antral stage, the use of Dehydroepiandrosterone, which decreases with age has been shown to produce adequate fertilized ova well after 40 years of age. At the other end of the spectrum, premature ovarian failure and its variants often display a short number of CAG repeats on the androgen receptor making further efforts useless.

- *Immunological issues:* Since the work of Peter Medewar it has been known that pregnancy is an immunological process with hormonal mechanisms. Labor is the final controlled sloughing of a partially compatible placental graft. Immunologically disorders are known to interfere with successful pregnancy, best described in the midtrimester pregnancy losses associated with antiphospholipid antibodies. It is claimed by some that lower levels, possibly by a inflammatory local effects, prevent adequate implantation and are hence listed as untreatable infertility. This is a developing field but is beyond the capabilities of most ART units. Other unrecognized problems are that the mucrosomal antibodies in thyroid autoimmunity are the causes of pregnancy failure and require high doses of steroids with their attendant problems to achieve a successful pregnancy. This requires informed individual management rather than application of guidelines.

  Finally, all autoimmune disease wax and wane but serious systemic involvement by Systemic Lupus Erythematosus (SLE), systemic sclerosis and rheumatoid arthritis in particular are a contraindication to further efforts at achievement of pregnancy because of a shortened lifespan, aggravation by pregnancy and the effects of toxic drugs on the conceptus.
- *Recurrent genetic problems:* Single gene dominant disorders are well described as a contraindication to further pregnancies and in recurrent miscarriages some 6 percent demonstrate a causal abnormality rather than the resultant of disordered pregnancy.

  This list now includes such biological disorders as the Fragile X Syndrome and mitochondrial abnormalities. This list is expanding rapidly as a result of Genome Wide Association Studies (GWAS), and in the not too distant future with costs reducing rapidly GWAS will probably become a routine screening test to prevent further futile efforts.
- *Obesity:* Obesity is considered a major factor in the developed world but is merely a fact of life in the developing often deprived world.

ECONOMIC AND FINANCIAL IMPLICATIONS

The biological drive of women to achieve motherhood (added to by family pressures) can make women (in particular) impervious to financial considerations to the detriment of their families, particularly in these days of economic downturn where 2/yrds of bankruptcies in a rich country such as the USA are due to medical debt.

This has led to a drive towards selective natural cycle treatments with their attendant lower costs. The other direction, as pointed out by Alan Trounson, who produced the first frozen embryo successful pregnancy and is a real world leader in reproductive biology, is that a no frills IVF pregnancy in developing countries can be achieved for as little as US $ 100. It is often forgotten that the super stimulation protocols of HMG were developed by the Seegar Jones's by simply doubling the normal levels of gonadotropins cyclically and that downregulation was introduced to prevent a 30 percent rate of premature ovulation and make the process more predictable. These protocols have made drug therapy a major burden on patients, so Alan Trounson must be taken seriously. This requires biological knowledge far beyond the usual guideline protocols.

Another stressful issue is repeated ART failures which again in our low socioeconomic group has a tremendous impact on the decision for another attempt as the genetic reasons are not very clear.

Pregnancy rate following one cycle of IVF and Embryo Transfer (ET) can be as high as 60 percent. But even in the very successful units, some couples fail repeatedly. The causes for Repeated Implantation Failure (RIF) maybe because of reduced endometrial receptivity, embryonic defects or multifactorial causes. Various uterine pathologies, such as thin endometrium, altered expression of adhesive molecules and immunological factors, may decrease endometrial receptivity, whereas genetic abnormalities of the male or female, sperm defects, embryonic aneuploidy or zona hardening are among the embryonic reasons for failure of implantation. Endometriosis and hydrosalpinges may adversely influence both. In this mini review, we discuss the suggested methods for evaluation and treatment of RIF: repeated hysteroscopy, myomectomy, endometrial stimulation, immunotherapy, Preimplantation Genetic Screening (PGS), assisted hatching, Zygote Intra-fallopian Transfer (ZIFT), coculture, blastocyst transfer, cytoplasmic transfer, tailoring stimulation protocols and salpingectomy for hydrosalpinges.

The use of ART, though often perceived to be discretionary and expensive, has important economic implications. Debate abounds regarding both the allocation of finite resources in this area and the appropriate balance of costs borne by individual patients and society, in France, IVF is fully reimbursed by the social security system, whilst in Belgium, Denmark and Norway the state bears most, but not all, of the cost of IVF. In contrast, there are wide variations in local provision of ART via the National Health Service (NHS) in England and Wales—the so-called 'postcode lottery' effect, which results in inequalities in access to NHS-funded ART (Brown, 1999). According to recent estimates, only one in four IVF cycles performed in the UK is funded by the NHS.

In Pakistan none of the ART centers are national funded and nor the insurance company directly take the responsibility of the technical support. I feel proud to mention the name of one center Baqai Institute of Reproduction and Developmental Sciences, the first center in Karachi and second center of Pakistan who is offering less then 600 dollar/cycle without medication and blood tests for the holy month of ramazan as a low cost package for low socioeconomic group of subfertile couples. In any case due to religious constrains an area where the unpreveliged and poor parents are selling their children or killing them due to poverty and having one man is earning for the extended family, it is advisable to adopt a child and spent the amount on his upbringing rather than to sell every asset on a chance ranging from 25 to 40 percent.

ALTERNATIVES TO ART IN OBTAINING A FAMILY, THE RELIGIOUS AND ETHICAL LIMITATIONS

There are many technically feasible successful processes other then ART. These include Artificial Insemination by Donar (AID), third party IVF/ Intracytoplasmic Sperm Injection (ICSI), surrogacy and adoption. These are limited by individual, social, moral, ethical and religious factors and are practiced to a varying degree worldwide. In general, the more conservative religious societies (particularly Islam and Catholics) forbid any intervention outside marriage or interference with potential life of the gametes.

It is noteworthy that a legal framework requires legalistic acrobatics and generally considers such pregnancies in the same light as adopted children but there are many loopholes with major legal sensationalism, e.g. frozen embryos.

IMPLICATIONS OF THE EXTENDED FAMILY IN INDO-PAKISTAN

It is wise therefore to remember that the family is the basis of all societies, and in conservative societies the rational approach is adoption although even here, Western liberalism creates problems of informing the children. In addition, the extended family influence in developing conservative societies is poorly dealt with in dominant Western literature because they can be very intrusive and often require more counseling then the couple themselves. This is usually simply accepted as a fact of life rather than acting as a true advocate of the distressed couple.

In Eastern culture and most commonly in Indo-Pak the hold of in-laws specially on the wife is too much focused for the reason of subfertility, more so that they will keep on marrying their sons for more than two to three times without even excluding azospermia or severe oligoasthenoteratospermia also if the treatment fails then the wife is blamed due to cultural taboos. Therefore breaking the news or advice for no more attempts need proper counseling and psychological support by the ART team.

Finally, to deal with this sad thwarted female and family, it is appropriate to remind them of Khalil Jibran in 4 the Prophet "your children are not your children. They are rather the affirmation of your belief in the continuation of life".

BIBLIOGRAPHY

1. Alviggi C, Humaidan P, Howles CM, Tredway D, Hillier SG. Biological versus chronological ovarian age: implications for assisted reproductive technology. Reprod Biol Endocrinol 2009;22:7:101.
2. 'Emotional facts' reproduced with kind permission of Kay Oke ed., from Taking Charge of your Infertility, Melbourne IVF, 1999.
3. Margalioth EJ, Chetrit Ben, Gal M, Eldar T. Investigation and treatment of repeated implantation failure following IVF-ET. Human Reproduction 21(12):pp. 3036-43.
4. Redmayne and Klein, 1993; Lieberman and Matson, 1995; Ledger and Skull, 2000).
5. Serour G. Bioethics in infertility management in the muslim world. The European Association of Gynaecologists and Obstetricians vol 2: 2 Available: http://www.obgyn.net/eago/art12.htm, 1996.
6. Vayena E, et al. International Working Group for Registers on Assisted Reproduction (online) Available: http://www.who.int/reproductive-health/infertility/3.pdf, 1997.
7. Wikipedia. Infertility (online) Avaliable: http://en.wikipedia.org/wiki/Infertility (6th September 2005).

Index

Page numbers followed by *f* refer to figure and *t* refer to table